Nanomaterials and Point of Care Technologies

Point of care (POC) diagnostic devices are predominantly used for the diagnosis and monitoring of diseases. To make these technologies scalable for manufacturing, user-friendly, inexpensive, sensitive, and rapid, a combination of such devices with nanomaterials is required. This book deals with new emerging fields such as POC technologies and advanced nanotheranostics using nanomaterials and their technologies and applications in diagnosis. In this book, current advances for the application of nanomaterials such as carbon nanotubes, graphene, and magnetic nanoparticles in POC devices and future directions are reviewed.

This book:

- Presents a comprehensive account of needs and challenges of POC diagnostics.
- Describes the fundamentals of rationale of nanomaterials as remarkable building blocks for biosensing.
- Discusses development of critical diagnosis in POC systems.
- Deals with the advantages of nanomaterial-based sensing strategies.
- Illustrates the challenges and breakthroughs of technologies for cost-efficient biosensing platform.

This book is aimed at researchers and professionals in nanotechnology and biomedical engineering.

Nanomaterials and Point of Care Technologies

Edited by
Sushma Dave, Jayashankar Das,
and Mika Sillanpää

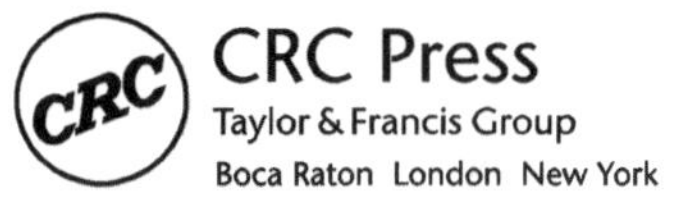

CRC Press is an imprint of the
Taylor & Francis Group, an informa business

First edition published 2025
by CRC Press
2385 NW Executive Center Drive, Suite 320, Boca Raton FL 33431

and by CRC Press
4 Park Square, Milton Park, Abingdon, Oxon, OX14 4RN

CRC Press is an imprint of Taylor & Francis Group, LLC

Library of Congress Cataloging-in-Publication Data
Names: Dave, Sushma, editor. | Das, Jayashankar, editor. | Sillanpää, Mika E. T., editor.
Title: Nanomaterials and point of care technologies / edited by Sushma Dave, Jayashankar Das and Mika Sillanpää.
Description: First edition. | Boca Raton, FL : CRC Press, 2025. | Includes bibliographical references and index.
Identifiers: LCCN 2024011015 (print) | LCCN 2024011016 (ebook) |
ISBN 9781032327280 (hardback) | ISBN 9781032327297 (paperback) |
ISBN 9781003316435 (ebook)
Subjects: MESH: Nanostructures | Point-of-Care Systems | Biosensing Techniques
Classification: LCC R857.B54 (print) | LCC R857.B54 (ebook) | NLM QT 36.5 |
DDC 610.285—dc23/eng/20240618
LC record available at https://lccn.loc.gov/2024011015
LC ebook record available at https://lccn.loc.gov/2024011016

ISBN: 9781032327280 (hbk)
ISBN: 9781032327297 (pbk)
ISBN: 9781003316435 (ebk)

DOI: 10.1201/9781003316435

Typeset in Times
by codeMantra

Contents

Acknowledgments

This work would not exist without the knowledge and assistance of the CRC Press Taylor & Francis group. Being the editor leader of great authors, which you have given us the chance to do, is a privileged position.

It's as challenging as it sounds to take an idea and convert it into a book. The experience is challenging and gratifying. I want to express my gratitude in particular to those who made this possible and stayed by us during the whole journey.

Foreword

The rapid increase in the number of deadly diseases and the limitations of existing diagnostic methods in developing countries are urgent issues in the health care industry. Fortunately, nanotechnology offers new possibilities in medical sciences, particularly through the use of nanomaterials, which have unique properties enabling the development of robust, affordable, efficient, portable, and user-friendly point of care (POC) diagnostic methods. Chapter 1 explores state-of-the-art, POC diagnostic tools, focusing on the synergistic effects of nanomaterials in enhancing the design, performance, and quality of these devices, while also discussing the advancements, advantages, disadvantages, and future trends of nano-based POC testing technologies. Chapter 2 discusses the use of nanotechnology in healthcare to create lighter and mechanically stronger materials with increased biocompatibility and bio-sorbability, enabling early disease detection through diagnostics, improved *in vivo* imaging, coatings for medical devices, and addressing genetic disorders. Chapter 3 explores the integration of therapy and diagnosis in medical approaches for personalized treatment, highlighting the importance of such techniques for early detection and treatment of diseases like cancer. Various nanomaterials with unique physio-chemical characteristics and high surface-to-volume ratio are being researched for theranostics, covering image-guided drug administration, optical imaging, magnetic resonance imaging, and magnetic hyperthermia, with a particular focus on nanoparticles enabling simultaneous diagnostic and therapeutic approaches. Chapter 4 presents the unique properties of graphene, a single sheet of graphite, and these properties make graphene a promising candidate in various fields, including sensor technology. However, to prevent aggregation and utilize its physicochemical properties, its functionalization with appropriate functional groups is necessary for the preparation of high-performance conducting materials. Chapter 6 shows that the increasing occurrence of infectious disease epidemics highlights the need for new and efficient techniques for both diagnosis and treatment, as the spread of diseases surpasses the rate of treatment development, emphasizing the importance of diagnostic technology as the first line of defense, and advancements in synthetic biology and nanotechnology offer effective, precise, and affordable platforms for identifying and preventing infectious diseases. The infectious disease outbreaks, including COVID-19, have highlighted the need for effective treatments, and the use of carbon-based nanomaterials, such as fullerenes, nanodiamonds, carbon nanotubes, graphene, and carbon-based quantum dots, shows promise in overcoming challenges associated with the treatment of pandemic and infectious diseases, providing potential diagnostic and therapeutic applications discussed in Chapter 7 for an alternative approach based on nanotechnology. Chapter 8 reports that an organic-based crystal, 4-(carboxymethoxy) anilinium bromide (4CMAB), is successfully grown and characterized for its versatile functions, including applications in electronics and biology, with single crystal XRD revealing the monoclinic crystal structure and the potential use in electronic and bio/pharma utilities supported by AD/AO data with IC50 values. One of the very exciting emerging areas is discussed in Chapter 9. This chapter provides an overview of highly sensitive wearable sensors that can be comfortably attached to human skin or integrated into clothes, utilizing nanomaterials as promising building blocks, and summarizes recent advances in nanomaterial-based wearable sensing devices for multipurpose sensing, including applications in medical care and sports activity monitoring, while also discussing future prospects, challenges, and opportunities in this field. In Chapter 10, the integration of diagnostic instruments with trustworthy and automated measurement evaluation, supported by POC devices and machine learning algorithms, enables accurate and affordable risk assessments for various ailments, leading to early disease detection and positive impacts on public health. By leveraging artificial intelligence algorithms, POC testing can be significantly enhanced, improving the performance and accuracy of POC sensors and facilitating the quantification of signals for improved diagnostics. From biological perspective, Chapter 11 explains that nanomaterials have significantly contributed to advancements in chronic disease diagnostics and therapeutics, particularly in the detection and treatment of diabetics by measuring patients' blood glucose levels, utilizing enzymatic and nonenzymatic glucose sensing based on nanomaterials with high sensitivity, selectivity, and wider linear range. Additionally, nanomaterials incorporated into polymeric matrices are explored for improved diabetic diagnostics and oral/pulmonary treatment, addressing challenges such as stability, degradation, pH sensitivity, and biostability. Chapter 12 explores recent advancements in droplet-based methods and the use of magnetic fluids and particles in the context of biomedical applications. Magnetism has long captivated interest, and its applications have extended to various fields. In the realm of microfluidics, droplet-based systems utilizing superparamagnetic nanoparticles or magnetic nanofluids have emerged as promising tools for biomedical applications, including biomarker detection, pathogen identification, and POC diagnostics, offering advantages of low cost and efficient resource utilization. By looking into the future, Chapter 13 summarizes recent advancements in wearable sensing devices and applications of nanomaterials, which have opened up new possibilities for monitoring physiological parameters and environmental conditions. This chapter explores the diverse applications of nanomaterial-based wearable sensors in medical care, including continuous health monitoring and tracking sports activity, while discussing future prospects and addressing challenges in this field.

Walter Z. Tang, PhD, PE,
Associate Professor,
Department of Civil & Environmental Engineering,
Florida International University, Miami, Florida 33174

About the Editors

Sushma Dave received her Master of Science and PhD degrees in Analytical Chemistry, Electrochemistry, and Environmental Chemistry from Biosensor Lab in the Chemistry Department of Jai Narayan Vyas University, Jodhpur. She has also completed a Bachelor of Law degree. She is involved continuously in the field of higher education teaching Pure, Applied Chemistry, Cheminformatics, Nanotechnology, Electrochemistry, Biology, Solid-Waste Management, Wastewater Treatment, and Environmental Chemistry to students of Engineering and Basic Sciences. She has also served as a Research Associate in Soil Biochemistry and Microbiology Division CAZRI, Jodhpur. Currently, she is a Professor and Head (administration) at Jodhpur Institute of Engineering & Technology, Mogra, Jodhpur, Rajasthan, India. She has published and presented over 50 papers in national and international journals and conferences, and participated in various workshops and training programs. Her areas of interest are Electrochemistry, Biosensors, Environmental Science, Nanotechnology, Biochemistry, Cheminformatics, Immunoinformatics, and Drug Repurposing. She has edited books and published a number of chapters with Elsevier and Springer. Currently she is working on a funded project in novel materials for environmental remediation, biosensor development, and repurposing of new drugs against infectious diseases.

Jayashankar Das is a young and dynamic technocrat and researcher from India dedicated to the development of an ecosystem of Science and Technology with strong Academia–Industry linkages. He received a gold medal for his master's degree in Biotechnology, and he is also a recipient of an honorary gold medal from former president Dr. A.P.J. Abdul Kalam in excellence in Biotechnology. He received his PhD in Biotechnology and served as a Scientist at IBSD, DBT, Government of India. He is the founder and CEO of a business portfolio named "Valnizen" which deals with regulatory documents and healthcare compliances and support services to African and southeast Asian countries. He has served as Joint Director to Gujarat State Biotechnology Mission, DST, Government of Gujarat and Joint Director to Gujarat Biotechnology Research Centre, DST, Government of Gujarat. His major agenda is development of key policies to drive the translational research and innovation in the globe. He has been served as the Director of Savli Technology Business Incubator, DST, GoG, India. He was actively involved in development and implementation of various policies and action plans like biotechnology policy, innovation policy, Interpol disaster management policy, and startup policy for many universities and government. Last but not least, he has been a member in advisory and governing bodies of many universities, institutions, and government departments, as well as many startup companies. In addition to his role as Senior Advisor to OSPF-NIAS, IISc Bangalore, his research team is also involved in addressing societal challenges via cutting-edge research, such as development of molecular diagnostics for infectious diseases, development of universal vaccine candidate for emerging diseases, development of miRNA-based targeted therapeutics, application of artificial intelligence in healthcare.

Mika Sillanpää received his MSc (Eng.) and DSc (Eng.) degrees from the Aalto University, where he also completed an MBA degree in 2013. He has published more than 850 articles in peer-reviewed international journals, including *Chemical Society Reviews*, *Advanced Materials*, *Environmental Science & Technology*, *Water Research*, *Applied Catalysis B: Environmental*, *Green Chemistry*, *Journal of Catalysis*, *Bioresource Technology*, *Renewable and Sustainable Energy Reviews*, *Analytical Chemistry*, *Journal of Physical Chemistry C*, *Mass Spectrometry Reviews*, *Chemical Engineering Journal*, and *Coordination Chemistry Reviews*. Having an h-index of 89, his publications have been cited over 40,000 times (Google Scholar). Also, he has been invited as an external examiner and opponent of several adjunct professorships and doctoral degrees, and participated in the evaluation of research proposals in over ten countries. He has supervised over 50 PhD students and been a reviewer of over 250 academic journals, many of which are top-ranked in their fields. He has received numerous awards for research and innovation. For example, he is the first Laureate of Scientific Committee on the Problems of the Environment's (SCOPE) Young Investigator Award, which was delivered at the UNESCO Conference in Shanghai 2010 for his significant contributions, outstanding achievements, and research leadership in environmental technological innovations to address present water pollution problems worldwide, especially with regard to wastewater treatment and reuse. In 2011, he was invited to act as a Principal Scientific Reviewer in the GEO-5 report of the United Nations Environmental Programme (UNEP). In 2012, he received Tapani Järvinen Environmental Technology Award and Publication Award of the University. In 2014, he received the Science Award of the Lappeenranta University of Technology and Pro Mikkeli Award. In 2018, he was invited as a Member of the Finnish Academy of Sciences and Letters and Academy of Technical Sciences. He also received a Literature Award from the Water Association of Finland in 2018. In 2017, 2018, 2019, and 2020, he was listed as a Highly Cited Researcher by Thomson Reuters.

Contributors

Mohammed Al Sibani
Department of Biological Sciences and Chemistry
University of Nizwa
Nizwa, Oman

Syed Nasimul Alam
National Institute of Technology Rourkela
Rourkela, India

Shimaa M. Ali
Department of Chemistry, Faculty of Science
Cairo University
Giza, Egypt

J.P. Borah
Nanomagnetism Lab., Department of Physics
National Institute of Technology Nagaland
Dimapur, India

Vaibhav Chaudhary
National Institute of Technology Rourkela
Rourkela, India

Abhay Chowdary Edara
National Institute of Technology Rourkela
Rourkela, India

Kajari Das
Department of Biotechnology, College of Basic Science and Humanities
Odisha University of Agriculture and Technology
Bhubaneswar, India

Aditya Dave
Department of Data Science
IIT Madras
Chennai, India

Sushma Dave
Department of Applied Sciences
JIET Jodhpur
Rajasthan, India

Vishakha Dave
Department of Physics
Maharaja Krishnakumarsinhji Bhavnagar University
Bhavnagar, India

Urja Desai
Department of Zoology, BMT, HG and WLBC, School of Sciences
Gujarat University
Ahmedabad, India

Khadijah M. Emran
Department of Chemistry, Faculty of Science
Taibah University
Madinah, Saudi Arabia

Saima Farooq
Department of Biological Sciences and Chemistry
University of Nizwa
Nizwa, Oman

Edara Arka Ghosh
National Institute of Technology Rourkela
Rourkela, India

Urvashi Gupta
Department of Chemical Engineering
University of Petroleum and Energy Studies
Dehradun, India

Sabtain Haider
Department of Chemistry
Quaid-i-Azam University
Islamabad, Pakistan

Muhammed Iqbal
Department of Chemistry
University of Calicut
Malappuram, India

Snehal Jani
Anant School for Climate Action
Anant National University
Ahmedabad 382115, India

Ganeshlenin Kandasamy
Department of Biomedical Engineering
Vel Tech Rangarajan Dr Sagunthala R&D Institute of Science and Technology
Chennai, India

Fahmida Khan
Department of Chemistry
National Institute of Technology
Raipur, India

Dhanalakshmi, M.
Research and Development Centre
Bharathiar University
Coimbatore, India

Dunaboyina Sri Maha Vishnu
Department of Biological Sciences and Chemistry
University of Nizwa
Nizwa, Oman

Dipak Maity
Integrated Nanosystems Development Institute
Indiana University Indianapolis
IN, 46202, USA
Department of Chemistry and Chemical Biology
Indiana University Indianapolis
IN, 46202, USA

Naveen Mindi
National Institute of Technology Rourkela
Rourkela, India

Shreya Modi
Department of Microbiology
Shri Sarvajanik Science College
Mehsana, India

Maheswata Moharana
Department of Chemistry
National Institute of Technology
Raipur, India

Nishant Nair
Laboratoire Rhéologie et Procédés
University of Grenoble Alpes
Grenoble, France

Zakira Naureen
Department of Biological Sciences and Chemistry
University of Nizwa
Nizwa, Oman

Rawda M. Okasha
Department of Chemistry, Faculty of Science
Taibah University
Madinah, Saudi Arabia

Medha Pandya
Department of Life Sciences
Maharaja Krishnakumarsinhji Bhavnagar University
Bhavnagar, India

Megha Pandya
Research Institute for Sustainable Humanosphere
Kyoto University
Uji, Japan

Subrat Kumar Pattanayak
Department of Chemistry
National Institute of Technology
Raipur, India

Mhonyamo M. Patton
Nanomagnetism Lab., Department of Physics
National Institute of Technology Nagaland
Dimapur, India

Gongotree Phukan
Nanomagnetism Lab., Department of Physics
National Institute of Technology Nagaland
Dimapur, India

Ankita Rai
School of Physical Sciences
Jawaharlal Nehru University
New Delhi, India

Vijai K. Rai
Department of Chemistry
University of Lucknow
Lucknow, India

Nityananda Sahoo
National Institute of Technology Rourkela
Rourkela, India

Farhat Saira
NanoSciences and Technology Department
National Centre for Physics
Islamabad, Pakistan

Pankaj Shrivastava
National Institute of Technology Rourkela
Rourkela, India

Uddeshya Shukla
National Institute of Technology Rourkela
Rourkela, India

Asima Siddiq
Nano Sciences and Technology Department
National Centre for Physics
Islamabad, Pakistan

Manorama Singh
Department of Chemistry
Guru Ghasidas Vishwavidyalaya
Bilaspur, India

Barkha Tiwari
Department of Organic and Nano Engineering
Hanyang University
Seoul, South Korea

Mohanan, V.P.
Department of Chemistry
University of Calicut
Malappuram, Kerala

1 Introduction to Nanomaterials for Point of Care Diagnostics

Technologies and Applications

Sabtain Haider, Farhat Saira, Asima Siddiq, Dunaboyina Sri MahaVishnu, Mohammed Al Sibani, Zakira Naureen, and Saima Farooq

1.1 INTRODUCTION

Today, we live in a society that is facing some critical problems like overpopulation, lack of basic resources, environmental pollution, health concerns, and much more. Among them, the rapid growth of health-related concerns is the major threat faced by the entire world. Although recent advancements in the field of medicine have achieved tremendous milestones to cure deadly diseases like tumors, tuberculosis, HIV, etc. [1], the efficient diagnostics play a key role to cure any disease. The diagnostics are predominantly performed at centralized laboratories by trained professionals and are costly, secluded, and require plenty of time (sometimes from days to weeks), which results in improper, ineffective, and late treatment [1,2]. According to the World Health Organization (WHO), every year about half a million people are victimized by some form of illness that will lead lethal progression [3]. The most probable reason is the improper diagnosis due to long durations and costly processes, non-availability, and lack of facilities, which lead to individual death. The accurate and precise diagnosis of human-related diseases (like infections, pathogens, genetic disorders, etc.) is of valuable importance to help patients interact with the most suitable therapeutic agent (physician) within a short time, which results in effective prognosis [4].

DOI: 10.1201/9781003316435-1

During the COVID-19 pandemic outbreak, developing countries not only faced a strong economic crisis, but every activity of humans throughout the world was also limited to home. The centralized laboratories were also under extreme burden due to their limited number of facilities with the growing rates in the number of patients. The patients having chronic disease like diabetes required regular follow-ups for the complete assessment of the disease [2–5]. These are the reasons that make us think about alternative solutions for conventional laboratories that are less fragmented and more patient-centered. This is only possible by treating patients through primary care facilities rather than expensive healthcare facilities at hospitals [6]. Therefore, the need of the hour is to develop technologies that diagnose the disease at the proximity of patient care, primarily known as point of care testing (POCT) [7].

1.2 WHAT IS POCT

The term "point of care testing" was first coined in 1994, which resulted in a rapid increase in the number of publications focusing on utilization of the POCT methods. The rate of increase in POCT application is 12% per year, which will account for nearly 50% of all *in vitro* testing conducted in the upcoming years [8]. The POCT market is the fastest growing, with a projected value from USD 36.4 billion (2022) to 52 billion (2029). The POCT majorly comprises non-professional testing devices such as glucose monitoring systems and pregnancy testing strips, with rapid growth in professional testing devices for infectious diseases, intensive care, cardiac biomarkers, hematology, lipid profiles, and coagulation [9]. The rapid development of new POCT molecular testing devices for the verification of critical diseases will attract more interest for the growth of POCT technology compared to conventional laboratories in the near future.

According to the College of American Pathologists, POCT is the on-site, economical, and effective diagnostic process that is carried out on the mobile devices and is easily accessible to patients and therapeutic agents within a short span of time [5,9]. In literature, POCT is defined as "testing samples from the patients swiftly at their locus to assist physicians with prompt diagnosis and surgical intervention" [8]. The efficient POCT must have key features that are summarized by the WHO in the acronym "ASSURED": affordable, specific, sensitive, user-friendly, rapid and robust, equipment free, and deliverable to end users [4,7]. POCT techniques are categorized into four main classes [10]:

1. Those with short assaying time, to reinforce treatment regimen to severity (e.g., meningitis).
2. Those for the quick measures, to prevent an outbreak (e.g., methicillin-resistant *Staphylococcus aureus* (MRSA)).
3. Those for the verification of pathogens.
4. Those for the self-monitoring by patients who do not attend follow-ups (e.g., patients suffering from sexually transmitted infections).

1.2.1 Advantages of POCT Technologies

Compact size, mobile and portable devices, short assaying time, and swift reporting, which lead to quick clinical decision-making and early treatments are the key advantages of POCT over traditional testing techniques [11]. In addition, POCT requires a small volume of sample, which is of key importance in the case of newborns and patients from whom collecting a sample is strenuous [2,12]. POCT also offers economical diagnostics, which result in improving and advancing healthcare facilities in low-economic countries [12]. It enhances patient management by improving the interaction between patients and their care takers, which reduces mortality and morbidity of patients [4,13]. POCT is much more helpful for patients who require follow-up on a regular basis by reducing clinical visits and avoiding hospital admission [14].

1.2.2 Categories of POCT Technologies

In centralized laboratories, first the sample is collected at venesection and then transferred for analysis, and the report is released in a certain turnaround time [12–14]. After the advent of POCT, the centralized laboratories reach patients at their bedside with fast diagnostics, which leads to swift prognosis. POCT techniques are displaying a promising future for diagnosis and the modernization of the medical field. POCT devices are categorized into two main classes [15,16].

1.2.2.1 Miniaturized POCT Devices

These are simply defined as devices that are able to automatically prepare, analyze, and detect samples to be used on a handheld basis [15,17]. These devices vary in range from dipsticks to small canisters used in blood gas analyses. These devices are in true sense portable and used by the patient themselves or by healthcare professional near the patient's bedside [18]. Most of these devices use a finger prick sampling technique in comparison to bench-top devices, which require sample containers, labeling, and even transport in some cases. A brief description of some of the common miniaturized devices is discussed below.

1.2.2.1.1 Dipstick POCT Devices

The dipstick endures as a cornerstone of the POCT technologies and is frequently employed by healthcare workers, physicians, and patients in various tests, e.g., urinalysis. In 1950, the first paper-based dipstick test was performed to measure glucose levels in urine samples [19]. The dipstick can analyze up to ten analytes and can be utilized in connection with a monitoring device to minimize possible errors [20]. The use of dipstick involves applying sample on a multilayer, porous pad containing reagents, membrane, and reflectance technology. The membrane obstructs red cells from entering into the portion of pad, where reflectance detects the presence of analytes [21]. Although these devices are successful in detecting a range of analytes in the blood and urine, their performance is widely dependent on the factors such as sample volume, membrane efficiency, and the elapsed time of the reading device [22].

1.2.2.1.2 Immunosensing Strips

Immunostrips are commonly based on immunosensors using optical, piezoelectric, electrochemical, and thermoelectric transducers, in which bioreceptors act as identifying agents that bind and detect analytes by fluorescence or reflectance spectrophotometry [23]. The optical immunosensors mostly work by absorbance, scattering, reflectance, and luminescence methods [24]. They are present in several different forms, e.g., the diffuse-through design using a porous matrix unit, in which diverse immunoassays are present that is able to estimate beta human chronic gonadotropin [25]. Lateral flow immunoassay (LFIA) is the most widely used microfluidic commercialized POCT devices. In LFIA, capillary action platforms is used which requires a small quantity of sample for the identification of bioreceptors such as antibody, antigen, and nucleic acid within 5–20 minutes [26]. The separation occurs as the sample passes through the solid phase in a lateral flow design, which is the most common and in fact leading technology in the POCT market. LFIA is a fast, compact, easy-to-operate, and simple method for the SARS-CoV-2 detection [27]. Multi-channel light detectors in reader devices can extend the usefulness of the lateral flow strips from qualitative to quantitative monitoring. Charge-coupled devices (CCDs) have cameras that are more sensitive to light and are used to assess lower light signals than reflectometers. Acute care metrics such as D-dimers are often measured using these devices [28].

1.2.2.1.3 Integrated Cartridges

The i-STAT gadget, known as "integrated cartridge," is a good example of handheld devices [29]. The cartridge is introduced into the reader after a sample of whole blood is placed. Thin-film sensors and micro-fluids are combined in the cartridge, which is present in a variety of forms for specific analytes [30]. The gadget has been used for more than two decades, and now, it is seen in a wide variety of POCT settings. Their popularity stems from the fact that they offer a wide range of critical care testing on a single device with a variety of cartridges [31]. As a result, when using several devices, users just need to become familiar with one operating technique rather than several techniques, which makes i-STAT a cost-effective option for performing a small number of crucial tests.

1.2.2.2 Bench-Top POCT Devices

The POCT devices are increasingly used near patients' bedside. But before, it occupied lot of floor space and so needed to be made in compact sizes and simplified to be easily operated by healthcare staff and even patients. However, recent advancements in computer processing power and shrinking of devices provide solution to this issue [16,32]. In recent years, bench-top POCT devices are robust devices having greater sensitivity over a wide range of analytes to be employed [4]. There are a number of similarities between the design of these devices and those used in centralized laboratories. Some of the well-known bench-top devices are discussed in detail in the following.

1.2.2.2.1 Blood Gas Analyzers

The most common type is blood gas analyzer which performs multi-spectral absorbance to analyze different components of blood, including levels of electrolytes, glucose, hemoglobin, indirect bilirubin, and lactate [33]. In the past decades, the design and capabilities of these devices have significantly evolved, and now they are referred to as critical care analyzers because they can now test the levels of creatinine, glucose, urea, bilirubin, and hemoglobin derivatives [34]. When compared to cartridges-based system in small handheld devices, here sensors here are designed to be reused. A single cartridge pack is placed in the instrument which contains required sensors and reagents for calibration and cleaning. The lifetime of cartridge in the machine depends on the number of samples being analyzed and the amount of time passed [35]. Such complicated sensors and reagents with longer shelf-lives are difficult to produce in the past, but now, cartridge-based systems are commonplace around the world, and reliable and routine manufacture of these systems is possible [34–36]. Althoughthese devices are easy to operate, their high production cost is still an issue.

1.2.2.2.2 Glucose Meters

Initially, laboratory equipment was used in outpatient clinic for the services like diabetes care management. To serve their intended therapeutic functions, all POCT devices must be highly accurate and exact. In past years, the development of an efficient POCT device which can measure HbA1c level in a convenient manner with high precision and accuracy has been a major challenge [37]. As a result, bench-top glucose analyzers are produced to achieve the analytical standard necessary for efficient POCT diagnostics, and due to the latest innovations in this area, they demonstrate great compactness and performance [38]. The Siemens Diabetes Control Analyzer (DCA Vantage analyzer), USA was the first of its kind to measure HbA1c levels in the blood as well as the albumin/creatinine concentration in the urine. In addition, Roche Cobas b101 system can efficiently offer HbA1c and complete lipid profile testing, and is also smaller in size as compared to the DCA. The later can perform both lipid and HbA1c tests in 15 minutes [9].

Other devices are LABGEO IB10, Samsung, South Korea which can be used as cardiac indicator in ambulance service, Alere POC PIMA CD4 analyzer used for the CD4 counts, etc.

1.2.3 Classification of POCT Technologies in Terms of Application

The POCT technologies mostly employ biosensors. The biosensor is a miniaturized analytical system used for the observation of analytes that interact with biological components immobilized in the solid-state component of a physicochemical detector [39]. These interactions are detected by using different chemical, physical, electrochemical, physicochemical, and optical methods to measure different characteristic parameters of specific biomolecules for certain disease

[40]. The POCT devices are also categorized on the basis of their practical use in term of sample matrix, detection principle, complexity, measuring mode, and sensor features.

1.2.3.1 Qualitative Strip-Based POCT Devices

These simple readout devices are mostly strip-based and perform qualitative analysis by optical detection to discriminate results as positive or negative. Their working principle varies from lateral flow immunological test to chemical indicator test [40,41]. The sample is put on the strip which consists of a mixture of porous matrix and a carrier element holding dried reagent. The analyses are performed by permeating and wetting the stick layer. Urine, serum, and swabs are the commonly used samples to measure different parameters such as pH, specific gravity, protein level, glucose level, ascorbic acid level and to identify the presence of viruses, MRSA, Group A Streptococcus, etc. The common examples of these tests are PCR (Polymerase Chain Reaction) test, urinalysis test, rectal bleeding, pregnancy testing, and detection of infectious agents [14]. The most interesting application is the drug detection test which is performed on sweat, saliva, blood, or swab with the help of drug-wipe device manufactured by Securetec, Germany.

1.2.3.2 Quantitative Unit Use Analyzer Devices

These devices perform quantitative analysis mostly on single-use test strips. The common examples of these tests are blood sugar analysis like hemoglobin A1C (HbA1C), albumen to creatine ratio (ACR), C-reactive protein (CRP), and i-STAT. The EPOC (Enterprise Point-of-Care) cards are handheld devices are widely used for rapid blood analysis. The Bio-Rad HbA1C analyzers are also widely used for the measurement of average sugar level over the time of 2–3 months [29,30].

1.2.3.3 Bench-Top Analyzer Devices

These devices include a range of analyzers working in different principles. The optical analyzers are work on the principle of spectroscopy or reflectometry for the detection of bioanalyses such as Piccolo blood analyzers, Abaxis, USA. The Sysmex pocH-100i, Japan is another bench-top analyzer device that primarily preforms hematological analyses which involve hydrodynamic forces with impedance technology [39]. Similarly, some devices use immunoassay systems such as Eurolyser smart 700/546, Japan and AQT 90 Radiometer, Denmark for CRP and troponin I analysis.

1.2.4 Challenges to Recent POCT Technologies

The rise of population, inflation, and limitations of conventional diagnostics process led to increase in the demand of POCT devices [42]. The accessibility, user-friendly nature, cost-effectiveness, sensitivity, specificity, and short processing time of POCT technologies make them not only an efficient substitutes to conventional laboratories but also help in improving healthcare facilities in developing nations [12]. The recent developments in POCT diagnostics make them easier to carry out in nursing units, ambulances, houses, military camps, and even in space shuttles [43]. Despite all these, there are numerous hurdles still present in their usage. Most of the POCT reagents are produced for single use, which makes them expensive [2]. Currently, 25% of diagnostics employ POCT technologies, which also rises the concern about the quality and risk associated with POCT devices [9]. These tests are analyzed by clinical staff who are not appraised to the parameters affecting all the three phases of analysis (i.e., pre-analytical, analytical, and post-analytical phase), thus increasing error rate [44]. Cantero et al. [45] used a quality indicator (QI) measurement to determine pre-analytical error rate in POCT devices in comparison to central laboratory testing. The highest QI difference in pre-analytical phase related to patient identification and for sampling was found to be 45.3% vs 0.02% ($p<0.001$) and 15.8% vs 3.3% ($p<0.001$), while in analytical phase, POCT show better results in comparison to CL (Clinical Lab) testing. The QI for unacceptable results in ICP (Inductively Coupled Plasma) and EQAP (External Quality Assessment Program) are 0.8% vs 22.5% ($p<0.001$) and 8.3% vs 16.6% ($p<0.13$), respectively. Similarly, the efficiency of LFIA test is poor in term of accuracy, sensitivity, selectivity, specificity, detection limit, and quantification [27]. Nearly 3200 cases including 16 deaths are reported by the Food and Drug Administration (FDA) against glucose monitoring devices commonly known as glucometer kits [8,37]. In addition, glucometer, urinometer, and blood gas analyzers are the reservoirs of communicable diseases like HIV, etc. [6,26,44]. Therefore, it is necessary to evaluate risks associated to POCT.

1.3 NANOTECHNOLOGY FOR POCT TECHNOLOGIES

Nanotechnology is an ever-changing outlook that offers us unconventional solutions to real-world problems. The researchers have made strenuous efforts to tackle the above-mentioned problems, which result in new innovations in the field of nanoscience, neuroscience, and artificial intelligence [46]. The nanotechnology in association with therapeutics, monitoring, treatment, and of medical diagnosis comes up with a unique interdisciplinary concept primarily known as medicine. Various researchers with great expertise in physics, chemistry, biochemistry, computational science, engineering, and mathematics collaborated for the advancement of healthcare facilities using nanomedicine [26]. The biosensors are most widely employed by POCT diagnostic technologies. A biosensor is an analytical device that involves in the detection of analytes by combining a transducer (such as nanomaterials) with immobilized biological recognition elements (such as enzymes, proteins, aptamers, antibodies, nucleic acids, ligands, and molecularly imprinted polymers) for the occurrence of biological reactions that give measurable signals for the qualitative and quantitative analyses [47]. The recent advancement in nanoscience provides a wide variety of materials and their composites with unique properties that revolutionize the bio-sensing-based POCT diagnostics [4]. Changes in physical and chemical properties of semiconductor materials at nanoscale (1–100 nm) such as increased surface area, good strength multi-functionality, enhanced catalytic activity, excellent biocompatibility, and greater stability make them promising candidates for developing a variety of nanomaterial-incorporated enzymatic sensing portable devices such as biosensor, immunosensors, and genosensors [48]. They are used as carriers for immobilized recognizing bioelements or as labels for signal production, transduction, and amplification. They are also useful due to their similarity in size with various biomolecules such as nucleic acid, viruses, and small proteins [49]. In recent decades, many publications have been reported on the application of nanomaterials and their composites for the development of nanodiagnostic technologies as shown in Figure 1.1. Nanodiagnostics have been extremely studied due to their low cost, user-friendly nature, rapidness, robustness, unique properties, sensitivity, and selectivity for the detection of various diseases [42]. Nanomaterials are classified based on their dimensions and physical and chemical properties.

1.3.1 Classification of Nanomaterials-Based POCT

Nanoparticles having diameters from 1 to 100 nm offer a wide range of applications because of their sizes, shapes, and properties [50]. Both organic and inorganic nanomaterials are used in the development of enzymatic biosensors. Organic nanomaterials, majorly consisting of carbon allotropes such as carbon nanotubes (CNTs), graphene, and carbon nanowires, are widely employed [51–53]. Inorganic nanoparticles, such as gold (Au), silver (Ag), iron (Fe), copper (Cu), platinum (Pt), nickel (Ni), cobalt (Co) and their mixtures as well as metal oxides, have been employed in the manufacturing of biosensors [54–58]. The nanostructures are classified into different categories on basis of their dimensions.

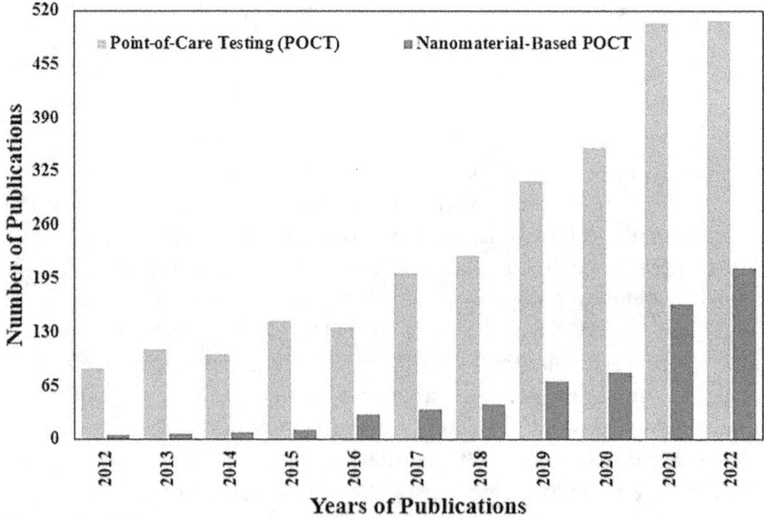

FIGURE 1.1 Number of publications per year for search keyword "Point of Care Testing (POCT)" and "Nanomaterial-Based POCT" on Science Direct. (Accessed on July 9, 2022.)

1.3.1.1 Types of Nanomaterials

1.3.1.1.1 Zero-Dimensional Spherical Nanomaterials

These particles are widely used owing to their strenuous properties and ease of preparation. They work as biological labels by simply attaching to the surface of biomarkers to give signal for the presence of analytes [59]. They involve a wide variety of mechanisms for detection of shift in absorption peak or any optical property (due to the quenching effect of adsorbed analytes), surface plasmon resonance effect (due to change in dielectric constant), and electrochemical changes (due to shift in conductance of nanomaterial or ohmic resistance of medium) [60]. Quantum dots and gold nanoparticles are most used zero-dimensional nanoparticles for the development of biosensors [61].

1.3.1.1.2 One-Dimensional Nanomaterials

These are nano-range materials in which growth is in one dimension. Their lengths and shapes have greater impacts on their properties such as mechanical strength, absorption, and surface area, which in turn determine their applications [62]. The preparation of these materials requires a meticulous method to control their homogeneity. Metal nanowires, metal rods, and single-walled carbon nanotubes are mostly employed for the advancement of biosensors [61].

1.3.1.1.3 Two-Dimensional Nanomaterials

These materials are made of single or ultra-thin layers of atoms expanded in two directions. These materials have unique properties such as excellent electrical conductivity, good mechanical strength, flexibility, thermal stability, large surface area, and biocompatibility, which make them promising candidates for the advancement of biosensors [63]. Graphene and carbon nanotubes are the major examples.

1.3.1.1.4 Three-Dimensional Nanomaterials

These particles have all three dimensions in nano range. Their properties are nearly like zero-dimensional nanoparticles, but their absorbance varies with the change in shape and size. Most of the metals and their oxides belong to this class, which are employed for the development of biosensors for POCT diagnosis [64].

1.3.1.2 Types of Nanomaterials Used in Biosensor-Based POCT Devices

In recent decades, different nanoparticles (such as metals, quantum dots, carbon allotropes, and conducting polymers) and their composites have gained much attention for the advancement of POCT diagnoses due to their unique chemical, electronic, magnetic, electrochemical, and physical properties in attribution to their dimensions.

1.3.1.2.1 Metal Nanoparticles

1.3.1.2.1.1 Gold Nanoparticles The precision, accuracy, and sensitivity are of more importance for analysis in clinical diagnostics. In past years, nanomaterials had been effectively employed for making sensitive biosensors for their application in immunochemistry, immunosensing, and bio-diagnostic assay [65]. Among all metal nanoparticles, colloidal gold nanoparticles have been most studied due to their high electron densities, extraneous catalytic activity, stability, and biocompatibility, and they found a wide range of applications in bioanalysis. Their size (1–100 nm), color (red), and shapes (nanorods, nanospheres, nanowires, nanocubes, etc.) strongly influence the way detection methods function like electrochemical, optical, etc. for rapid POCT diagnostics [66]. The surface plasmon resonance (SPR) in gold nanoparticles gives rise to unique optical properties which are helpful in colorimetric bioanalysis. The change in absorption or refractive index of gold nanoparticles occurs either due to induced aggregation caused by some bioanalytes or by the adsorption of specific bioanalytes [67]. Researchers have employed various synthesis strategies to modify the microenvironment for the bio-receptor on the surface of the gold electrode by simply adjusting its size and morphology [68]. These modifications aim to enhance the sensitivity and specificity of biosensors for improved bioanalysis. The gold nanoparticles are deposited on the surface of electrode to modify the biotransducer [69]. Due to large surface-to-volume ratio, a large number of sites are available for the bio-receptor and analytes [70]. In addition to the large surface area, the enhanced catalytic activity due to quantum dimension results in improved measurable signals [71]. Bikkarolla et al. [68] reported a lateral flow immunoassay (LFIA) based on gold nanoshells with a limit of detection value (LOD) of 0.6 ppm for thyroid-stimulating hormones, which is 26 times higher than conventional gold nanoparticles–based LFIA.

Recently, a hybrid of gold nanoparticles and other biocompatible molecules was introduced with improved biocompatibility and stability [72–74]. Jia et al. [72] developed a lateral flow immunoassay (LFIA) biosensor of high sensitivity and specificity using silica and gold nanoparticles (SiO_2/AuNPs) for the detection of botulinum neurotoxin type A (BoNT/A), staphylococcal enterotoxin B (SEB), and ricin with LOD values of 0.1, 0.5, and 0.1 ppb, respectively. Chiu et al. [51] reported the gold nanoparticles and graphene oxide hybrid–based label-free immunoassay for the detection of anti-BSA with an LOD value of 145 fM. Li et al. [73] reported a good specificity and detection of protein tyrosine phosphate 1B (PTP1B) at relatively an LOD value of 44 ppb with lateral flow immunoassay (LFIA) using biotin-peptide functionalized gold particles. Choi et al. [74] developed a biosensor using fluorescein isothiocyanate (FITC)/peptide–conjugated gold (Au) nanoparticle complexes (FPANs) for the detection of prostate-specific antigen (PSA) as a function of its concentration (10 pM–100 nM). In the absence of PSA, FPANs were not fluoresce due to the gold quenching effect. The biosensor involves the site-specific enzymatic cleavage reaction between PSA and FPANs to produce FTIC and Au nanoparticles, which results in strong emission in spectral region.

1.3.1.2.1.2 Other Metal Nanoparticles In addition to gold, platinum (Pt), silver (Ag), cobalt (Co), nickel (Ni), and other metals and their oxides are also incorporated in biosensors [54–59]. Gao et al. [55] prepared silver nanoparticles

(AgNPs) by using ascorbic acid and $NaBH_4$, and employed it for the ultra-sensitive colorimetric detection of carbohydrate antigen (CA125) and alkaline phosphate (ALP) with LOD values of 1.75 UmL^{-1} and 0.003 UL^{-1}, respectively. $NaBH_4$ acted as pre-reducing agent and promoted the surface plasmonic resonance, while ascorbic acid mediated the controlled growth of AgNPs. Gevaerd et al. [56] developed a nickel (Ni)-modified, screen-printed electrode coupled with microfluidic electrochemical devices for the detection of the level of cortisol in salivary samples having quantification and LOD values of 240 and 70 nM, respectively. Ali et al. [57] introduced a colorimetric portable device using smartphone application for the detection of uric acid on cellulose fiber strip by synthesizing citric-capped platinum nanoparticles (PtNPs) via a reduction method that showed greater selectivity, sensitivity, and an LOD value of 4.3 μM. Yang et al. [58] reported a copper oxide nanoparticles–based lateral flow strip biosensor (LFSB) for the detection of human papillomavirus type 16 (HPV 16). HPV 16 is a highly dangerous type of HPV which is transmitted sexually and responsible for nearly 50% of cervical cancer throughout the world. The CuO-based LFSB was successful in detecting of HPV 16 with an LOD value of 1 nM within 20 minutes.

The electrocatalytic ability of electrode materials is of great importance as non-enzymatic glucose sensor primarily concentrates on the electrocatalytic oxidation of glucose on electrode surface, which determines selectivity and sensitivity toward biological molecules [59,75,76]. For this purpose, different metals and their alloys or oxides are used. Vadlamani et al. [75] introduced an electrochemical biosensor based on cobalt-functionalized titania nanotubes (Co-TNTs) for the detection of receptor binding domain (RBD) of spike glycoprotein on the surface of severe acute respiratory syndrome coronavirus 2 (SARS-CoV-2) having an LOD value of 0.7 nM at a time period of 30 s. Karimi-Maleh et al. [59] reported an electrochemical sensor (non-enzymatic glucometer) based on palladium–nickel nanoparticles decorated on functionalized multi-wall carbon nanotubes (Pd-Ni@*f*-MWCNT) electrode having a great sensitivity of 71 $\mu A/mM\ cm^2$ and an LOD value of 0.026 μM for glucose detection at the potential of 0.5 V. Wei et al. [76] developed a carbon cloth hybrid button sensor (Co-MF/CC) modified by the cobalt metal organic framework employed for the detection of glucose with an LOD value of 0.15 nM.

1.3.1.2.2 Quantum Dots

Quantum dots (QDs) are the inorganic semiconductor nanostructures with diameter in the range of 1–10 nm. In 1980, L.E. Brus first synthesized QDs at AT&T Bell laboratories, USA [77]. Due to the quantum size effect, these particles have unique optical and electronic properties that lie somewhere between single atom and bulk material [78]. When semiconductor size falls below of Bohr radius, it experiences quantum confinement and turns into QDs. The quantum confinement creates more discrete energy levels, which results in increase in the bandgap. As the bandgap of QDs varies inversely with its size, which in turn determines the energy of emitted photon, small-size quantum dots show hypsochromic shift, while large size represents bathochromic shift [79]. The colloidal semiconductor quantum dots (QDs) are phosphors mainly synthesized from atoms belonging to groups II–VI, IV–VI, or III–V. Group II–VI compounds such as CdS and CdSe gained much attention as alternative florescent label in the field of biosensing for detection of influenza and *in vitro* and *in vivo* cancer due to fluorescence quantum yield, tunable size, and high absorbance [80].

Wu et al. [81] reported a paper-based lateral flow immunoassay (LFIA) for the detection of CRP. The LFIA employed CdSe/ZnS QDs which were synthesized by an environment-friendly phosphine-free method and later modified by amphiphilic oligomers. The QDs-based LFIA performed CRP detection test within 3 minutes with an LOD value of 0.30 ppb. GuO et al. [80] synthesized magnetic florescent beads (MFBs) by encapsulating iron nanoparticles modified by oleic acid encapsulated with octadecyl amine-CdSe/ZnS QDs as distinct core/shell structure. The MFBs are employed to purify aflatoxin B_1 (AFB) from dark soya sauce and serve as fluorescent ICA reporter to detect AFB with LOD values of 3 and 51 pg/mL in sauce extract and dark soy sauce, respectively. Wang et al. [78] developed a fluorescent immunochromatographic assay (ICA) using CdSe/ZnS-MPA QD nano beads adsorbed at the surface of silica (QDs@SiO_2) and employed them as luminescent ICA labels for the detection of SARS-CoV2 antigen and influenza A virus (FluA H1N1) simultaneously. The single test completes in 15 minutes with LOD values of 5 pg/mL and 50 pfu/mL for SARS-CoV2 antigen and influenza A virus (FluA H1N1), respectively. Fu et al. [82] designed a ratio-metric fluorescence system (FL) by using Ti_3C_2 QDs and Eu^{+3} ions for the detection of tetracycline. The FL works on the foster resonance energy transfer and antenna effect for the detection of tetracycline with an LOD value of 48.79 nM.

1.3.1.2.3 Carbon Allotropes

The carbon nanomaterials are of significance importance due to their strenuous physiochemical properties which expand their applications in the field of engineering, environmental sustainability, analytical chemistry, electrochemical storage, and nanodiagnostics [83]. In 1991, carbon nanotubes (CNTs) were first synthesized, which opened new doors in the field of medicine. Besides gold and magnetic nanoparticles, CNTs are extensively incorporated in enzymatic biosensors and immunosensors owing to their superior conductivity, greater tensile strength, excellent chemical stability, biocompatibility, and large surface area [84]. In CNTs, each carbon is sp^2 hybridized, forming a cylindrical shape having a length of hundreds of microns and diameter in nano range. The properties of CNTs vary with different structures as the tensile strength of CNTs is 50 folds than that of steel, its conductivity 1000 folds than that of copper wires, and it is thermally stable up to 3,000°C [54]. CNTs are widely employed as electroactive species or intermediate between metal electrodes in biosensors owing to their electrochemical inertness, high conductivity, and fast electron transfer [52].

Both single- and multi-walled CNTs (SWCNTs and MWCNTs) are employed for the development of POCT technologies. Shumeiko et al. [83] designed a paper dipstick biosensor based on peptide-encapsulated SWCNTs for the detection of trypsin (protease) in urine samples. The peptide/SWCNTs-based biosensor showed efficient sensitivity with an LOD value of 1 ppm. Veeralingam et al. [85] developed a biosensor based on MWCNT-coated paper substrate by employing novel strategy of wax deposition and later modified it by vacuum filtration to design hydrophilic and hydrophobic microchannels for highly sensitive and selective detection of cholesterol with the Michaelis-Menten constant (K_m) and LOD value of 9.3 and 3.2 nM, respectively. Ning et al. [86] reported highly sensitive dual-signals electrochemical biosensors based on both potential and current signals, consisting of platinum and β-cyclodextrin loaded polypyrrole coated chiral CNTs hybrid (Pt-β-CD@L/D-CNT@PPy) for the detection of tyrosine and tryptophan. Platinum and polypyrrole were used to enhance conductivity, while L/D-CNTs and β-cyclodextrin were used as chiral selectors, which results in excellent performance with LOD values of 0.107 and 0.133 nM for tyrosine and tryptophan, respectively.

In addition to CNTs, graphene is widely used for biosensor development since its discovery. Graphene is a flat hexagonal sheet made of two-dimensional sp^2-hybridized carbon atoms [17]. Graphene's structure and properties such mechanical, thermal, and electrical strength are similar to CNTs [87]. It has large surface area, which provides a greater number of redox sites and makes easier immobilization of bioreceptors than on cylindrical CNTs [88]. Wan et al. [89] prepared a nitrogen-doped porous graphene electrochemical biosensor via the laser reduction method and employed it for the detection of microRNA. The N-doped graphene biosensor showed high conductivity and sensitivity with an LOD value of 10 fM. Mattioli et al. [90] introduced a graphene-based electric electrochemical vertical device (EEVD) POCT biosensor which uses serologic IgG quantification for immobilized SARS-CoV-2 RBD bioconjugates. The several advantages of EEVD are as follows: it requires only 40 μL of human sample, it takes a time period of 15 minutes for analysis, and it has an LOD value of 1 pg/mL. Yoon et al. [91] fabricated a sweat glucose biosensor by immobilization of chitosan glucose oxidase on the surface of platinum nanoparticles (Pt) loaded on porous laser-induced graphene (LIG) electrode (Pt/LIG) which possesses a sensitivity of 4.622 μA/mM and an LOD value of 300 nM.

1.3.1.2.4 Conducting Polymers

Conducting polymers are organic macromolecules that have conjugated pi-electrons in their backbone structure and partially filled molecular orbitals those overlap to create a strong resonance effect throughout the lattice due to electron delocalization, which enhance electronic and optical properties [92]. The mechanical and electronic properties can be varied based on the synthesis approach and the chemical modeling [54]. The nanomaterials based on conducting polymers are thermally stable, conductive, soluble, and easy to process and have enhanced performance of biosensors by improving signal [93]. The electrode activity can be improved by growing nano conducting polymers which enhance immobilization of bioreceptors due to large surface area and biocompatibility [94]. Their electrical conductivity can be adjusted by optimizing pH, applied potential, and other environmental variables [95]. Polypyrrole, polyaniline, and polyacetylene are some widely used conducting polymers for biosensor development owing to their high conductivity and fast charge transfer properties. Ozkan et al. [96] prepared an electrochemical biosensing electrode by electropolymerization of thienyl pyrrole on chitosan (CS/pTP/GOx) and an electrode modified by chitosan-reduced graphene oxide (CS-rGO/pTP/GOx), and later employed them for glucose detection. The N^1, N^4-bis(2,5-di(thiophene-2-yl)-1H-pyrrol-1-yl) terephthalamide monomer was polymerized to synthesized poly thienyl pyrrole. The CS/pTP/GOx represents good selectivity, a higher sensitivity value of 0.322 $\mu A.\mu M^{-1}.cm^{-2}$ and a better LOD value of 0.097 μM in comparison to CS-rGO/pTP/GOx with a sensitivity and LOD value of 0.531 $\mu A/\mu M^1.cm^2$ and 0.159 μM, respectively. The former also retain a sensitivity of 98.6% over 9 weeks. Vais et al. [97] designed a label-free electrochemical sensor based on poly(ortho-aminophenol) thin film fabricated by electropolymerization on glassy carbon electrode (pOAP/GC electrode) for the detection of *Trichomonas vaginales* (TV). The pOAP/GC-based DNA biosensor showed a high sensitivity of 0.0113 $\mu A/\mu M^1.cm^2$ and an LOD value of 3.9×10^{-21} M.

1.4 APPLICATION OF NANODIAGNOSTIC TOOLS FOR POINT OF CARE TESTING (POCT) DEVICES

Commendable advancement has been made in the previous few years in the medical field. Still people are losing their lives because of respiratory infections, ischemic heart diseases, diabetes, and bacterial infections such as diarrheal diseases and tuberculosis. Reasons behind this are the lack of equipment, especially in the developing countries, and the time frame between the detection and treatment. POCT refers to medical diagnostic tests executed in the proximity of patient care within a minimal time. This is in contradictory to the traditional setup where testing is carried out in central laboratories and takes days to conclude results. Nanodiagnostics confer to diagnostic applications of nanotechnology, which offers earlier detection along with high sensitivity for multiple diseases [98]. The high surface-to-volume ratio of nanostructures offers a huge possibility for target molecules to attach and improve detection sensitivity [99,100]. The synthetic nanomaterials serve as transducers and offer a wide range of possibilities due to their unique properties, such as size, shape, biocompatibility, fluorescence, magnetism, and thermal and electrical conductivity. These properties confer upon nanodiagnostics platforms the ability to rapidly and accurately detect samples from patients at very low levels in real-time [100]. A flowchart of nanomaterials-based POCT diagnostics is presented in Figure 1.2.

Innovative POCT systems are expected from synergy of nanomaterials with a variety of biosensing systems and communication technologies from research labs to fulfill WHO standards referred to as ASSURED for applications in diagnostics. Currently, the POCT diagnostics are under high focus for diagnosis of infectious diseases because of their rapidness, low cost, and portability [101]. These are highlighted characteristics which are very crucial to the detection

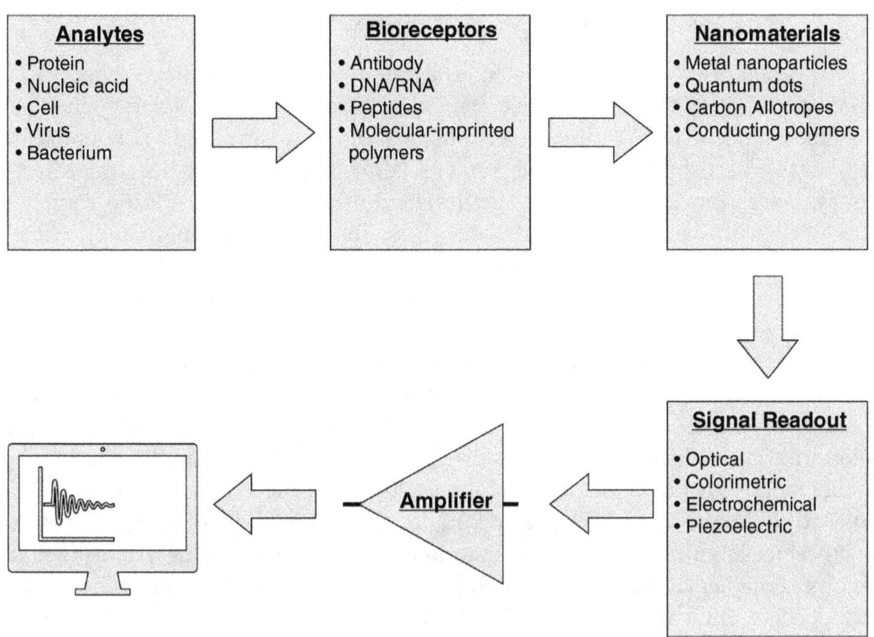

FIGURE 1.2 Flowchart of nanomaterial-based POCT diagnostics.

TABLE 1.1
Summary of POCT Nanodiagnostic Tools with Advantages [102,103]

POCT Nanodiagnostic Tools	System Components	Advantages
Diagnostic magnetic resonance platform	Magnetic nanoparticles NMR system	Rapid technique Sensitivity
Magnetic barcode assay systems	Magnetic nanoprobes Microfluidic system	Fast technique Good sensitivity and specificity
Cell phone dongle platform	Cell phone A dongle system with plastic cassettes Gold nanoparticles and silver ions	Prompt Handy Inexpensive User-friendly
Paper-based POCT platforms	Silver nanoparticles Lateral flow system	Quick Handy inexpensive equipment User-friendly

and control of infectious diseases, especially in under-developed countries. The advantages of different POCT nanodiagnostic tools over the conventional laboratory are summarized in Table 1.1.

1.4.1 Cell Phone–Based Dongle Platform

Cell phones offer a user-friendly interface and wireless data processing POCT diagnostics [104]. Recently, a novel nanodiagnostic platform replicating classical laboratory immunoassay into a cell phone setup was furnished. This could be effectively used in clinical environments [105]. Replicating ELISA microplate assay, a small and light dongle was designed using disposable plastic cassettes equipped with reagents. Instead of enzymes, silver ions and gold nanoparticles were cast off for the signal amplification steps [106]. All the functions were operated using the power from a cell phone. This system was fully controlled by optical, mechanical, and electronic features of nanomaterials distinguishing them from previous nanodiagnostic platforms that are dependent upon an external source. Blood collected through finger prick from 96 patients having potential infectious diseases was used to test the efficiency of the cell phone–based dongle platform. Three different infectious diseases were monitored simultaneously. The final reading can be obtained in 15 minutes, by which a detecting specificity from 79% to 100% and a sensitivity from 92% to 100% were verified. Recently, colorimetric measurement of silver precipitation on gold nanoparticles was utilized in another dongle platform based on cell phone system for the detection of hemoglobin concentration and measurement of HIV antibodies successfully [107]. These dongle platforms based on cell phone open a new window for the development of novel nanodiagnostic tools with amalgam of nanotechnology, microtechnology, and end-user electronics for POCT diagnosis of infectious diseases in the future.

1.4.2 Paper-Based POCT Platform

Paper being low-cost, disposable, and portable is a very suitable candidate for the POCT diagnosis. For the detection of infectious diseases, multiple paper-based POCT platforms with visible readouts have been extensively investigated [10]. Recently, a novel paper-based POCT diagnostic, in combination with multicolored silver nanoplates, displayed a platform for multiplexed detection of infecting pathogens [108]. The paper-based POCT platforms detect multiple infecting pathogens at a rapid testing speed using a single strip [109]. Paper-based POCT nanodiagnostic platform has the ability to fulfill the ASSURED criteria for diagnosis applications, but there are certain limitations, like less detection sensitivity which needs more work to improve.

1.4.3 Nano-Magnetic Resonance Imaging (Nano-MRI)

The MRI process being noninvasive is documented to have clinical potential [110]. Nanoscale-magnetic resonance imaging (nano-MRI) is an innovative technique with possibilities to bring the resolution of MRI measurements down to nanometric scale otherwise limited to micrometers for a single biomolecule. Nano-MRI research includes multiple applications of quantum mechanics and nanotechnologies like magnetic resonance force microscopy (MRFM) and optically detected magnetic resonance (ODMR) using nitrogen-vacancy (NV) centers.

A pH-sensitive MRI contrast agent based on Cap nanoparticles was engineered to release Mn ions in the cancerous environment, targeting for early recognition of millimetric liver metastases [111]. A pH-sensitive anticancer drug release was offered by graphene-based nanocomposite for enhancement of T2 contrast in MRI [112]. On the other hand, a composite of graphene and Fe_3O_4 nanoparticles demonstrated excellent stability, biocompatibility, and enhanced cellular MRI signal [113].

1.5 CONCLUSIONS AND FUTURE PERSPECTIVES

Nanodiagnostics aims at bringing POCT at fingertips. Reducing the time of diagnosis can help limit the spread of life-threatening infectious diseases and prevent other serious health conditions. The combination of POCT-based devices and electronic medical records provide healthcare-related information rapidly. Nanodiagnostics-based POCT can bring revolution to mankind by taking advantages of unique structural, optical, and electronic properties of nano-based materials.

The growing trend in the application of POCT in medical diagnostics is widely depends on its pros and cons related to patient health. The risk management associated with POCT is addressed by using unique approaches like error-grid analysis to evaluating the difference between POCT results and the central laboratory. The use of nanotechnology not only reduces risk in using POCT devices through enhanced sensitivity and selectivity, and broadens its application in disease detection. Nanotechnology opens up new doors for the development of economical, efficient, robust, rapid, user-friendly, and smart POCT devices, which will help advance medical facilities in less-developed countries. In the near future, nanomaterial-based POCT could employ smartphones to perform complete clinical diagnostics at remote locations including military camps, space shuttles, refugee camps, and remote adventure sites.

ACKNOWLEDGMENT

The authors are highly thankful to all the contributors.

CONFLICT OF INTEREST

No conflict of interest to declare.

REFERENCES

1. Pandey CM, Augustine S, Kumar S, Kumar S, Nara S, Srivastava S, et al. Microfluidics based point-of-care diagnostics. *Biotechnology Journal.* 2018;13(1):1700047.
2. Manocha A, Bhargava S. Emerging challenges in point-of-care testing. *Current Medicine Research Practice.* 2019;9(6):227–30.

3. Pashchenko O, Shelby T, Banerjee T, Santra S. A comparison of optical, electrochemical, magnetic, and colorimetric point-of-care biosensors for infectious disease diagnosis. *ACS Infectious Diseases*. 2018;4(8):1162–78.
4. Cordeiro M, Ferreira Carlos F, Pedrosa P, Lopez A, Baptista PV. Gold nanoparticles for diagnostics: Advances towards points of care. *Diagnostics*. 2016;6(4):43.
5. Singh P, Singh D, Sa P, Mohapatra P, Khuntia A, Sahoo SK. Insights from nanotechnology in COVID-19: Prevention, detection, therapy and immunomodulation. *Nanomedicine: Nanotechnology, Biology Medicine*. 2021;16(14):1219–35.
6. Farmer S, Razin V, Peagler AF, Strickler S, Fain WB, Damhorst GL, et al. Don't forget about human factors: Lessons learned from COVID-19 point-of-care testing. *Cell Reports Methods*. 2022;2(5):100222.
7. Clerico A, Zaninotto M, Plebani M. High-sensitivity assay for cardiac troponins with POCT methods. The future is soon. *Clinical Chemistry Laboratory Medicine*. 2021;59(9):1477–8.
8. Plebani M. Does POCT reduce the risk of error in laboratory testing? *Clinica Chimica Acta*. 2009;404(1):59–64.
9. St John A, Price CP. Existing and emerging technologies for point-of-care testing. *The Clinical Biochemist Reviews*. 2014;35(3):155.
10. Wang H, Sugiarto S, Li T, Ang WH, Lee C, Pastorin G. Advances in nanomaterials and their applications in point of care (POC) devices for the diagnosis of infectious diseases. *Biotechnology Advances*. 2016;34(8):1275–88.
11. Jung W, Han J, Choi J-W, Ahn CH. Point-of-care testing (POCT) diagnostic systems using microfluidic lab-on-a-chip technologies. *Microelectronic Engineering*. 2015;132:46–57.
12. Park H, Park Y, Lakshminarayana S, Jung H-M, Kim M-Y, Lee KH, et al. Portable all-in-one electroanalytical device for point of care. *IEEE Access*. 2022. doi: 10.1109/ACCESS.2022.3186678.
13. Shimetani N. Current status of POCT and its future challenges. *The Japanese Journal of Clinical Pathology*. 2011;59(9):864–8.
14. Luppa PB, Müller C, Schlichtiger A, Schlebusch H. Point-of-care testing (POCT): Current techniques and future perspectives. *TrAC Trends in Analytical Chemistry*. 2011;30(6):887–98.
15. Lopes LC, Santos A, Bueno PR. An outlook on electrochemical approaches for molecular diagnostics assays and discussions on the limitations of miniaturized technologies for point-of-care devices. *Sensors Actuators Reports*. 2022;4:100087.
16. Sharma A, Tok AIY, Alagappan P, Liedberg B. Point of care testing of sports biomarkers: Potential applications, recent advances and future outlook. *TrAC Trends in Analytical Chemistry*. 2021;142:116327.
17. Rawat P, Sharma PK, Malik V, Umapathi R, Kaushik N, Rhyee J-S. Emergence of high-performing and ultra-fast 2D-graphene nano-biosensing system. *Materials Letters*. 2022;308:131241.
18. Ranjan P, Singhal A, Sadique MA, Yadav S, Parihar A, Khan R. Scope of biosensors, commercial aspects, and miniaturized devices for point-of-care testing from lab to clinics applications. In *Biosensor Based Advanced Cancer Diagnostics*: Elsevier; 2022. pp. 395–410. doi: 10.1016/B978-0-12-823424-2.00004-1.
19. Park J, Shin JH, Park J-K. Pressed paper-based dipstick for detection of foodborne pathogens with multistep reactions. *Analytical Chemistry*. 2016;88(7):3781–8.
20. Queiroz SC, Dela Cruz C, Casalechi M, Nery SF, Reis FM. Seminal protein levels assessed with dipstick test correlate with sperm recovery after cryopreservation. *Human Fertility*. 2022;25(2):349–55.

21. Merrelaar AE, Bögl MS, Buchtele N, Merrelaar M, Herkner H, Schoergenhofer C, et al. Performance of a qualitative point-of-care strip test to detect DOAC exposure at the emergency department: A cohort-type cross-sectional diagnostic accuracy study. *Thrombosis Haemostasis.* 2022. doi: 10.1055/s-0042-1750327.
22. Latour K, De Lepeleire J, Catry B, Buntinx F. Nursing home residents with suspected urinary tract infections: a diagnostic accuracy study. *BMC Geriatrics.* 2022;22(1):1–10.
23. Shahdeo D, Chauhan N, Majumdar A, Ghosh A, Gandhi SJAABM. Graphene-based field-effect transistor for ultrasensitive immunosensing of SARS-CoV-2 Spike S1 antigen. *ACS Applied Bio Materials.* 2022;5:3563–3572.
24. Xu D, Huang X, Guo J, Ma X. Automatic smartphone-based microfluidic biosensor system at the point of care. *Biosensors Bioelectronics.* 2018;110:78–88.
25. Apilux A, Ukita Y, Chikae M, Chailapakul O, Takamura Y. Development of automated paper-based devices for sequential multistep sandwich enzyme-linked immunosorbent assays using inkjet printing. *Lab on a Chip.* 2013;13(1):126–35.
26. Syedmoradi L, Daneshpour M, Alvandipour M, Gomez FA, Hajghassem H, Omidfar K, et al. Point of care testing: The impact of nanotechnology. *Biosensors Bioelectronics.* 2017;87:373–87.
27. Fortunati S, Giliberti C, Giannetto M, Bolchi A, Ferrari D, Donofrio G, et al. Rapid quantification of SARS-Cov-2 spike protein enhanced with a machine learning technique integrated in a smart and portable immunosensor. *Biosensors.* 2022;12(6):426.
28. Kumar A, Parihar A, Panda U, Parihar DS. Microfluidics-based point-of-care testing (POCT) devices in dealing with waves of COVID-19 pandemic: The emerging solution. *ACS Applied Bio Materials.* 2022;5:2046.
29. Xu Y, Wang T, Chen Z, Jin L, Wu Z, Yan J, et al. The point-of-care-testing of nucleic acids by chip, cartridge and paper sensors. *Chinese Chemical Letters.* 2021;32:3675–3686.
30. Kulinsky L, Noroozi Z, Madou M. Present technology and future trends in point-of-care microfluidic diagnostics. *Microfluidic Diagnostics.* 2013;949:3–23. doi: 10.1007/978-1-62703-134-9_1.
31. Gubala V, Harris LF, Ricco AJ, Tan MX, Williams DE. Point of care diagnostics: Status and future. *Analytical Chemistry.* 2012;84(2):487–515.
32. Sluss PM. Quantitative benchtop analyzers, estradiol, and parathyroid hormone: 3 wishes for future point-of-care testing. *Point of Care.* 2008;7(3):88–91.
33. Parupudi T, Panchagnula N, Muthukumar S, Prasad S. Evidence-based point-of-care technology development during the COVID-19 pandemic. *Biotechniques.* 2020;70(1):58–67.
34. Lopez-Barbosa N, Gamarra JD, Osma JF., The future point-of-care detection of disease and its data capture and handling. *Analytical Bioanalytical Chemistry.* 2016;408(11):2827–37.
35. Wilson S, Steele S, Adeli KJB, Equipment B. Innovative technological advancements in laboratory medicine: Predicting the lab of the future. *Biotechnology Biotechnological Equipment.* 2022;36(supl):S9–S21.
36. Hutter T, Collings T, Kostova G, Frankl FEK. Point-of-care and self-testing for potassium: Recent advances. *Sensors Diagnostics.* 2022;1:614–626.
37. Teo E, Hassan N, Tam W, Koh S. Effectiveness of continuous glucose monitoring in maintaining glycaemic control among people with type 1 diabetes mellitus: A systematic review of randomised controlled trials and meta-analysis. *Diabetologia.* 2022;65:1–16.
38. Zhang M, Cui X, Li N. Smartphone-based mobile biosensors for the point-of-care testing of human metabolites. *Materials Today Bio.* 2022;14:100254.

39. Chinnadayyala SR, Park J, Le HTN, Santhosh M, Kadam AN, Cho S, et al. Recent advances in microfluidic paper-based electrochemiluminescence analytical devices for point-of-care testing applications. *Biosensors Bioelectronics.* 2019;126:68–81.
40. Henihan G, Schulze H, Corrigan DK, Giraud G, Terry JG, Hardie A, et al. Label-and amplification-free electrochemical detection of bacterial ribosomal RNA. *Biosensors Bioelectronics.* 2016;81:487–94.
41. Bayoumy S, Martiskainen I, Heikkilä T, Rautanen C, Hedberg P, Hyytiä H, et al. Sensitive and quantitative detection of cardiac troponin I with upconverting nanoparticle lateral flow test with minimized interference. *Scientific Reports.* 2021;11(1):1–9.
42. Wang Y, Yu L, Kong X, Sun L. Application of nanodiagnostics in point-of-care tests for infectious diseases. *International Journal of Nanomedicine.* 2017;12:4789.
43. Doern CD, Miller MB, Alby K, Bachman MA, Brecher SM, Casiano-Colon A, et al. Proceedings of the clinical microbiology open 2018 and 2019-a discussion about emerging trends, challenges, and the future of clinical microbiology. *Journal of Clinical Microbiology.* 2022;60:e00092–22.
44. Buño A, Oliver P. POCT errors can lead to false potassium results. *Advances in Laboratory Medicine.* 2022;3(2):142–6.
45. Cantero M, Redondo M, Martín E, Callejón G, Hortas ML. Use of quality indicators to compare point-of-care testing errors in a neonatal unit and errors in a STAT central laboratory. *Clinical Chemistry.* 2015;53(2):239–47.
46. Li S. Development and research of health examination and nursing technology based on nanotechnology. *Journal of Nanomaterials.* 2022;2022:1–9.
47. Yun Y-H, Eteshola E, Bhattacharya A, Dong Z, Shim J-S, Conforti L, et al. Tiny medicine: Nanomaterial-based biosensors. *Sensors.* 2009;9(11):9275–99.
48. Wang X, Li F, Guo Y. Recent trends in nanomaterial-based biosensors for point-of-care testing. *Frontiers in Chemistry.* 2020;8:586702.
49. Lyberopoulou A, Efstathopoulos EP, Gazouli M. Nanotechnology-based rapid diagnostic tests. In *Proof Concepts in Rapid Diagnostic Tests Technologies.* 2016:89–105. doi: 10.5772/63908.
50. Nehra A, Singh KP. Current trends in nanomaterial embedded field effect transistor-based biosensor. *Biosensors Bioelectronics.* 2015;74:731–43.
51. Chiu N-F, Chen C-C, Yang C-D, Kao Y-S, Wu W-R. Enhanced plasmonic biosensors of hybrid gold nanoparticle-graphene oxide-based label-free immunoassay. *Nanoscale Research Letters.* 2018;13(1):1–11.
52. Sireesha M, Jagadeesh Babu V, Kranthi Kiran AS, Ramakrishna S. A review on carbon nanotubes in biosensor devices and their applications in medicine. *Nanocomposites.* 2018;4(2):36–57.
53. Dai B, Zhou R, Ping J, Ying Y, Xie L. Recent advances in carbon nanotube-based biosensors for biomolecular detection. *TrAC Trends in Analytical Chemistry.* 2022;154:116658.
54. Ronkainen NJ, Okon SL. Nanomaterial-based electrochemical immunosensors for clinically significant biomarkers. *Materials.* 2014;7(6):4669–709.
55. Gao J, Jia M, Xu Y, Zheng J, Shao N, Zhao M. Prereduction-promoted enhanced growth of silver nanoparticles for ultrasensitive colorimetric detection of alkaline phosphatase and carbohydrate antigen 125. *Talanta.* 2018;189:129–36.
56. Gevaerd A, Watanabe E, Belli C, Marcolino-Junior LH, Bergamini MF. A complete lab-made point of care device for non-immunological electrochemical determination of cortisol levels in salivary samples. *Sensors Actuators B: Chemical.* 2021;332:129532.

57. Ali M, Khalid MAU, Shah I, Kim SW, Kim YS, Lim JH, et al. based selective and quantitative detection of uric acid using citrate-capped Pt nanoparticles (PtNPs) as a colorimetric sensing probe through a simple and remote-based device. *New Journal of Chemistry*. 2019;43(20):7636–45.
58. Yang Z, Yi C, Lv S, Sheng Y, Wen W, Zhang X, et al. Development of a lateral flow strip biosensor based on copper oxide nanoparticles for rapid and sensitive detection of HPV16 DNA. *Sensors Actuators B: Chemical*. 2019;285:326–32.
59. Karimi-Maleh H, Cellat K, Arıkan K, Savk A, Karimi F, Şen F, et al. Palladium-Nickel nanoparticles decorated on Functionalized-MWCNT for high precision non-enzymatic glucose sensing. *Materials Chemistry Physics*. 2020;250:123042.
60. Sahoo S, Nayak A, Gadnayak A, Sahoo M, Dave S, Mohanty P, et al. Quantum dots enabled point-of-care diagnostics: A new dimension to the nanodiagnosis. In *Advanced Nanomaterials for Point of Care Diagnosis and Therapy*: Elsevier; 2022. pp. 43–52. doi: 10.1016/B978-0-323-85725-3.00005-2.
61. Rahman BA, Viphavakit C, Chitaree R, Ghosh S, Pathak AK, Verma S, et al. Optical fiber, nanomaterial, and thz-metasurface-mediated nano-biosensors: A review. *Biosensors*. 2022;12(1):42.
62. Sen D, Patil V, Smriti K, Varchas P, Ratnakar R, Naik N, et al. Nanotechnology and nanomaterials in dentistry: Present and future perspectives in clinical applications. *Engineered Science*. 2022;20:14–24.
63. Chen P, Tang Z, Huang K, Wei Y, Li D, He Y, et al. Immunofluorescence and two-dimensional visual analysis of HIV-1 p24 antigen in clinical samples enhanced by poly-T templated copper nanoparticles and QDs. *Sensors Actuators B: Chemical*. 2022;354:131209.
64. Purohit B, Kumar A, Mahato K, Srivastava A, Chandra P. Engineered three-dimensional Au-Cu bimetallic dendritic nanosensor for ultrasensitive drug detection in urine samples and in vitro human embryonic kidney cells model. *Microchemical Journal*. 2022;176:107239.
65. Omidfar K, Khorsand F, Azizi MD. New analytical applications of gold nanoparticles as label in antibody based sensors. *Biosensors Bioelectronics*. 2013;43:336–47.
66. Choi DH, Lee SK, Oh YK, Bae BW, Lee SD, Kim S, et al. A dual gold nanoparticle conjugate-based lateral flow assay (LFA) method for the analysis of troponin I. *Biosensors Bioelectronics*. 2010;25(8):1999–2002.
67. Della Ventura B, Gelzo M, Battista E, Alabastri A, Schirato A, Castaldo G, et al. Biosensor for point-of-care analysis of immunoglobulins in urine by metal enhanced fluorescence from gold nanoparticles. *ACS Applied Materials Interfaces*. 2019;11(4):3753–62.
68. Bikkarolla SK, McNamee SE, Vance P, McLaughlin J. High-sensitive detection and quantitative analysis of thyroid-stimulating hormone using gold-nanoshell-based lateral flow immunoassay device. *Biosensors*. 2022;12(3):182.
69. Zhan F, Wang T, Iradukunda L, Zhan J. A gold nanoparticle-based lateral flow biosensor for sensitive visual detection of the potato late blight pathogen, *Phytophthora infestans*. *Analytica Chimica Acta*. 2018;1036:153–61.
70. Borse VB, Konwar AN, Jayant RD, Patil PO. Perspectives of characterization and bioconjugation of gold nanoparticles and their application in lateral flow immunosensing. *Drug Delivery Translational Research*. 2020;10(4):878–902.
71. Meenakshi MM, Annasamy G, Sankaranarayanan M. Green synthesis of graphene gold nanocomposites for optical sensing of ferritin biomarker. *Materials Letters*. 2021;303:130446.

72. Jia X, Wang K, Li X, Liu Z, Liu Y, Xiao R, et al. Highly sensitive detection of three protein toxins via SERS-lateral flow immunoassay based on SiO_2@ Au nanoparticles. *Nanomedicine: Nanotechnology, Biology Medicine.* 2022;41:102522.
73. Li X, Zhu Q, Xu F, Jian M, Yao C, Zhang H, et al. Lateral flow immunoassay with peptide-functionalized gold nanoparticles for rapid detection of protein tyrosine phosphatase 1B. *Analytical Biochemistry.* 2022;648:114671.
74. Choi JH, Kim HS, Choi J-W, Hong JW, Kim Y-K, Oh B-K, et al. A novel Au-nanoparticle biosensor for the rapid and simple detection of PSA using a sequence-specific peptide cleavage reaction. *Biosensors Bioelectronics.* 2013;49:415–9.
75. Vadlamani BS, Uppal T, Verma SC, Misra M. Functionalized TiO_2 nanotube-based electrochemical biosensor for rapid detection of SARS-CoV-2. *Sensors.* 2020;20(20):5871.
76. Wei X, Guo J, Lian H, Sun X, Liu B. Cobalt metal-organic framework modified carbon cloth/paper hybrid electrochemical button-sensor for nonenzymatic glucose diagnostics. *Sensors Actuators B: Chemical.* 2021;329:129205.
77. Efros AL, Brus LE. Nanocrystal quantum dots: From discovery to modern development. *ACS Nano.* 2021;15(4):6192–210.
78. Wang C, Yang X, Zheng S, Cheng X, Xiao R, Li Q, et al. Development of an ultrasensitive fluorescent immunochromatographic assay based on multilayer quantum dot nanobead for simultaneous detection of SARS-CoV-2 antigen and influenza A virus. *Sensors Actuators B: Chemical.* 2021;345:130372.
79. Singh S, Dhawan A, Karhana S, Bhat M, Dinda A. Quantum dots: An emerging tool for point-of-care testing. *Micromachines.* 2020;11(12):1058.
80. Guo L, Shao Y, Duan H, Ma W, Leng Y, Huang X, et al. Magnetic quantum dot nanobead-based fluorescent immunochromatographic assay for the highly sensitive detection of aflatoxin B1 in dark soy sauce. *Analytical Chemistry.* 2019;91(7):4727–34.
81. Wu R, Zhou S, Chen T, Li J, Shen H, Chai Y, et al. Quantitative and rapid detection of C-reactive protein using quantum dot-based lateral flow test strip. *Analytica Chimica Acta.* 2018;1008:1–7.
82. Fu C, Ai F, Huang J, Shi Z, Yan X, Zheng X, et al. Eu doped Ti_3C_2 quantum dots to form a ratiometric fluorescence platform for visual and quantitative point-of-care testing of tetracycline derivatives. *Spectrochimica Acta Part A: Molecular Biomolecular Spectroscopy.* 2022;272:120956.
83. Shumeiko V, Paltiel Y, Bisker G, Hayouka Z, Shoseyov O. A paper-based near-infrared optical biosensor for quantitative detection of protease activity using peptide-encapsulated SWCNTs. *Sensors.* 2020;20(18):5247.
84. Justino CIL, Rocha-Santos TAP, Duarte AC. Advances in point-of-care technologies with biosensors based on carbon nanotubes. *TrAC Trends in Analytical Chemistry.* 2013;45:24–36.
85. Veeralingam S, Badhulika S. Enzyme immobilized multi-walled carbon nanotubes on paper-based biosensor fabricated via mask-less hydrophilic and hydrophobic microchannels for cholesterol detection. *Journal of Industrial Engineering Chemistry.* 2022;113:401–410.
86. Ning G, Wang H, Fu M, Liu J, Sun Y, Lu H, et al. Dual signals electrochemical biosensor for point-of-care testing of amino acids enantiomers. *Electroanalysis.* 2022;34(2):316–25.
87. Arshad F, Nabi F, Iqbal S, Khan RH. Applications of graphene-based electrochemical and optical biosensors in early detection of cancer biomarkers. *Colloids Surfaces B: Biointerfaces.* 2022;212:112356.

88. Alhazmi HA, Ahsan W, Mangla B, Javed S, Hassan MZ, Asmari M, et al. Graphene-based biosensors for disease theranostics: Development, applications, and recent advancements. *Nanotechnology Reviews.* 2022;11(1):96–116.
89. Wan Z, Umer M, Lobino M, Thiel D, Nguyen N-T, Trinchi A, et al. Laser induced self-N-doped porous graphene as an electrochemical biosensor for femtomolar miRNA detection. *Carbon.* 2020;163:385–94.
90. Mattioli IA, Castro KR, Macedo LJ, Sedenho GC, Oliveira MN, Todeschini I, et al. Graphene-based hybrid electrical-electrochemical point-of-care device for serologic COVID-19 diagnosis. *Biosensors Bioelectronics.* 2022;199:113866.
91. Yoon H, Nah J, Kim H, Ko S, Sharifuzzaman M, Barman SC, et al. A chemically modified laser-induced porous graphene based flexible and ultrasensitive electrochemical biosensor for sweat glucose detection. *Sensors Actuators B: Chemical.* 2020;311:127866.
92. Minisy I. Nanostructured conducting polymer composites. Univerzita Karlova, Přírodovědecká fakulta: Univerzita Karlova, Přírodovědecká fakulta; 2022.
93. Hosseini SS, Salimi A, Adeli M. Nanoscale sensors based on conductive polymers. In *Conductive Polymers in Analytical Chemistry*: ACS Publications; 2022. pp. 219–54. doi: 10.1021/bk-2022-1405.ch009.
94. Rebelo TS, Miranda IM, Brandão AT, Sousa LI, Ribeiro JA, Silva AF, et al. A disposable saliva electrochemical MIP-based biosensor for detection of the stress biomarker α-amylase in point-of-care applications. *Electrochem.* 2021;2(3):427–38.
95. Beitollahi H, Dourandish Z, Tajik S, Jahani PM. Application of conductive polymer nanocomposites. In *Conductive Polymers in Analytical Chemistry*: ACS Publications; 2022. pp. 313–44. doi: 10.1021/bk-2022-1405.ch012.
96. Özkan BÇ, Aras TS, Turhan H, Ak M. Highly stable and reproducible biosensor interface based on chitosan and 2, 5-Di (thienyl) pyrrole based conjugated polymer. *Materials Chemistry Physics.* 2022;288:126397.
97. Vais RD, Heli H, Sattarahmady N, Barazesh A. A novel and ultrasensitive label-free electrochemical DNA biosensor for *Trichomonas vaginalis* detection based on a nanostructured film of poly (ortho-aminophenol). *Synthetic Metals.* 2022;287:117082.
98. Li D, Müller MB, Gilje S, Kaner RB, Wallace G. Processable aqueous dispersions of graphene nanosheets. *Nature Nanotechnology.* 2008;3(2):101–5.
99. Paredes J, Villar-Rodil S, Martínez-Alonso A, Tascon JMD. Graphene oxide dispersions in organic solvents. *Langmuir.* 2008;24(19):10560–4.
100. Arfin T, Rangari SN. Graphene oxide-ZnO nanocomposite modified electrode for the detection of phenol. *Analytical Methods.* 2018;10(3):347–58.
101. Scardino PT, Hay AM. Point of care testing: A welcome advance? *Nature Clinical Practice Urolog.* 2007;4(8):401.
102. Chung HJ, Castro CM, Im H, Lee H, Weissleder R. A magneto-DNA nanoparticle system for rapid detection and phenotyping of bacteria. *Nature Nanotechnology.* 2013;8(5):369–75.
103. Gish RG, Gutierrez J, Navarro-Cazarez N, Giang K, Adler D, Tran B, et al. A simple and inexpensive point-of-care test for hepatitis B surface antigen detection: serological and molecular evaluation. *Journal of Viral Hepatitis.* 2014;21(12):905–8.
104. Zurovac D, Sudoi RK, Akhwale WS, Ndiritu M, Hamer DH, Rowe AK, et al. The effect of mobile phone text-message reminders on Kenyan health workers' adherence to malaria treatment guidelines: a cluster randomised trial. *The Lancet.* 2011;378(9793):795–803.

105. Laksanasopin T, Guo TW, Nayak S, Sridhara AA, Xie S, Olowookere OO, et al. A smartphone dongle for diagnosis of infectious diseases at the point of care. *Science Translational Medicine*. 2015;7(273):273re1.
106. Chin CD, Laksanasopin T, Cheung YK, Steinmiller D, Linder V, Parsa H, et al. Microfluidics-based diagnostics of infectious diseases in the developing world. *Nature Medicine*. 2011;17(8):1015–9.
107. Guo T, Patnaik R, Kuhlmann K, Rai AJ, Sia SK. Smartphone dongle for simultaneous measurement of hemoglobin concentration and detection of HIV antibodies. *Lab on a Chip*. 2015;15(17):3514–20.
108. Yen C-W, de Puig H, Tam JO, Gómez-Márquez J, Bosch I, Hamad-Schifferli K, et al. Multicolored silver nanoparticles for multiplexed disease diagnostics: Distinguishing dengue, yellow fever, and Ebola viruses. *Lab on a Chip*. 2015;15(7):1638–41.
109. Fenton EM, Mascarenas MR, López GP, Sibbett SS. Multiplex lateral-flow test strips fabricated by two-dimensional shaping. *ACS Applied Materials Interfaces*. 2009;1(1):124–9.
110. Pohlmann A, Cantow K, Hentschel J, Arakelyan K, Ladwig M, Flemming B, et al. Linking non-invasive parametric MRI with invasive physiological measurements (MR-PHYSIOL): Towards a hybrid and integrated approach for investigation of acute kidney injury in rats. *Acta Physiologica*. 2013;207(4):673–89.
111. Mi P, Kokuryo D, Cabral H, Wu H, Terada Y, Saga T, et al. A pH-activatable nanoparticle with signal-amplification capabilities for non-invasive imaging of tumour malignancy. *Nature Nanotechnology*. 2016;11(8):724–30.
112. Ramachandra Kurup Sasikala A, Thomas RG, Unnithan AR, Saravanakumar B, Jeong YY, Park CH, et al. Multifunctional nanocarpets for cancer theranostics: Remotely controlled graphene nanoheaters for thermo-chemosensitisation and magnetic resonance imaging. *Scientific Reports*. 2016;6(1):1–14.
113. Dinh C-T, Nguyen T-D, Kleitz F, Do T-O. A new route to size and population control of silver clusters on colloidal TiO_2 nanocrystals. *ACS Applied Materials Interfaces*. 2011;3(7):2228–34.

2 Nanotechnology-Based Diagnostics for Healthcare

Arka Ghosh, Pankaj Shrivastava, Uddeshya Shukla, Vaibhav Chaudhary, Naveen Mindi, Nityananda Sahoo, Abhay Chowdary Edara, and Syed Nasimul Alam

2.1 INTRODUCTION

Humanity has always sought miracle cures and means to put an end to the suffering caused by diseases. According to researchers, the use of nanotechnology in medicine could be our first great step in achieving this dream. The integration of nanotechnology with healthcare promises a bright prospect for healthcare. Nanomedicines use nanotechnology for the treatment and diagnosis of diseases. Nanotechnology has the potential to transform the healthcare industry in terms of identifying diseases, assessing damage, and treating diseases. The development of devices and procedures that use nanomaterials and other nanotechnology has seen immense progress in the last decade [1–5]. A lot of research is going on in this field either to find new ways of diagnosis and treatment, or to improve the existing method and techniques. Incredible developments in the concepts that were envisioned a few decades ago may very soon turn into realities. Nanotechnology is dedicated to designing and developing advanced structures and structure composed systems by changing the atomic and molecular arrangement of the material at nano level. Majorly, the diseases in a body occur when there is a change occurs critically at molecular and cellular levels. Nanotechnology can be very effectively used to cure diseases by reaching down to the cells. Nanotechnology deals with the fabrication and application of nanoscale systems and has brought about a revolution. It can have a huge impact on the diagnosis, treatment, and prevention of diseases. Nanotechnology has brought about a major technological advancement that is capable of providing precise and effective therapy. Nanomaterials and nanotechnology together contribute in a large scale to the field of disease diagnosis, imaging, and various applications like targeted drug delivery. Nanotechnology can provide personalized, tailored medicine and therapy depending on the patient's genetic and disease profile. The term "nanotechnology" refers to the design and

DOI: 10.1201/9781003316435-2

manipulation of materials at the atomic and molecular scale. Nanotechnology is the science and engineering of things that are less than 100 nm in size in any one of their dimensions. The prefix "nano" resembles dwarf taken from a Greek word "nanos." For instance, a DNA double helix formed by two complementary strands of nucleotides held together by hydrogen bonds between guanine-cytosine (G-C) and adenine-thymine (A-T) base pairs is only 2 nm in diameter, and the diameter of an atom is less than 1 nm. Figure 2.1 shows the classification of nanomaterials [6–10].

Nanotechnology, along with instrumentation and telecommunication, helps improve the preciseness of diagnostic and therapeutic problems and could very effectively improve the care and management of diseases like cancer. Nanotechnology has the potential for application in areas like molecular diagnostics and drug delivery. The use of nanotechnology in diagnostic techniques promises to provide rapid testing, potentially in the office of the doctor. This will allow rapid diagnosis and can enable the immediate start of medicines. Early detection with the help of nanotechnology will also enable us to detect the disease at an early stage, which would help us prevent its spread, causing less damage to the patient. Nanotechnology-based medical diagnosis techniques are already under development. Nanotechnology has had a great impact on disease diagnostics by making use of the unique characteristics of nanomaterials such as their mechanical, thermal, optical, fluorescent, and magnetic properties. These properties of

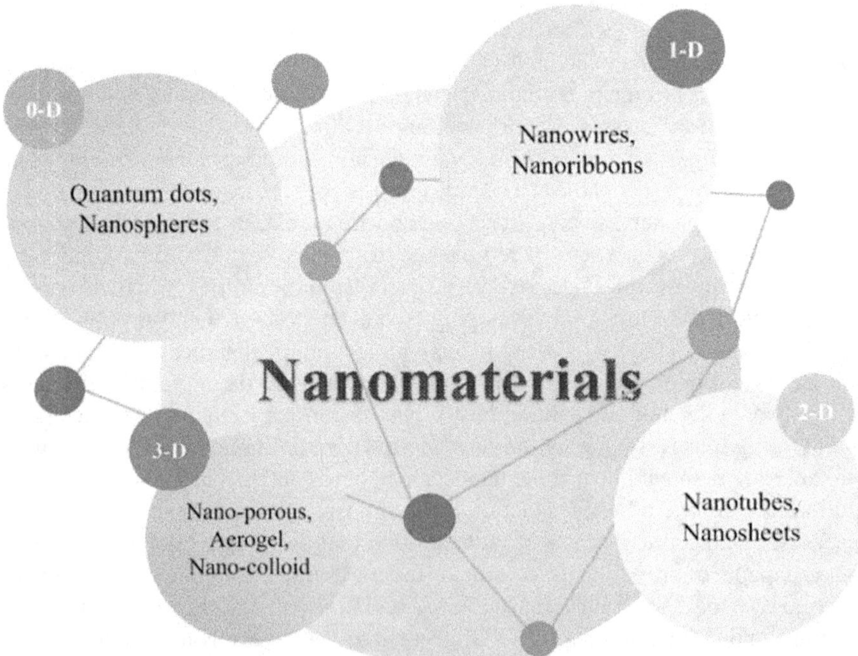

FIGURE 2.1 Classification of nanomaterials.

nanomaterials have been used in developing innovative devices. Nanomedicines are highly effective in drug delivery. It is also effective in treating other therapeutic treatments to specify tumor sites. It targets cells with minimum or no side effects as compared with regular chemotherapy and radiation. Normal chemotherapy and radiation cause damage to healthy blood cells during the treatment [11–14]. Figure 2.2 shows the medical applications of nanotechnology.

Nanotechnology is already making a huge impact in healthcare and diagnostics. Nanoparticles are being used to treat various stomach and intestinal tumors helping in delivering drugs at appropriate locations and improving diagnosis through medical imaging. There are different 0D to 3D nanomaterials like carbon nanotubes (CNTs), fullerenes, nanoparticles, graphene and its derivatives, quantum dots (QDs), and several others being used in the fabrication of diagnostic tests based on nanotechnology [15]. Nanocoatings are advanced and one of the prominent applications that nanotechnology has to offer. Suitable nanocoatings can increase the biocompatibility of medical devices and make it easier to integrate them with tissues in the vicinity of the place installed. Some examples are stent coating in cardiology, coating on substrate joint implants in orthopedics, and in dentistry as dental implant coatings. Furthermore, some nanomaterial coatings have anti-microbial properties that are used in medical textiles and wound care. Nanomaterials are also used to mimic and replace naturally existing structures in the body for optimized physical, biological, and mechanical properties of the implanted medical devices. Another set of applications utilize the unique magnetic and electrical properties of nanoscale materials. This feature is especially useful for medical devices in fields like cardiology and neurology; for

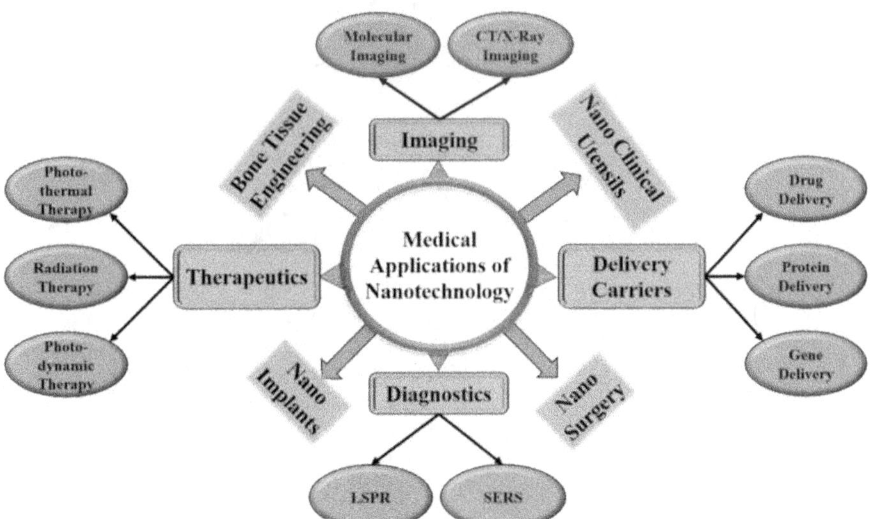

FIGURE 2.2 Medical applications of nanotechnology.

example, improving current cardiac arrhythmia treatment. Nanotechnology also enables the advancement of batteries to have significantly longer lifespans for the continuous operation of implantable medical devices [16,17]. Numerous applications of nanotechnology are exclusive to oncology; for example, early detection of cancer using diagnostic tests and devices for determining the precise periphery of a tumor or material growth during surgical operations. Also, the effectiveness of the treatments like chemotherapy/radiation therapy can be improved by nanomaterials by locally raising temperatures so that tumor cells can be directly destroyed at high temperatures. Nanoparticles can be used as contrast agents for popular *in vivo* imaging systems like magnetic resonance imaging (MRI), computed tomography (CT) scanning, positron emission tomography (PET), and ultrasound. Nanoparticles are capable of circulating in confined regions of individual organs, tissues, or cells. This allows us to produce a high-contrast image resulting in greater sensitivity imaging, which can be useful in studying pharmacokinetics or diagnosis of visual diseases [18,19]. Figures 2.3 and 2.4 illustrate the applications of nanotechnology in healthcare and diagnostics.

Nanotechnology has paved the way for very effective healthcare and provides new insights into the area of drug usage. It has the potential to increase life expectancy by providing novel and highly innovative technologies in the areas of diagnostics and healthcare. QDs are a form of nanoparticles composed of semiconductor material, mainly sulfides of metals like cadmium (Cd) and zinc (Zn) having a diameter of 2–10 nm. It is made up of a metalloid crystalline core and a cap or shell that protects the core while also making the QDs biocompatible.

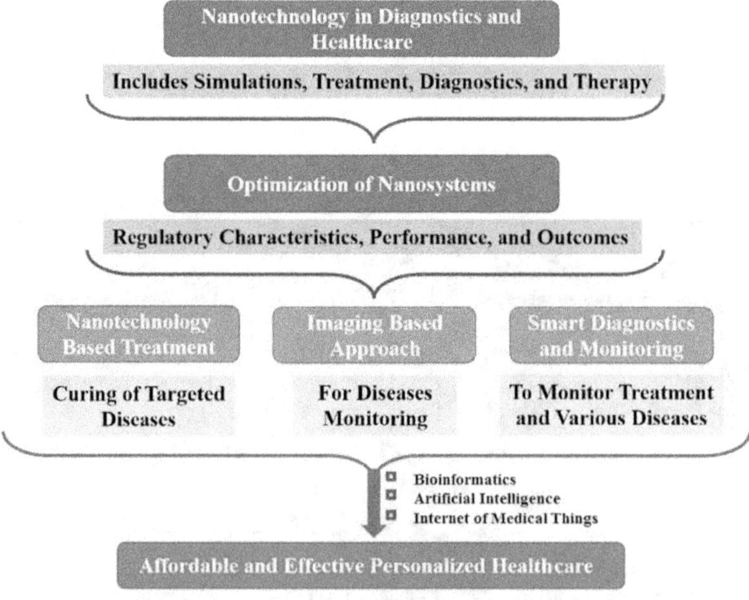

FIGURE 2.3 Nanotechnology in diagnostics and healthcare.

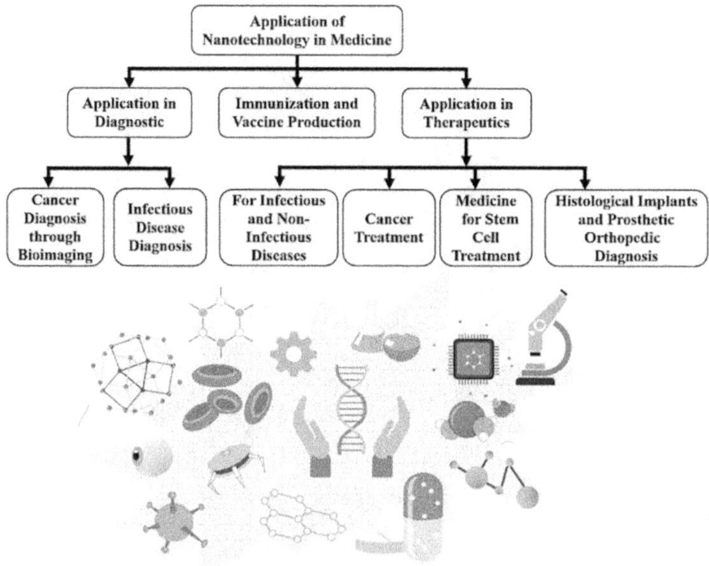

FIGURE 2.4 Applications of nanotechnology in healthcare.

To improve the durability and suspension qualities, as well as achieve the desired aim such as medication delivery or molecular imaging, biocompatible coatings or functional groups are applied to the core shell. It should be noted that any flaw in the coating material or technique could expose a metalloid core *in vivo*, which could be harmful as a composite. QDs are used for viral infections, treatments, and various imaging techniques. Combined QD has been found to be effective in the treatment of AIDS and may transport saquinavir via BBB [20]. Chemotherapeutic drugs containing essential lung toxins are usually delivered using carbon nanoformulations. The use of protoporphyrin IX with multidrug nanotube to treat colds has also been shown to be effective. The flu virus is blocked by this chemical due to the breakdown of RNA strands and protein oxidation. Antibacterial properties can be obtained from a variety of natural and microbiological sources. They come from a variety of sources, including frog skin, marine resources, plants, animals, and bacteria. HIV, H1N1, DENV, and HCV are all treated with it. Drug withdrawal is faster with nanospheres. Acyclovir-loaded chitosan nanospheres are more effective than acyclo viral one in treating herpes. Nanocapsules are used to increase drug loading and delivery of complementary drugs. The drug is delivered directly to the cytoplasm using only core nanocapsules with capturing azidothymidine triphosphate (AZT-TP) [21,22]. Dendrimers possess a high level of cell absorption, extended cycle duration, and targeted delivery. Recently, glycol dendropeptide has been introduced as an anti-viral medicament. Dendrimers having blocking properties are also available. Viral entry fusion has proven very effective in the treatment of HIV and AIDS. HSV2 is a herpes simplex virus. Polyanionic carbosilane, for example, is one of them. Dendrimers are repetitively branched

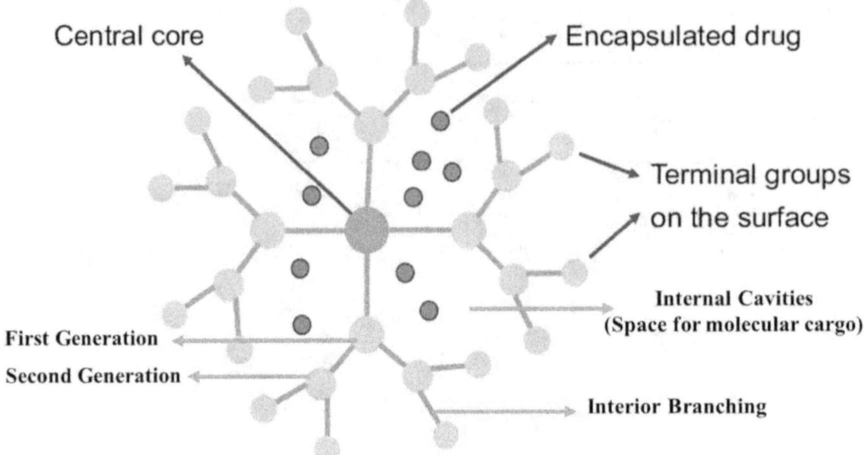

FIGURE 2.5 Dendrimer.

molecules. The word "dendrimer" comes from the Greek word "Dendron", which means "tree". They are a family of nanosized, highly branched three-dimensional molecules. Dendrimers are highly defined nanoparticles. Figure 2.5 illustrates the molecular structure of a dendrimer [23].

2.2 NANOBOTS AND SMART PILLS

Nanobots are nearly 100 nm wide in size and are artificially made nanosized robots that execute very critical yet specific functions and are developed from molecular components. The science behind nanobots is termed "nanorobotics" and deals with designing and fabricating nanobots and their accessories at the atomic or nanosized level. They are capable of traveling inside the human bloodstream and are often used during drug injection and drug delivery. In general, the drug when given through injections or through medicines initially goes throughout the body before reaching the destined infected area. Nanobots can release the drug at targeted sites, and this effectively reduces any chances of possible side effects. Nanobots have sensors that can target molecules. In medical science and healthcare, there is only a tiny room for error. There are certain tasks in medical science, like eliminating defective parts in a DNA structure or pinpointing cancer cells, that require extremely high precision. These tasks that are almost impossible can be done using nanobots and nanomachines. The section that takes care of holding and releasing the small quantity of the drug is called payload [24,25]. Nanobots are miniature surgeons, which are at a micro-scale. Nanobots are still in the development stage. Intracellular structures can be repaired and replaced by nanobots. By replicating themselves, nanobots correct the defect in genetics. They eradicate the disease by replacing DNA molecules with them. Figure 2.6 lists the various functions of nanobots and shows the cross section of a nanobot. The advancement in the medical sector through nanotechnology is possible in

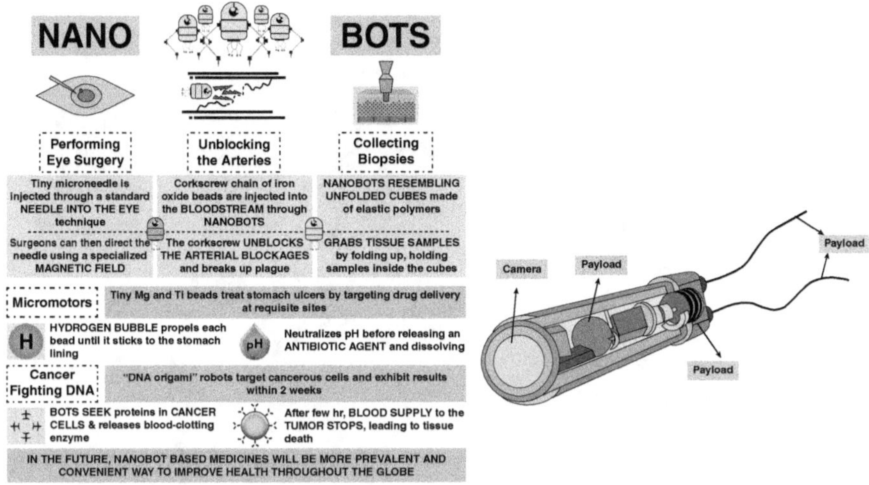

FIGURE 2.6 Nanobots.

the near future in a few years. Eye surgeries are also going to be performed by nanobots. This process is done with the help of a microscopic needle by inserting it into the retina of the eye. This needle can be directed using a specific magnetic field that is operated by the surgeons. Artery blockages can be cleared by the nanobots by drilling into them. Nanobots that contain carbon nanotubes (CNTs) are being developed by researchers at Michigan State University and Stanford University. These nanobots carry a drug that erodes the arterial plaque gradually. In this way, the risk of heart attacks is reduced. Scientists at Toronto University have developed nanobots that resemble unfolded cubes. They perform quick biopsies of suspected malignant masses. After these cubes reach the target tissue, they fold up and take a sample of it. The operations done by human surgeons are slower and less accurate than the biopsies.

Nanobots have the potential to change the future of medical treatment. The Food and Drug Administration (FDA) of the USA has already approved the ingestible camera (PillCam) which is a smart pill equipped with a camera. Another smart pill which is a vibrating capsule (Vibrant Capsule) promotes muscle contractions to jumpstart digestion. It can very effectively treat constipation with the use of laxatives and thus avoid side effects. Smart pills, like Dose Tracking Pills, have a sensor that releases the drug through a patch worn by the patient. App can now track drugs, dosage, and time. A smart pill can improve drug adherence and patient outcomes. Another smart pill, the Atmo Gas capsule, has a permeable membrane that allows gases to enter the capsule. Sensors in the capsules can detect the levels of O_2, H_2, and CO_2. A Smart Sensor capsule developed by MIT can unfold into a Y-shaped lodging in the stomach for about a month (Figure 2.7). These capsules reduce the necessity of drug injection inside the stomach. When it is delivered orally, it lodges itself on the organ after unfolding itself automatically. The sensors detect the viral signals released from the ill parts of the body and

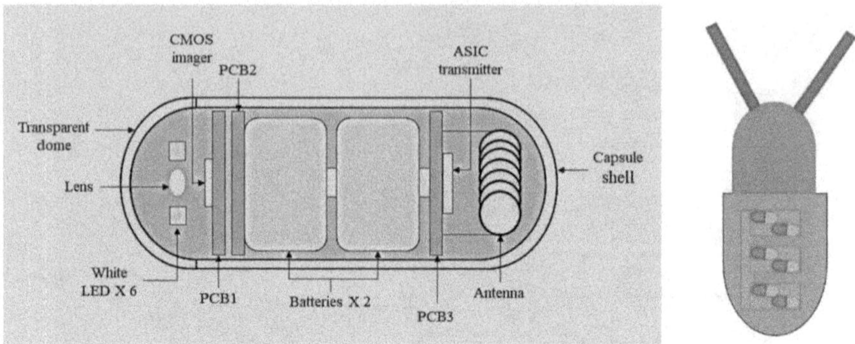

FIGURE 2.7 Smart capsule.

diagnose the problem regarding and act accordingly. This act of signal detecting and diagnosing the problem is called treatment monitoring. The drug-containing counterparts can then release the medications according to the requirement. These medicines can be ejected at target parts of the body [26,27].

Smart pills are electronic devices at the nanoscale. They look similar to pharmaceutical pills, but they are ahead of them by doing the functions like sensing, imaging, and drug delivery. We can say that nanotechnology is a boon because it helps the medicine sector a lot. Examples are PillCam (the tablet which has a minute camcorder) explained in Figure 2.8a and Dose Tracking Pill shown in Figure 2.8b. The Dose Tracking Pill is a highly useful device as treatment nonadherence costs have risen up to $290 billion in the US. One more example of smart pills is the Atmo Gas capsule. Its function is to examine the gases present inside the human gut when it is consumed. Its main motive is to report any disorders. Sensors in the capsule detect the levels of H_2, O_2, and CO_2 along with the presence

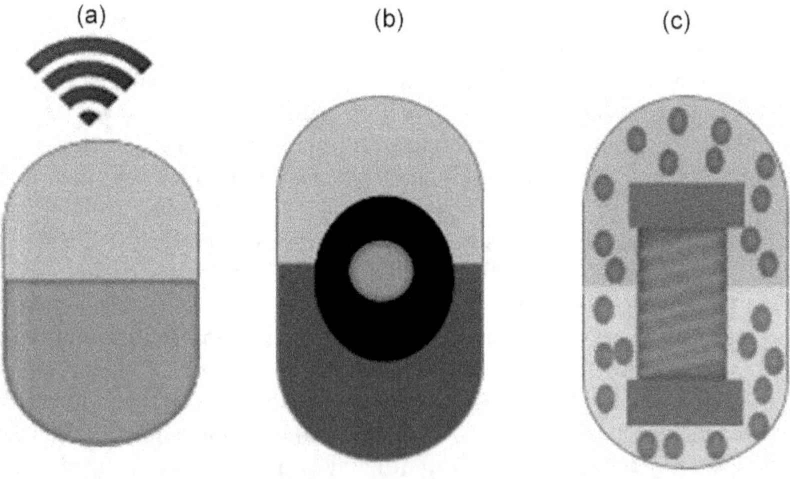

FIGURE 2.8 (a) Pill cam, (b) Dose Tracking Pill, and (c) Atmo Gas capsule.

of harmful substances in the body with the help of its sensors. O_2 levels allow researchers to point the capsule's location to the gut microbiome. Figure 2.8c is the schematic diagram of an Atmo Gas capsule. It helps in giving abrupt information on personalized diet and nutrition plans. It diagnoses disorders in the intestinal part, especially the gastrointestine, detects infectious organs of the digestive systems, and tracks food sensitivities.

2.3 NANOTECHNOLOGY-BASED PROSTHETICS

Tan et al. [28] reported on the manufacturing of an intelligent prosthetic limb. Carbon-based nanomaterials have been used for the development of prosthetic limbs. Carbonaceous materials either in form of reinforcements or bulk materials exhibit strong material stability and a very simple mechanism of transmission. It has been seen earlier also that hybrid nanomaterials exhibit better material characteristics. Hence, there is a strong need for new hybrid nanomaterials that can provide higher performance to prosthetic devices and remarkably improve the quality of life of the disabled. The biosensing properties exhibited by the prosthetic limbs manufactured using nanomaterials give rise to the designing and production of various other nanocomposites that can be used as advanced functioning prosthetic limbs. Researchers at Oak Ridge National Laboratory (ORNL) are collaborating with researchers from NASA to develop multifunctional, highly flexible, light-weighted, integrated skins (also called FILM skin) that can be employed for next-generation prosthetic hands, legs, and arms. The team is trying to develop a revolutionary skin that can outperform the current prosthetic coverings in properties as well as functionality. This will allow the prosthetic wearer to feel heat, cold, and touch. The researchers are trying to develop a material that can match the properties of the natural skin. This artificial skin will be able to sense both temperature and pressure. The researchers are trying to develop a unit square-sized FILM skin patch that will be light in weight and highly durable made up of polymer composite reinforced with CNT nanoreinforcement which can be used for the covering of prosthetics and function as the natural skin. Figure 2.9 illustrates the advantages of using nanotechnology in prosthetics.

2.4 DNA NANOTECHNOLOGY

Over the past few decades, the DNA molecule has been used to develop a variety of nanoscale materials. DNA, which is a genetic material, serves as a platform to develop chemical, mechanical, and physical devices. DNA has shown its excellence as a fabrication technique of different nanosized structures and instruments that are used in biological applications. Due to the advancement in the field of nanotechnology, it is possible to design and fabricate instruments and structures using DNA to be used in different biomedical applications such as delivering drugs to desired locations and creating new and advanced vaccines. DNA nanotechnology could be highly effective in diagnosing diseases like cancer in very early or developing stages. DNA nanotechnology has been used for tissue generation, disease diagnosis and prevention, biosensing and bioimaging, inflammation

Fast
Integration
Better Bio-
compatibility
Greater
Strength
Less
Toxicity
Better
Morphological
Properties
Advantages of
Nanotechnology
on Prosthetics
Enhanced
Durability
Better
Mechanical
Performance
Optimal and
Accurate
Design
Better
Hygiene
High
Failure
Resistance
High
Fatigue
Resistance

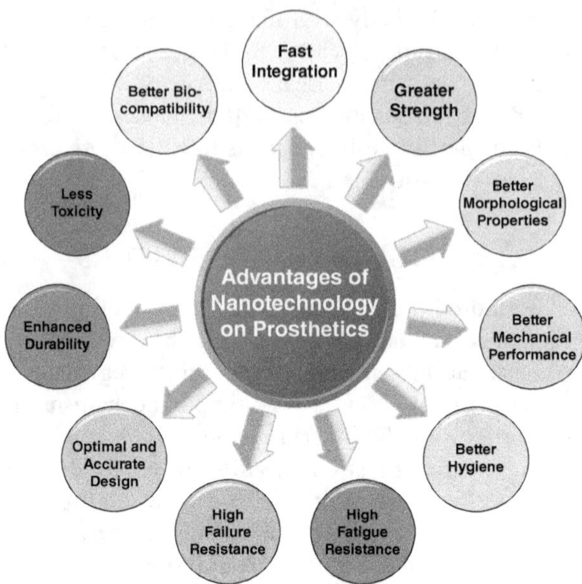

FIGURE 2.9 Advantages of nanotechnology in prosthetics.

restriction, drug delivery, and therapeutics. The DNA-based nanoscale structure and devices are extremely efficient to diagnose cancer-growing viruses at a particular location of a body due to their predictable secondary structures, small sizes, high biocompatibility, and programmability. The rapid growth in the DNA-based nanotechnology like signal amplification has led to enormous functionalization of DNA-based nanomaterials. With the evolution in the field of DNA nanotechnology, various DNA nanomaterials are designed and brought into production that has simple to complex shapes and sizes based on Watson-Crick base pairing for molecular self-assembly. DNA-based nanomaterials exhibit great potential to overcome the limitations like reduced dosing due to cardiotoxicity, vascular permeability issues, low payload efficiency to target cells, and unpredictable drug release rates related to the current nanotechnologies available to us. DNA nanomaterials have given plentiful delicate bio-recognition components for target detecting, and they have been utilized as acceptable supplements or substitutes for the current detecting components. A very precise methodology is exhibited to diagnose various premature, temporary, and catastrophic diseases via DNA-based diagnostic routes. DNA-based diagnostic approaches utilize *in vitro* DNA manipulations like restriction analysis, PCR, DNA hybridization, SNPs, and or short tandem repeat (STR) detection. In order to target specific disease cells, scientists are creating nanobots based on DNA. To transport a molecular payload, an origami nanobot out of DNA has been developed by researchers at Harvard Medical School. They have demonstrated the way how these nanobots kill specific disease cells by delivering molecules [29,30]. Figure 2.10 shows the double-helix structure of DNA and the various applications of DNA nanotechnology.

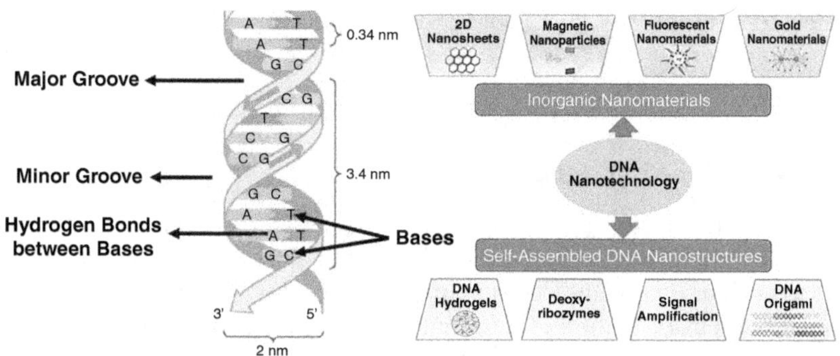

FIGURE 2.10 Double-helix structure of DNA and different applications associated with DNA nanotechnology.

2.5 APPLICATION OF MICELLES IN DIAGNOSTICS

Another class of organic nanoparticles utilized in diagnosis is micelles. This hydrophobic core-hydrophilic self-assembling colloidal nanoparticle is made of surfactants like sodium lauryl sulfate. There may also be medications and are functionalized with polymers and targeting compounds. In locations with leaky vasculatures, such as those with tumors, inflammation, and infection, these can passively collect. Micelles have been utilized successfully in the pharmaceutical industry to transport water-soluble medications. Due to their great stability and superior biocompatibility, polymer micelles have recently attracted more and more attention for tumor imaging. Liquids and soluble copolymers can be combined to create a specific kind of polymeric micelles. The modified micelles may work as imaging probes for multi-modal tumor diagnosis since they can carry a variety of specific target moieties on their surface [31,32].

2.6 NON-IMPLANTABLE MEDICAL DEVICES

Nano-structuration has already found application in needles, catheters, bandages, scalpels, and other diagnostic devices. For a very long time, silver (Ag) has been well renowned for its anti-microbial properties along with a broad activity spectrum, due to which it is added in bandages. This anti-infectious property arises from the synergetic interaction between nanoparticles and silver ions through catalytic, Fenton-like processes. These ions come from corrosion/dissolution of nanoparticles when extracellular water and exudates come into contact [33–35]. In comparison to salt, the colloidal form provides for a longer and more effective action. This approach is utilized to avoid infections in surgical masks as well as to prevent nosocomial infections by catheter coatings. Additional research on catheters aims to incorporate polymeric matrices comprised of ceramic or clay nanoparticles, or possibly carbon nanotubes (CNT), to strengthen the currently used materials and enhance physical and mechanical qualities. Nanometric diamond coating is done on scalpels, which allows for finer and more precise incisions due to the low coefficient of friction leading to less invasive surgery. The coating formed also reduces tissue adherence on the scalpel's surface, making penetration easier.

2.7 IMPLANTABLE MEDICAL DEVICES

Stents, synthetic grafts, implants for organs, and even artificial organs are some of the developed implantable medical devices that contain nanoparticles. Synthetic grafts are primarily used as a substitute for vessels for developing *in silico* organs. Nanofibers are made this way, for instance, by electrospinning. We can tailor these nanofibers in terms of size (depending upon the polymer used), shape, and density to generate extracellular matrices that are very much comparable to the biological surroundings. Coronary stents are devices having a tubular shape that are used to treat patients with arterial occlusion. They are inserted inside a coronary blood vessel via a catheter. They are also one of the most commonly used medical devices. Stents support a section of arteries/veins or any other tubular body part to restore and maintain its patency. Patients with peripheral artery disease, such as narrowing of blood vessels in the upper and lower leg, are also treated with stents. There are many types of stents available, like drug-eluting, bare metal, and bio-resorbable vascular scaffolds. Polyzene-F (a derivative of polyphosphazene) is a nanocoating for stents that has good hemocompatibility and promotes rapid and total vessel-healing due to an anti-platelet impact at the implantation site [36–38]. After clinical testing, it was seen that this coating outperformed other routes such as new biodegradable or metallic alloy stents in terms of benefit/risk balance. Aside from vascular applications, there are a large variety of implants available for joints, bones, eyes, and teeth. Such implants are designed to last for up to 10–15 years, and the metal alloys used have excellent mechanical properties and corrosion resistance. The nanostructure surface of the implant material as well as its nature (hydroxyapatite/calcium phosphate for bones) has been demonstrated to improve cell adhesion and differentiation resulting in increased long-period biocompatibility. Nanoparticles have aided in the advancement and development of artificial organs such as the kidney, heart, and retina. In 2013, the Carmat Company implanted the first completely artificial heart. This revolutionary heart has benefited ten patients thus far. In this approach, synthetic or hydrophobic biomaterials are used to coat internal surfaces and near the valves which are in direct contact with the bloodstream to prevent blood cell adhesion and coagulation, while the arteries and veins have deposition of nano-porous surface biomaterials in their interface. Besides these, other miniaturized systems are also used to reproduce the physical activity of the heart. It is essential to note that the problems that occurred after the artificial heart was implanted (bacterial infection/power failure leading to patient's death) were not due to nanomaterials present in the device. Artificial kidneys are made up of thousands of nano-porous structures that can particularly select toxins to adsorb [39–41]. The main concept is to replicate the endocrine, immunological, and metabolic activities of the organ by the combination of a bio-reactor built from human kidney tubule cells and an ultra-filtration membrane.

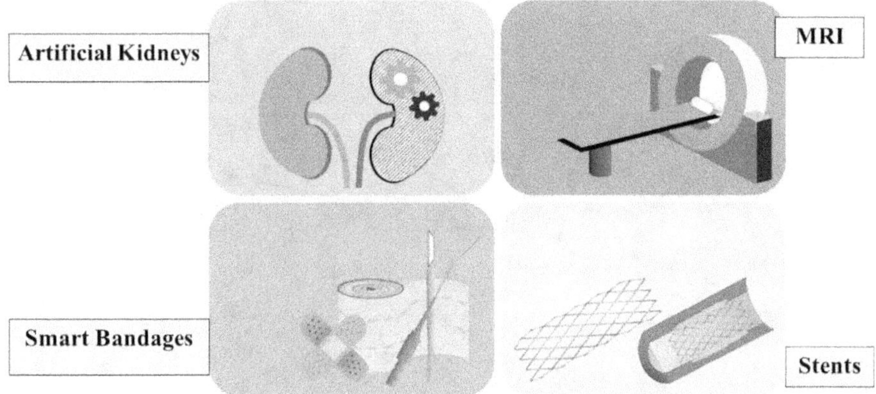

FIGURE 2.11 Nanomaterials in various medical devices.

To imitate renal action, cells are grown on a nano-porous silicon thin film, which prevents protein deposition and limits blood protein loss. Artificial retina implants ($3\times3\,mm^2$) are being tested that can send information from a camera to the optic nerve via miniaturized nanoelectrodes (up to 1,500). New methodologies for developing artificial retinas were recently published in a few studies. Figure 2.11 shows some of the devices in which nanotechnology has been used.

Another area where nanotechnology is being applied to develop tools and devices is *in vivo* imaging. MRI and ultrasound produce images with better contrast and distribution when nanoparticle contrast agents are used. Nanoparticles can assist cardiovascular imaging for the visualization of blood pooling, atherosclerosis, ischemia, angiogenesis, and focal regions of inflammation. Nanoparticle qualities are also helpful in imaging for oncology. QDs, when used in combination with MRI, can give outstanding images of tumor spots. Cadmium selenide nanoparticles (QDs) illuminate under the exposure of UV light. They can seep into a cancer tumor after being injected. Therefore, the surgeon can distinctively see the glowing tumor and remove it with more precision. Such nanoparticles are significantly brighter than organic dyes, and just a single source of light is sufficient to excite them. This suggests that using fluorescent QDs, instead of organic dyes, as a contrast medium could result in images of higher contrast at a lesser cost. However, QDs are often made from hazardous elements, but this problem can be dealt with by using fluorescent dopants [42–45].

2.8 NANOFIBERS

Nowadays, the hospitals are using nanofibers in wound dressings, surgical textiles, implants, tissue engineering, and artificial organ parts. Smart badges absorb themselves into the tissue once the wound heals when they are left on the wound site. Scientists are trying to develop these smart bandages. Infection is detected by the sensors in these smart bandages. Besides these sensors, it also contains

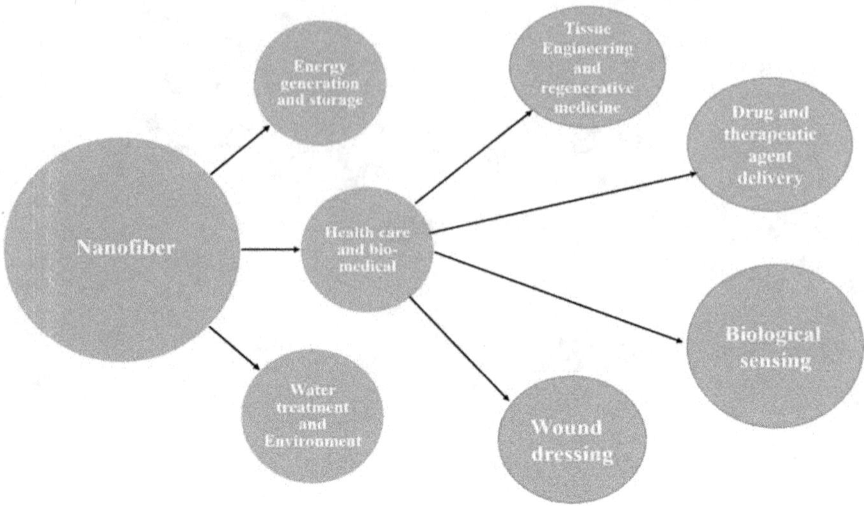

FIGURE 2.12 Application of nanofiber in the medical industry.

clotting agents and antibiotics. A pH-sensitive smart bandage was developed by the Institute of Advanced Studies in Science and Technology, India. These bandages can supply the medicine that is needed for the wound at that particular pH. These bandages are made with a nanotechnology-based cotton patch that uses common materials like cotton and jute. In order to achieve the desired therapeutic effects, nanofibers-based drug delivery systems are being used for specific drug release, that too at a specific target location and set time. Nanofibers use a suitable polymer with increased efficiency in order to achieve immediate drug release. Nanopatch vaccines, a nanofiber patch that uses nanoparticles to impose vaccine directly into the immune system lying under the skin, is being developed by Vaxxas. The motive is to reduce the risk of bacterial attack and eliminate the need for the chilling of the vaccine [46–48]. Figure 2.12 illustrates the applications of nanofibers in the medical industry.

2.9 WEARABLES DEVELOPED USING NANOTECHNOLOGY

Nowadays, nanotechnology-based clothes are being used because of the advantage of monitoring the health of patients. These clothes contain sensors that collect data about our blood pressure and heartbeat. It saves lives by altering the conditions in serious situations of the patients. Figure 2.13 shows the nano wear that was widely used during the Covid-19 pandemic. This nano wear was invented by a US-based start-up. They launched NanoSENSE in 2019 which works on heart failure management and diagnosis with a closed-loop machine learning platform. It uses nanosensors to collect data about cardiac output as well as records phonocardiography, pulse pressure ratio, and rate of flow in the heart. It also has the technology which assesses the multi-channel ECG. In order to identify the

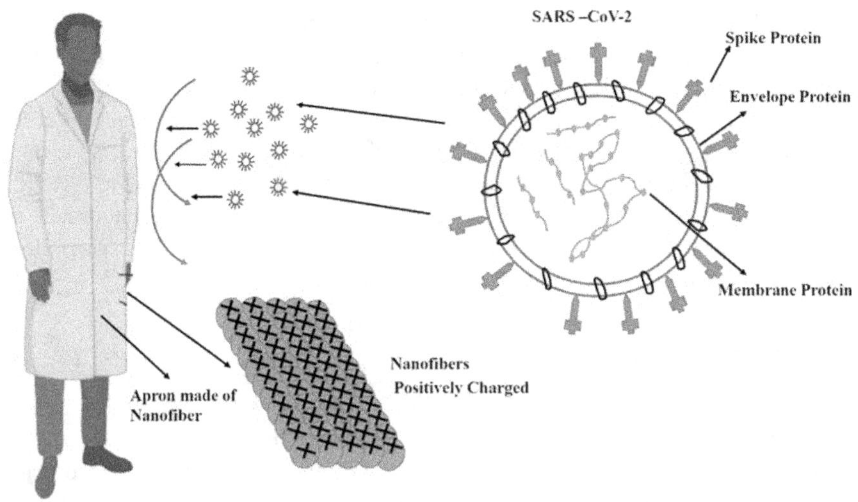

FIGURE 2.13 Wearables developed by using nanotechnology for SARS-CoV-2.

Covid-19 patients with its nanosensors using nano wear cloth, Nano wear collaborated with Hackensack Meridian Health Systems in July 2020. These cloth wear detect physiological and biomarker changes [49–51].

2.10 NANO SOLUTIONS FOR COVID-19

COVID-19 can also be treated with stimulating nanomedicine, such as the secretome of mesenchymal stem cells. In patients infected with COVID-19, *in vitro* evidence of secreted extracellular material sowed numerous therapeutic effects. Mesenchymal stem cells (MSCs) can treat acute respiratory distress syndrome (ARDS), fight fibrosis, and regenerate and repair lung damage by secreting IL-10, a factor in hepatocyte growth, and VEGF. T lymphocytes and macrophages can be incorrectly assembled by MSCs, leading to their subdivision into subcutaneous T cells and anti-inflammatory macrophages. MSCs are the best choice of existing COVID-19 cell phone treatment drugs because of their functional properties. Exosomes are also an effective treatment option for COVID-19. Exosomes are small packets produced by stem cells containing biological proteins and nucleic acid molecules. They exhibit stimulating, immune, and anti-inflammatory properties similar to those of their own mesenchymal stem cells [52–56].

2.11 DRAWBACKS AND CHALLENGES

Nanotechnology in healthcare has the ability to drastically transform medical science and benefit developing countries as part of beneficial nanotechnology. However, it will open up a whole new domain which is set to pose many profound and complex ethical doubts in front of medical professionals. There is a thin line between non-medical and medical applications of nanotechnology for therapeutic, diagnostic, and preventive functions. The fact that nanotechnology should be applied to make purposeful alterations inside the body even when there is no medical requirement is just one heated issue in a large number of concerns. In nanotechnology-based medical devices, the undiscovered aspect is whether the manufacturing methods, exposure, and handling of products would have any significant negative influence on health. Also, the long-term influence of these nano-devices on humans is still uncertain, and their large-scale direct or indirect manufacturing in the environment is not yet known.

2.12 SUMMARY

Nanotechnology helps us detect early indications of sickness and assess genetic prepositions more quickly and accurately. Traditional tests take long time and are costlier. Doctors have to rely on sophisticated instruments and elaborate protocols. A huge number of tests must be sent to centralized laboratories. Nanotechnology, on the other hand, is revolutionizing the field of medicine in a variety of ways. So, in terms of diagnostics, it will provide a highly accurate and sensitive tool that enables point of care diagnostics. At the nanometric scale, the earliest signs of disease occur. A human body is comprised of hundred trillion living cells that communicate with one another to exist. The messages are made up of very tiny molecules. DNA fragments are small, complicated proteins with a diameter of a few nanometers. These molecular messengers set off reaction cascades, which are the languages of the most intimate form of communication. When a cell becomes ill, it sends out several messages. They are referred to as biomarkers by a biologist. They are the disease's molecular hallmark as well as the cues, or indicators, on which even the most advanced diagnostic tool is based. It turns out that practically every disease has a distinct genetic marker and, in many cases, a unique protein marker. The world has gotten very excellent at recognizing what these markers are in the last couple of decades, and now it has begun to build tests for all kinds of different indicators that allow us to quickly access, establish the stage of the disease, and then follow up with a course of therapy. The machine exemplifies many of the advancements advocated by nanoscientists, such as being simple, entirely automated, and using disposable cartridges. Doctors can determine the existence of many diseases, genetic predispositions, or viruses in the blood with just one sample. Researchers can use fundamental characteristics of molecular messengers to explore illness biomarkers. According to a lock-and-key logic, they are only attached to specific other molecules. If the diseases are present, these bonding chemicals, known as ligands, can be employed to locate and capture the target. The researchers need to see if bonding has occurred at a molecular level to detect the disease. In conclusion, it can be claimed that the development of nanotechnology has raised the diagnostic methods used in medical science to a new level. The nanoparticles can deeply permeate all biological components because of their incredibly small size. Diverse biomarkers like antibodies, oligonucleotides, peptides, and fluorophores can be functionalized on the surface of the nanoparticles. A timely diagnosis of an illness is considered to result in its cure. Therefore, diagnostic methods based on nanomaterials aid in the early identification and diagnosis of any disease state.

REFERENCES

1. Gomez-Marquez J, Hamad-Schifferli K. Local development of nanotechnology-based diagnostics. *Nat Nanotechnol.* 2021 May 12;16(5):484–6.
2. Alharbi KK, Al-sheikh YA. Role and implications of nanodiagnostics in the changing trends of clinical diagnosis. *Saudi J Biol Sci.* 2014 Apr;21(2):109–17.
3. Yin HQ, Langford R, Burrell RE. Comparative evaluation of the antimicrobial activity of ACTICOAT antimicrobial barrier dressing. *J Burn Care Rehabil.* 1999 May;20(3):195–200.
4. Meetoo D. Nanotechnology: The revolution of the big future with tiny medicine. *Br J Nurs.* 2009 Oct 1;18(19):1201–6.
5. Ma W, Zhan Y, Zhang Y, Mao C, Xie X, Lin Y. The biological applications of DNA nanomaterials: Current challenges and future directions. *Signal Transduct Target Ther.* 2021 Oct 8;6(1):351.
6. Sami A, Mahmood RT, Shah SH, Iqbal MU. Nanotechnology in human health care system: A review. *J Pub Health Bio Sci.* 2012;1(4):121–6.
7. Laroui H, Rakhya P, Xiao B, Viennois E, Merlin D. Nanotechnology in diagnostics and therapeutics for gastrointestinal disorders. *Dig Liver Dis.* 2013 Dec;45(12):995–1002.
8. Shrivastava P, Alam SN, Biswas K. Ex situ fabrication of multiwalled carbon nanotube-reinforced aluminum nanocomposite via conventional sintering and SPS techniques. *Arab J Sci Eng.* 2022 Jul 29;47(7):8643–62.
9. Paules CI, Marston HD, Fauci AS. Coronavirus infections-more than just the common cold. *JAMA.* 2020 Feb 25;323(8):707.
10. Mainardes RM, Diedrich C. The potential role of nanomedicine on COVID-19 therapeutics. *Ther Deliv.* 2020 Jul;11(7):411–4.
11. Mukherjee S, Ray S, Thakur R. Solid lipid nanoparticles: A modern formulation approach in drug delivery system. *Indian J Pharm Sci.* 2009;71(4):349.
12. Edagwa B, Zhou T, McMillan J, Liu X-M, Gendelman H. Development of HIV reservoir targeted long acting nanoformulated antiretroviral therapies. *Curr Med Chem.* 2014 Oct 24;21(36):4186–98.
13. Sharma A, Kakkar A. Designing dendrimer and miktoarm polymer based multi-tasking nanocarriers for efficient medical therapy. *Molecules.* 2015 Sep 17;20(9): 16987–7015.
14. Anu Mary Ealia S, Saravanakumar MP. A review on the classification, characterisation, synthesis of nanoparticles and their application. *IOP Conf Ser Mater Sci Eng.* 2017 Nov;263:032019.
15. Shrivastava P, Alam SN, Maity T, Biswas K. Effect of graphite nanoplatelets on spark plasma sintered and conventionally sintered aluminum-based nanocomposites developed by powder metallurgy. *Mater Sci.* 2021 Sep 1;39(3):346–70.
16. Geertsma R, Park M, Puts C, Roszek B, van der Stijl R, de Jong W. Nanotechnologies in medical devices. Rijksinst voor Volksgezond en Milieu. 2015;86.
17. Yadavalli T, Shukla D. Role of metal and metal oxide nanoparticles as diagnostic and therapeutic tools for highly prevalent viral infections. *Nanomed Nanotechnol Biol Med.* 2017 Jan;13(1):219–30.
18. Guo H, MacKay JA. A pharmacokinetics primer for preclinical nanomedicine research. In: *Nanoparticles for Biomedical Applications.* Elsevier; 2020. pp. 109–28. doi: 10.1016/B978-0-12-816662-8.00008-4.

19. Chen Y-T, Kolhatkar AG, Zenasni O, Xu S, Lee TR. Biosensing using magnetic particle detection techniques. *Sensors*. 2017 Oct 10;17(10):2300.
20. Tiwari PK, Sahu M, Kumar G, Ashourian M. Pivotal role of quantum dots in the advancement of healthcare research. *Comput Intell Neurosci*. 2021 Aug 6;2021:1–9.
21. Jung JH, Park BH, Oh SJ, Choi G, Seo TS. Integration of reverse transcriptase loop-mediated isothermal amplification with an immunochromatographic strip on a centrifugal microdevice for influenza A virus identification. *Lab Chip*. 2015;15(3):718–25.
22. Kumar A, Mazinder Boruah B, Liang X-J. Gold nanoparticles: Promising nanomaterials for the diagnosis of cancer and HIV/AIDS. *J Nanomater*. 2011;2011:1–17.
23. Mittal P, Saharan A, Verma R, Altalbawy FMA, Alfaidi MA, Batiha GE-S, et al. Dendrimers: A new race of pharmaceutical nanocarriers. *Biomed Res Int*. 2021 Feb 15;2021:1–11.
24. Viswanathan SM. Nanobots in medical field: A critical overview. *Int J Eng Res*. 2019 Dec 11;8(12):65–68.
25. Prabhu S, Poulose EK. Silver nanoparticles: Mechanism of antimicrobial. *Int Nano Lett*. 2012;2:32–41.
26. Poduval RK, Noimark S, Colchester RJ, Macdonald TJ, Parkin IP, Desjardins AE, et al. Optical fiber ultrasound transmitter with electrospun carbon nanotube-polymer composite. *Appl Phys Lett*. 2017 May 29;110(22):223701.
27. Dunn K, Edwards-Jones V. The role of Acticoat™ with nanocrystalline silver in the management of burns. *Burns*. 2004 Jul;30:S1–9.
28. Tan Q, Wu C, Li L, Shao W, Luo M. Nanomaterial-based prosthetic limbs for disability mobility assistance: A review of recent advances. *J Nanomater*. 2022 Mar 31;2022:1–10.
29. Lucas CR, Halley PD, Chowdury AA, Harrington BK, Beaver L, Lapalombella R, et al. DNA origami nanostructures elicit dose-dependent immunogenicity and are nontoxic up to high doses in vivo. *Small*. 2022 Jul 28;18(26):2108063.
30. Alt V, Bechert T, Steinrücke P, Wagener M, Seidel P, Dingeldein E, et al. An in vitro assessment of the antibacterial properties and cytotoxicity of nanoparticulate silver bone cement. *Biomaterials*. 2004 Aug;25(18):4383–91.
31. Jhaveri AM, Torchilin VP. Multifunctional polymeric micelles for delivery of drugs and siRNA. *Front Pharmacol*. 2014 Apr 25;5:77.
32. Erdemir A, Donnet C. Tribology of diamond-like carbon films: Recent progress and future prospects. *J Phys D Appl Phys*. 2006 Sep 21;39(18):R311–27.
33. Pallotta A, Clarot I, Sobocinski J, Fattal E, Boudier A. Nanotechnologies for medical devices: Potentialities and risks. *ACS Appl Bio Mater*. 2019 Jan 22;2(1):1–13.
34. El-Sayed A, Kamel M. Advances in nanomedical applications: Diagnostic, therapeutic, immunization, and vaccine production. *Environ Sci Pollut Res*. 2020;27(16):19200–13.
35. Wicki A, Witzigmann D, Balasubramanian V, Huwyler J. Nanomedicine in cancer therapy: Challenges, opportunities, and clinical applications. *J Control Release*. 2015 Feb;200:138–57.
36. Mrowietz C, Franke RP, Seyfert UT, Park JW, Jung F. Haemocompatibility of polymer-coated stainless steel stents as compared to uncoated stents. *Clin Hemorheol Microcirc*. 2005;32(2):89–103.
37. Shahriar S, Mondal J, Hasan M, Revuri V, Lee D, Lee Y-K. Electrospinning nanofibers for therapeutics delivery. *Nanomaterials*. 2019 Apr 3;9(4):532.
38. Hathout RM, Kassem DH. Positively charged electroceutical spun chitosan nanofibers can protect health care providers from COVID-19 infection: An opinion. *Front Bioeng Biotechnol*. 2020 Aug 18;8:885.

39. Divya Rani VV, Vinoth-Kumar L, Anitha VC, Manzoor K, Deepthy M, Shantikumar VN. Osteointegration of titanium implant is sensitive to specific nanostructure morphology. *Acta Biomater.* 2012 May;8(5):1976–89.
40. Fissell WH, Fleischman AJ, Humes HD, Roy S. Development of continuous implantable renal replacement: Past and future. *Transl Res.* 2007 Dec;150(6):327–36.
41. Fissell WH, Manley S, Westover A, Humes HD, Fleischman AJ, Roy S. Differentiated growth of human renal tubule cells on thin-film and nanostructured materials. *ASAIO J.* 2006 May;52(3):221–7.
42. Henn C, Satzl S, Christoph P, Kurz P, Radeleff B, Stampfl U, et al. Efficacy of a polyphosphazene nanocoat in reducing thrombogenicity, in-stent stenosis, and inflammatory response in porcine renal and iliac artery stents. *J Vasc Interv Radiol.* 2008 Mar;19(3):427–37.
43. Wang H, Zhao Q, Ni Z, Li Q, Liu H, Yang Y, et al. A ferroelectric/electrochemical modulated organic synapse for ultraflexible, artificial visual-perception system. *Adv Mater.* 2018 Nov;30(46):1803961.
44. Muthusubramaniam L, Lowe R, Fissell WH, Li L, Marchant RE, Desai TA, et al. Hemocompatibility of silicon-based substrates for biomedical implant applications. *Ann Biomed Eng.* 2011 Apr 2;39(4):1296–305.
45. Vasita R, Katti DS. Nanofibers and their applications in tissue engineering. *Int J Nanomedicine.* 2006 Jan;1(1):15–30.
46. Maillard L, Vochelet F, Peycher P, Ayari A, Barra N, Billé J, et al. MAPT (Mono Antiplatelet Therapy) as regular regimen after COBRA PzFTM nanocoated coronary stent (NCS) implantation. *Cardiovasc Revasc Med.* 2020 Jun;21(6):785–9.
47. Nedjari S, Hébraud A, Eap S, Siegwald S, Mélart C, Benkirane-Jessel N, et al. Electrostatic template-assisted deposition of microparticles on electrospun nanofibers: Towards microstructured functional biochips for screening applications. *RSC Adv.* 2015;5(102):83600–7.
48. Stendahl JC, Sinusas AJ. Nanoparticles for cardiovascular imaging and therapeutic delivery, Part 2: Radiolabeled probes. *J Nucl Med.* 2015 Nov;56(11):1637–41.
49. Venkatraman G, Ramya R, Shruthilaya M, Akila K, Ganga B, Suresh Kumar R, et al. Nanomedicine: Towards development of patient-friendly drug-delivery systems for oncological applications. *Int J Nanomedicine.* 2012 Feb;7:1043.
50. Wu P, Yan X-P. Doped quantum dots for chemo/biosensing and bioimaging. *Chem Soc Rev.* 2013;42(12):5489.
51. Ivanoska-Dacikj A, Oguz-Gouillart Y, Hossain G, Kaplan M, Sivri Ç, Ros-Lis JV, et al. Advanced and smart textiles during and after the COVID-19 pandemic: Issues, challenges, and innovations. *Healthcare.* 2023 Apr 13;11(8):1115.
52. Harding CV, Heuser JE, Stahl PD. Exosomes: Looking back three decades and into the future. *J Cell Biol.* 2013 Feb 18;200(4):367–71.
53. Kumar V, Lee D-J. Effects of thinner on RTV silicone rubber nanocomposites reinforced with GR and CNTs. *Polym Adv Technol.* 2017 Dec;28(12):1842–50.
54. Tournebize J, Sapin-Minet A, Bartosz G, Leroy P, Boudier A. Pitfalls of assays devoted to evaluation of oxidative stress induced by inorganic nanoparticles. *Talanta.* 2013 Nov;116:753–63.
55. Simone G, Di Carlo Rasi D, de Vries X, Heintges GHL, Meskers SCJ, Janssen RAJ, et al. Near-infrared tandem organic photodiodes for future application in artificial retinal implants. *Adv Mater.* 2018 Dec;30(51):1804678.
56. Perez JM, Simeone FJ, Saeki Y, Josephson L, Weissleder R. Viral-induced self-assembly of magnetic nanoparticles allows the detection of viral particles in biological media. *J Am Chem Soc.* 2003 Aug 1;125(34):10192–3.

3 Biomaterials for Theranostic Nanosystems

Gongotree Phukan, Mhonyamo M. Patton, and J.P. Borah

3.1 INTRODUCTION

One of the significant challenges in clinical trials is overcoming differences in medication response caused by genetic diversity in large patient populations, which can be addressed with the help of personalised treatment. But when it comes to such kinds of treatments, the pharmacokinetic heterogeneity of medications in patients appears as one of the main obstacles. Therefore, it is crucial to diagnose the ailment and administer the necessary therapy at the same time in order to realise the vision of personalised treatment. This makes the real-time pharmacokinetic monitoring of patients possible, which may also help reduce the frequency of adverse medication reactions as well as pave the way for providing information for creating new treatment regimens. Such materials that unite therapeutic and diagnostic imaging modalities are what Funkhouser termed a "theranostic" when he first used the term in 2002 [1]. Describing the concept of the theranostic approach in a single sentence "offers the potential to address unwanted discrepancies in biodistribution that now exist in various imaging and therapeutic agents by combining therapy and diagnosis into one 'package' as opposed to the development and use of separate materials".

Cancer theranostics, which combines diagnostic and therapeutic methods in the treatment of cancer, seems like a great way to expedite therapy and simplify patient care. This is especially important now since, despite the availability of supportive care and therapeutic techniques, the number of cancer diagnoses and associated mortality rates around the world continue to be serious issues. The two essential foundations for success in the cancer battle continue to be an earlier and more accurate cancer diagnosis and better therapies, particularly those that strive for tailored treatment. It looks to be important for the development of individualised cancer treatments. Additionally, theranostics is essential for evaluating chemotherapy since it can visualise the size of the tumour and provide feedback on the effectiveness of the treatment. Furthermore, it has the capacity to examine and track the effectiveness of anticancer medications against tumours in patients followed by therapy.

 DOI: 10.1201/9781003316435-3

Different nanomaterials have recently become an interesting tool in cancer theranostics due to their inherent molecular properties that help with successful diagnosis and therapy applications [2]. Figure 3.1 illustrates many application areas for nanoparticles in cancer theranostics [3]. Nanoparticles have a high surface-to-volume ratio, which makes it possible to simultaneously co-functionalise the surface with diagnostic and therapeutic formulations. There are different ways to accomplish theranostics using nanomaterials: (i) combining nanoparticles to various imaging modalities to develop photo-sensitive compounds, (ii) using the inbuilt properties of nanomaterials to apply them in therapies, or (iii) integrating small drug molecules or any biological entity to the nanoparticle for drug delivery approach. To give an instance, many nanoparticles, including semiconductor quantum dots, have inherent fluorescence capabilities which can be directly used or combined with other imaging modalities. Iron oxide nanoparticles, meantime, have inherent magnetic and imaging features that can be enhanced to create theranostic nanoparticles. Researchers are also exploring the use of metal nanoparticles like gold, silver, zinc, platinum, etc. as theranostic particles, either naturally or through surface modification [4]. Carbon nanotubes (CNTs) and polymer-based nanomaterials are other materials that researchers are interested for usage as theranostic particles in addition to these. Figure 3.2 presents a schematic representation to help with comprehension of the fundamental idea of cancer detection and treatment using nanoparticles.

This chapter highlights the various therapy and diagnostic modalities that, when used together, can be used as theranostic tools for the treatment of cancer, with a special focus on several kinds of nanomaterials that are either applied or have strong potential for theranostics. Image-guided medication administration is also covered, along with therapeutic techniques like magnetic hyperthermia,

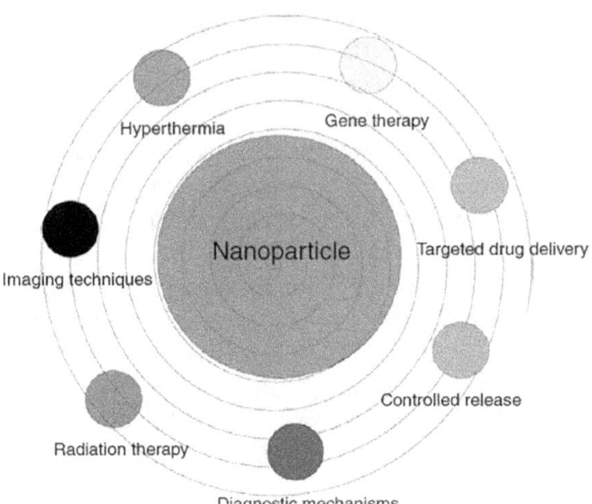

FIGURE 3.1 Different application areas of nanoparticles in cancer theranostics. Copyright 2022. Drug Discovery Today. Elsevier: Reproduced with permission.

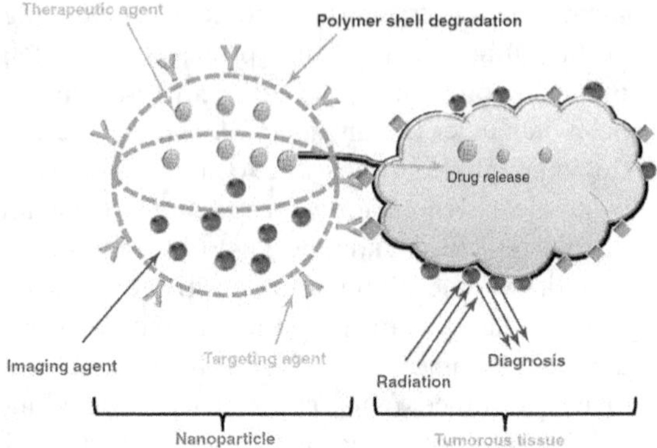

FIGURE 3.2 Use of nanoparticles for theranostic approach. Copyright 2022. Drug Discovery Today. Elsevier: Reproduced with permission.

molecular imaging modalities like magnetic resonance imaging (MRI), optical imaging, etc. This chapter also discusses a variety of potential candidates with extraordinary chemical and physical properties, in particular metal and metal oxide nanoparticles, semiconductor quantum dots, carbon nanotubes, and nanomaterials based on polymers.

3.2 SOME APPLICATIONS OF THE THERANOSTIC APPROACH

3.2.1 Magnetic Hyperthermia Therapy

In recent years, targeted hyperthermia treatment using magnetic nanoparticles (MNPs) was the main focus of treatment in cancer therapy. MNPs provide the necessary heat in magnetic hyperthermia to elevate the temperature to a therapeutic level. When subjected to a certain alternating magnetic field (AMF), these MNPs generate heat that raises the temperature to a certain limit (41°C–46°C), which can promote apoptosis/necrosis in cancer cells. A particular class of magnetic nanoparticles, such as ferrimagnetic, ferromagnetic, and superparamagnetic states, have been able to monitor the mechanism by which the MNPs convert magnetic energy to thermal energy.

The MNPs must be cell-accepting, non-immunogenic, biocompatible, and able to produce efficient heating profiles when exposed to AMF in order to be used in the treatment of hyperthermia. The proper design of MNPs is necessary for *in vivo* application in the treatment of cancer via hyperthermia. In addition to adjusting the size of MNPs and the magnetic field characteristics, the heating efficiency can be adjusted by a number of factors, including magnetic anisotropy and saturation magnetisation [5,6]. In general, a magnetic field with sufficiently high frequency may result in heating of the magnetic material by independent mechanism: eddy current, hysteresis loss, and relaxation loss. The single domain

MNPs that behave as a paramagnetic material with extremely high magnetic susceptibility shows a unique class of magnetic nature, known as superparamagnetism. When the external magnetic field is removed from a superparamagnetic material, remanence magnetisation disappears. This property makes superparamagnetic nanoparticles a promising choice for *in vivo* applications, as the lack of remanence in these substances lowers the risk of blood vessel embolism [7]. Heat is produced in single-domain MNPs as a result of superspin alignment in the direction of the applied magnetic field. When the magnetic moment rotates inside the MNPs, it exhibits the Néel relaxation, and the Brown relaxation occurs during the physical rotation of the MNPs to align its superspin in the direction of the applied field.

In magnetic hyperthermia therapy, the heating efficiency must be as high as possible with less treatment time duration and a low concentration of injected MNPs [8]. The minimum amount of MNPs that can be utilised in living organs is one of the main problems being investigated in magnetic hyperthermia. Magnetic hyperthermia therapy is often used as an adjunct to amplify the effects of chemotherapy and radiotherapy.

3.2.2 Image-Guided Therapy

The primary goal of the theranostic field is to create innovative strategies to facilitate imaging tools for *in vivo* picturing of drug delivery, drug release, and therapy monitoring. An essential inference of this idea is the use of imaging in surgical treatment, which seems to represent one of the applications which are closest to a practical translation. Thereby, theranostic is a subclass of image-guided therapies (IGTs), where both therapy and imaging facilities are possible on a single platform.

Molecular imaging enables the analysis and measurement of biological processes in organisms at the cellular or subcellular level. Imaging can monitor and describe the progression of the disease in a clinically useful manner by using specific molecular probes or contrast agents. MRI, optical imaging (fluorescent and luminescent imaging), X-ray computed tomography (CT), ultrasound (US), photoacoustic tomography (PAT), single-photon emission computed tomography (SPECT), and positron emission tomography (PET) are examples of current imaging modalities.

3.2.2.1 Magnetic Resonance Imaging

MRI is a technique that utilises magnetism, radiofrequency (RF) pulses, and a computer to create images of tissues or organs. It is reasonably a safe medical imaging modality that is especially used to detect and characterise soft tissue pathologies. The term "MRI" generally indicates the proton (^{1}H) MRI, which is based on the nuclear properties of protons of water content inside the body, but there are also other MRI techniques that are based on heteroatoms like fluorine (19F), carbon (13C), etc. The basic principles are similar for both heteroatom and proton MRI, which are detailed in various pieces of literature before [9]. In a few words, magnetic field exposure makes the alignment of the nuclear spin moment of water protons present in the body along the longitudinal plane. Application of radiofrequency pulses after that "flips" the moment towards the transverse plane. Upon turning the RF pulse off, the transverse magnetisation decays over time by a process known as relaxation. The relaxing process of the nuclei to their original aligned states is recorded and converted into three-dimensional (3D) images which have high resolution, penetration, and contrast. MRI signal can be improved by reducing T1 (longitudinal) and T2 (transverse) relaxation times in water protons when contrast agents are used. Although the MRI contrast agents substantially increase tissue contrast and are therefore a valuable diagnostic tool, MRI's inherent low sensitivity continues to be a problem. Gd_2O_3, Fe_3O_4, and FeCo alloys are some popularly studied nanomaterials as MRI contrast agent [10].

3.2.2.2 Optical Imaging

One of the low-cost, non-ionising radiation imaging techniques for non-intrusively looking into a patient's body to obtain images at the cellular level is optical imaging. Photons emitted in the visible and near-infrared (NIR) ranges by bioluminescent or fluorescent probes after they absorb light are detected using this technique. Furthermore, optical imaging lends itself well to multimodal imaging because it spans a wide resolution (0.3 μm) [11] and wavelength range, and it is frequently used in conjunction with other imaging techniques. Unfortunately, optical imaging has some drawbacks like high background noise because of tissue autofluorescence. However, using light in the second near-infrared window (NIR-II, having a wavelength between 1,000 and 1,700 nm) has been shown to overcome this limitation [12]. Unlike the imaging in the visible range (wavelength between 400 and 700 nm) or in the first NIR range (i.e., NIR-I, wavelength 700–900 nm) that is utilised conventionally, NIR-II biological imaging has several advantages, including deeper penetration depth, higher spatial resolution, and reduced optical absorption as well as reduced scattering from biological substances with minimal tissue autofluorescence. In recent times, NIR fluorescence imaging in conjunction with novel fluorescent probes has received considerable attention. NIR fluorescent probes with high sensitivity and efficiency can be functionalised by targeting ligands, and therapeutic agents offer new possibilities for clinical diagnostics and therapies, and will undoubtedly play an important role in cancer therapy.

3.2.3 Drug Delivery

A drug delivery system (DDS) is a device or a formulation that allows a therapeutically active ingredient to reach its site of action while avoiding non-target cells, organs, or tissues. Traditionally used DDSs, such as tablets, capsules, syrups, and ointments, have poor bioavailability as well as incapability in achieving sustained release. Controlled DDSs are being developed to address the issues associated with traditional drug delivery.

Image-guided drug delivery (IGDD), which combines the strength of optical imaging with drug targeting, has emerged as an intriguing research domain for realising the vision of personalised medical treatment [13]. This technology is primarily used in preclinical research to noninvasively visualise and quantify the behaviour of nanocarriers after administration. IGDD detects the particle *in vivo* to determine the best-suited drug delivery route and dosage, to initiate drug release, and to ascertain treatment effectiveness. As a result, one of its primary goals is to create platforms for multifunctional and combined DDSs for cancer treatments. This has been made possible through the development of multifunctional nanoparticles containing image-contrast agents such as dyes, quantum dots (QDs), or magnetic/radioactive particles. The key benefit of IGDD technologies, whether related to image-localised drug release from non-targeted particles or targeted nano-based molecular imaging and therapy, is deeper particle penetration into the disease site.

3.3 NANOMATERIALS FOR THERANOSTIC APPROACH

3.3.1 Metal and Metal Oxide Nanoparticles

In recent years, nanoparticles like metal and metal oxide have been a great focus in research to gain more precise diagnostic equipment and therapies that are more effective. Developing a new material with superior biological functionality and little toxicity is the key challenge scientists often face for positive therapeutic effects. The ability to produce, characterise, and specifically adjust the functional characteristics of nanoparticles for theranostic applications has been made possible by the progress of nanotechnology.

Metal nanoparticles are useful for the construction of molecular contrast devices due to their capable optical absorption connected to the surface plasmon resonance of noble metals [14]. Metal nanoparticles are a promising candidate for diagnostics and sensing because of characteristics like visible and near-infrared region scattering and absorption. Gold nanoparticles deposited on appropriate substrates can enhance the luminescence properties [15]. In photoacoustic imaging, gold nanorods were used to track the blood flow in real time [16]. Gold nanoparticles modified with some bio-specific compounds can enhance binding to specific tissues as claimed by researchers [17]. Many researchers have reported using silver nanoparticles (AgNPs) as an anticancer agent and have emphasised their potential in the field of anticancer therapy [18]. A fraction of the impinging light can be absorbed and scattered by plasmonic structures in AgNP. After being selectively absorbed by cancer cells, absorbed light can be employed for thermal death, while dispersed light can be used for imaging. Furthermore, the visible-spectrum plasmon resonance of AgNPs can be tailored to any wavelength [19].

Metal oxide NPs are useful for magnetic separation of biological products and cells, diagnostics, and as a tool for specific-site medication administration due to their magnetic properties [20]. Iron oxide nanoparticles (mostly, magnetite) have been approved for drug delivery [21]. For therapeutic and diagnostic applications, the magnetic characteristics of iron oxide have been used in contrast agents for MRI, magnetic particle imaging, ultrasonic methods, photoacoustic imaging, and magnetic hyperthermia [22]. Fe_3O_4 magnetic nanomaterials can be directed, manipulated, and concentrated by an applied external magnetic field [23]. The inherent fluorescence of ZnO nanowires is used to image cancer cells, and the electrical characteristics of zinc oxide (ZnO) are beneficial for biomedical applications [24]. Functionalised surfaces of ZnO nanowires have higher water solubility and biocompatibility, which lowers their toxicity. There are numerous biological applications for titanium oxide (TiO_2). The use of TiO_2 for photo-killing treatment of malignant cancer cells was first reported by Fujishima et al. [25]. Due to its capacity to promote cell adhesion and osseointegration, TiO_2 is utilised in bone and tissue engineering [26].

3.3.2 Quantum Dots

Luminescent semiconductor nanocrystals, commonly referred to as QDs, are one of the most fascinating developments in research tools in chemistry, physics, and biology. QDs are zero-dimensional nanomaterials that display the three-dimensional (3D) quantum confinement effect, and their sizes range from 2 to 10 nm [27]. They have a Bohr radius similar to an exciton. Because QDs limit the 3D mobility of electrons, their electrical structure resembles that of atoms, earning them the moniker "artificial atoms". These inorganic fluorescent nanocrystals are often made of periodic groups of semiconductors in the II–VI or III–V range, such as CdSe or InP, respectively. These semiconductors have either cubic or hexagonal crystalline structures, as opposed to the mixed crystalline structure seen in the nanoscaled particles. When a photon with the appropriate energy strikes a semiconductor, an electron is excited from the valence band to the conduction band, forming an exciton (electron–hole pair) that is weakly bound by Coulomb forces. The energy levels are quantised due to the quantum confinement effect, and the crystal sizes determine how far apart they are from one another. Because of the ensuing event, QDs have exceptional optical properties, such as narrow, symmetric, and size-tunable emission spectra in addition to broad excitation spectra, which makes them particularly advantageous in multicolour fluorescent applications. Two further characteristics of QDs that are usually cited as advantages over organic fluorophores or fluorescent proteins include stronger fluorescence (10–100 times brighter) and improved anti-photobleaching fluorescence stability (100–1,000 times more stable). These characteristics make it simpler to continuously observe intra- and intermolecular interactions in living cells and animals.

The main aspects of building effective medication delivery systems are the tracking of nanocarriers in the cells and their potential interactions there. The ability of QDs to self-report their fluorescence and the possibility of drug attachment on their surface make them both simple to track and capable of targeted therapeutic activity against preferred targets. Through carefully chosen literature that focuses on their effectiveness as carriers/vehicles for therapeutic chemicals as well as on genes that kill or change malignancies, Tripathi and his colleagues' [28] review gives readers a bird's-eye view of QD applications in theranostics. For enhancements in bioimaging and drug delivery, Wang et al. [29] reviewed the literature based on the fabrication and use of liposomes coupled with QDs. When phospholipids are spread in water, they create vesicles called liposomes, which have a bilayer structure. They noted that by combining QD with a therapeutic agent in a liposome-based delivery system, it is possible to monitor the payload's biodistribution *in vivo*, which lowers the risk of drug toxicity having unwanted side effects in healthy tissues. Multifunctional CdSe/ZnS semiconductor QDs were synthesised by Gillies [30], who also examined them for potential *in vitro* and *in vivo* anticancer theranostics. Highly fluorescent Mn-doped ZnS quantum dot nanocrystals (quantum yield: ~80%) were synthesised by Ang et al. [31]. HeLa cell labelling and anticancer medication release investigations have demonstrated the potential use of these materials for cancer theranostics. Additionally, integrating fluorescent QDs with magnetic nanoparticles creates new nanocomposites that could serve as multifunctional, multi-targeting, and multi-treating two-in-one tools [32]. A nanocomposite comprised of CdTe QDs and amino acid–coated Fe_3O_4 magnetic nanoparticles that exhibit magnetic and fluorescent characteristics was synthesised by Arturo et al. [33]. They drew the conclusion that the fabricated nanosystem could well be employed as a drug delivery medium and as a linker for antibodies, functional compounds, and fluorophores. Optical bioimaging, diagnostics, and therapy are further areas where the nanocomposite can offer tremendous potential.

3.3.3 Carbon Nanotubes

Carbon nanotubes are nanoscale hollow tubes made up of one or more seamless, cylindrical graphene sheets of sp^2 carbon atoms bonded together in a honeycomb structure. This unique structure is a member of the fullerene family, another allotropic form of carbon after diamond and graphite. Based on the number of rolled-up graphene sheets concentrically, CNTs are classified into single-walled (SWNT), double-walled (DWNT), and multi-walled (MWNT). CNTs are manufactured using a variety of methods, including the arc discharge method, the laser method, chemical vapour deposition, and ball milling. Since Iijima discovered them in 1991 [34], these carbon allotropes have sparked intense interest due to their special physical and chemical characteristics and potential applications in a wide range of fields, ranging from sensors, electronic devices to nanocomposite materials with high strength and low weight. Their combination of electrical, mechanical, thermal, and optical properties has piqued biomedical researchers' interest. CNTs are being used to develop new technologies for the detection, treatment, and monitoring of diseases like cancer [35]. There are two sides to every coin, and CNTs have unique structural characteristics that make them more hydrophobic in water and give them built-in cytotoxicity [36]. The door to CNT bio-applications doesn't open until techniques for functionalising these molecules with organic groups and enhancing hydrophilicity to reduce cytotoxicity are developed. Because of their large surface area, they can adsorb or conjugate with a wide range of therapeutic molecules. CNTs can thus be surface engineered (i.e., functionalised) to improve their aqueous phase dispersibility or to provide the appropriate functional groups that can attach to the intended therapeutic material or target tissue to induce a therapeutic effect.

Thermal tumour ablation therapies based on nanotechnology that are minimally invasive, rapidly administered, and highly selective are being developed using a variety of nanomaterials. Carbon nanotubes are one such material. Significant efforts are currently being made to develop CNT-based clinical treatments. As per Gannon et al. [37], RF field exposure causes significant heat release by SWNTs. Cancer cells were demonstrated to be thermally destroyed in the presence of SWNTs when exposed to radiofrequency fields in both *in vitro* and *in vivo* experiments. SWNTs have a substantial intrinsic optical absorbance in NIR (700–1,100 nm) spectral window, which can be exploited to optically stimulate nanotubes inside living cells to create multifunctional nanotube biological transporters. Due to SWNT's high local heating caused by continuous NIR light, cell death may result [38]. Since carbon nanotubes make excellent chemotherapeutic drug carriers, their combination with magnetic nanoparticles offers a fresh opportunity for multimodal thermo-chemotherapy. To produce magnetic carbon nanotubes, Zuo et al. bonded magnetic nanoparticles ($Zn_{0.54}Co_{0.46}Cr_{0.6}$-$Fe_{1.4}O_4$) in a low Curie temperature to the surface of carbon nanotubes [39]. Under the clinically applied magnetic field of frequency 100 kHz and intensity: 200 Oe, these MCNTs exhibit a Curie temperature of 43°C and a self-heating temperature of 42.7°C, which makes them appropriate for use in hyperthermia. Similarly, Dalal et al. synthesised $Li_{0.3}Zn_{0.3}Co_{0.1}Fe_{2.3}O_4$ (LZC) nanoparticles in the matrix of MWCNTs and successfully achieved a hyperthermia temperature of 42°C for an AC magnetic field with 300 kHz frequency and having the intensity of 420 Oe [40]. There is evidence that adding spinel ferrite nanoparticles with the chemical formula MFe_2O_4 (M=Mn, Co, Ni, Mg, or Zn) to pristine CNTs can enhance their optical, magnetic, and electrochemical properties [41]. In a recent study, solvothermal-produced Fe_3O_4 was formed into a composite with polyethylene glycol (PEG) and amine-functionalised MWCNT [42]. An evaluation of the specific absorption rate revealed that nanocomposites are just as effective at generating heat under an oscillating magnetic field as bare Fe_3O_4, and even more so at larger field amplitudes for tailoring with magnetic anisotropy.

Imaging investigations with CNTs have increased during the past few years [43]. Hua Gong and colleagues reviewed the recent developments in the use of carbon nanotubes, including single-walled and multi-walled carbon nanotubes, as multifunctional nanoprobes for biomedical imaging [44]. Ultrasound, CT scan, and MRI can all be used to track and monitor functionalised carbon nanotubes that include gold and magnetic nanoparticles [45]. Because of this, the nanocomposite with different features can be utilised for both imaging and treatment at the same time as a multimodal tool. Multi-walled carbon nanotubes functionalised with magnetic Fe_3O_4 and gold nanoparticles were investigated by Saghatchi et al. [46]. They found that the nanocomposites increase the effectiveness of radiation and thermotherapy in the destruction of cancer cells by being X-ray and radio wave absorbent. Additionally, given their capacity as a contrast agent in CT scan and ultrasound imaging, they contribute to simultaneously tracking and visualising the therapeutic process. In order to diagnose and treat metastatic lymph nodes, Sheng et al. [47] produced MWNTs for a lymphatic theranostic system by coating MWNTs with manganese oxide and PEG. The effectively synthesised theranostic drug demonstrated strong dual-modality lymphatic tracking capabilities, high tumour ablation efficiency, and outstanding photothermal therapy (PTT) security to surrounding tissues.

Additionally, many other useful compounds, including medicines, peptides, and nucleic acids, can be incorporated into the walls and tips of CNTs thanks to their exceptional features, particularly their ultrahigh surface area. According to research, functionalised CNTs can enter mammalian cells by endocytosis or other ways [48]. They are excellent candidates for drug delivery because they can transport therapeutic medications more securely and effectively into the cells by recognising cancer-specific receptors on the cell surface with the aid of particular peptides or ligands on their surface. Recently, some researchers have already created innovative SWNT-based, tumour-targeted DDS. Functionalised SWNTs, tumour-targeting ligands, and anticancer medications often make up these delivery systems.

3.3.4 Polymer-Based Nanomaterials

Theranostic biomaterials including iron oxide, gold nanoparticles, and CNTs have all been the subject of extensive research. However, it has been noted that all of these substances have the potential to generate oxidative stress and membrane damage, which might result in cell death. Theranostic probes connected to a polymeric substance will solve this issue. Because of this reason, theranostic nanomedicine has seen a lot of interest in polymer-based materials. Large numbers of smaller molecules, or repeating units, known as monomers, are covalently conjugated to produce macromolecules known as polymers. Both natural and synthetic polymers have been employed in theranostic applications to transport genes, medicines, and imaging agents. There should be at least three primary components to a polymer-based theranostic material: (i) the polymeric component, which typically gives biocompatibility and solubility, (ii) an imaging-friendly chemical group or component (such as a contrast agent), and (iii) a "therapeutic" component that contains medicine or a gene or initiates therapy. A unique type of macromolecules known as conjugated polymers (CPs) have massive pi-conjugated backbones. CPs have a special ability to absorb and release light energy, which may be successfully transformed into fluorescence, heat, and other energies thanks to their highly electron-delocalised architectures and effective coupling between optoelectronic segments. They have been demonstrated to be prospective theranostic agents since they are materials that are both optically and electrically active.

Polymeric materials with various functions and qualities for producing theranostic nanoparticles are addressed and compared in the review article by Peng et al. [49]. They stated that polymeric multifunctional nanoparticles could be used in conjunction with therapy to exhibit unique magnetic, electrical, and optical properties enabling concurrent imaging. The various kinds of nanoscale polymer carriers utilised for the administration of chemotherapeutic drugs and the mechanisms that promote their targeted distribution to tumour cells were explored in another review by Parveen et al. [50]. In the biomedical field, polymer-based superparamagnetic iron oxide nanoparticles (SPIONs) have become increasingly popular as multipurpose drug delivery methods in addition to macromolecular MRI contrast enhancement agents. There have been many polymer-based SPION-containing DDSs created thus far, including liposomes, micelles, and nanoparticles of various sizes. In order to stabilise SPION in biological conditions and to lower oxidation during theranostic applications, polymers are utilised to coat them. Dextran, chitosan, polyethylene glycol (PEG), polyvinyl pyrrolidone (PVP), and polyvinyl alcohol (PVA) are a few examples of natural and synthetic polymers that have been utilised to coat various kinds of SPION in recent years.

3.4 CHALLENGES AND FUTURE PERSPECTIVES

Nanomaterials, when combined with several capabilities, have the huge potential to dramatically improve disease diagnosis and treatment. The fundamental benefits of nanomedicine come from its ability to include a variety of functionalities, such as targeting, imaging, and therapy. Researchers' interest in the synthesis and usage of these materials is quickly expanding as a result of their adaptability and future applications. Since the methods and designs for their synthesis have been well established, the development of such agents appears to be a logical continuation from particles created exclusively for therapy or imaging. The high surface to volume ratio of nanoparticles offers extra benefits when functionalising with extra targeted ligands or any other surface modifiers. Theranostic nanomaterials have many benefits from a therapeutic perspective, one of which being their ultimate usefulness in the concomitant diagnosis and treatment of disease. It also includes a mechanism to monitor and determine the location and appropriate control over the release of therapeutic agents. In order to improve the effectiveness and safety of drugs, theranostics also monitor the patient's response to the treatment and reduce unnecessary treatment of patients which may result significantly in the comprehensive system of healthcare [51]. As a result, theranostics, as an emerging science, offers a chance for pharmaceutical and diagnostics businesses to comply with the FDA's strict financial and regulatory requirements [52].

In an effort to solve these issues, many nanomaterials have been developed. Nanomedicines were first coined by the National Institutes of Health (NIH) [53], and nanomedicine is defined as nanoparticle-based treatments made up of various organic or inorganic nanomaterials used for biological system diagnostics, therapy, imaging, monitoring, and control.

Numerous developments in the biological use of nanoparticles have been reported in recent years. The most encouraging feature of these recent advancements is that some of the research projects are beginning to use the most recent theories about cancer, i.e., theranostics is expanding to encompass elements of both molecular imaging and customised cancer therapy [54,55].

Despite these achievements, theranostic nanomedicine also faces many challenges. The nano–bio interaction is one of the main obstacles to implementation of theranostic nanomedicine in clinical settings. Nanomedicine's possible toxicity or incompatibility with biological material has the potential to cause diseases including immunoreaction, inflammation, or other unidentified ailments. The toxicity of the nanoparticle relies on a number of factors, including size, ζ-potential, and solubility of nanoparticles [56]. The complexity of developing a predictable and repeatable synthesis process is another significant obstacle. Synthesis of nanoparticles in a larger scale varies in physical and chemical characteristics and hence affects the yield of reproducibility. Additionally, since theranostic nanoparticles are multifunctional, a more accurate chemistry, synthesis control, and good manufacturing practises are essential for making the arduous transition from the laboratory to clinical trials [40]. The disconnect between the scientific community and government regulatory agencies is another problem that has to be addressed. Numerous government laws focused on regulatory elements linked to quality control, manufacturing methods, safety profiles, and patent protection are keeping an eye on the commercialisation of nanomedicine [57]. Although the already available nanomedicines may have met general regulatory standards, it may still be necessary to revise the standards in order to validate the quality, control, safety, and efficacy of other theranostic nanoparticles for human use.

3.5 CONCLUSION

Theranostic nanomedicine has considerably evolved and has immense potential advancement, yet there is certain field it has to revolutionise for further use in clinical trials. In the past decade, the engineering of diverse theranostic nanoparticles for cancer imaging and treatment has grown at an unparalleled rate. It is obvious that, despite the potential of nanotheranostics, more research is needed to expand our knowledge of the ways in which therapeutic and diagnostic chemicals interact. Presently innovative solutions are being extensively studied and identified which will one day allow nanoparticles to carry out their full potential as the best option for theranostic nanomedicine.

REFERENCES

1. Kelkar SS, Reineke TM. Theranostics: Combining imaging and therapy. *Bioconjug Chem.* 2011;22(10):1879–903.
2. Sharmiladevi P, Girigoswami K, Haribabu V, Girigoswami A. Nano-enabled theranostics for cancer. *Mater Adv.* 2021;2(9):2876–91.

3. Ahmed N, Fessi H, Elaissari A. Theranostic applications of nanoparticles in cancer. *Drug Discov Today*. 2012;17(17–18):928–34. Available from: https://doi.org/10.1016/j.drudis.2012.03.010.
4. Sharma H, Mishra PK, Talegaonkar S, Vaidya B. Metal nanoparticles: A theranostic nanotool against cancer. *Drug Discov Today*. 2015;20(9):1143–51. Available from: https://doi.org/10.1016/j.drudis.2015.05.009.
5. Hergt R, Dutz S, Zeisberger M. Validity limits of the Néel relaxation model of magnetic nanoparticles for hyperthermia. *Nanotechnology*. 2010;21(1):015706.
6. Hergt R, Dutz S, Röder M. Effects of size distribution on hysteresis losses of magnetic nanoparticles for hyperthermia. *J Phys Condens Matter*. 2008;20(38):385214.
7. Laurent S, Dutz S, Häfeli UO, Mahmoudi M. Magnetic fluid hyperthermia: Focus on superparamagnetic iron oxide nanoparticles. *Adv Colloid Interface Sci*. 2011;166(1–2):8–23. Available from: https://doi.org/10.1016/j.cis.2011.04.003.
8. Hervault A, Thanh NTK. Magnetic nanoparticle-based therapeutic agents for thermo-chemotherapy treatment of cancer. *Nanoscale*. 2014;6(20):11553–73.
9. Grover VPB, Tognarelli JM, Crossey MME, Cox IJ, Taylor-Robinson SD, McPhail MJW. Magnetic resonance imaging: Principles and techniques: Lessons for clinicians. *J Clin Exp Hepatol*. 2015;5(3):246–55. Available from: https://doi.org/10.1016/j.jceh.2015.08.001.
10. Shokrollahi H. Contrast agents for MRI. *Mater Sci Eng C*. 2013;33(8):4485–97. Available from: https://doi.org/10.1016/j.msec.2013.07.012.
11. Quek CH, Leong KW. Near-infrared fluorescent nanoprobes for in vivo optical imaging. *Nanomaterials*. 2012;2(2):92–112.
12. Kenry, Duan Y, Liu B. Recent advances of optical imaging in the second near-infrared window. *Adv Mater*. 2018;30(47):1–19.
13. Lanza GM, Moonen C, Baker JR, Chang E, Cheng Z, Grodzinski P, et al. Assessing the barriers to image-guided drug delivery. *Wiley Interdiscip Rev Nanomed Nanobiotechnol*. 2014;6(1):1–14.
14. Liao H, Nehl CL, Hafner JH. Biomedical applications of plasmon resonant metal nanoparticles. *Nanomedicine*. 2006;1(2):201–8.
15. Bhattacharya R, Mukherjee P. Biological properties of "naked" metal nanoparticles. *Adv Drug Deliv Rev*. 2008;60(11):1289–306.
16. Wang H, Huff TB, Zweifel DA, He W, Low PS, Wei A, et al. In vitro and in vivo two-photon luminescence imaging of single gold nanorods. *Proc Natl Acad Sci USA*. 2005;102(44):15752–6.
17. Faraji AH, Wipf P. Nanoparticles in cellular drug delivery. *Bioorganic Med Chem*. 2009;17(8):2950–62. Available from: https://doi.org/10.1016/j.bmc.2009.02.043.
18. Zhang XF, Liu ZG, Shen W, Gurunathan S. Silver nanoparticles: Synthesis, characterization, properties, applications, and therapeutic approaches. *Int J Mol Sci*. 2016;17(9):1534.
19. Evanoff DD, Chumanov G. Synthesis and optical properties of silver nanoparticles and arrays. *ChemPhysChem*. 2005;6(7):1221–31.
20. Estelrich J, Escribano E, Queralt J, Busquets MA. Iron oxide nanoparticles for magnetically-guided and magnetically-responsive drug delivery. *Int J Mol Sci*. 2015;16(4):8070–101.
21. Prilepskii AY, Fakhardo AF, Drozdov AS, Vinogradov V V., Dudanov IP, Shtil AA, et al. Urokinase-conjugated magnetite nanoparticles as a promising drug delivery system for targeted thrombolysis: Synthesis and preclinical evaluation. *ACS Appl Mater Interfaces*. 2018;10(43):36764–75.
22. Gupta AK, Gupta M. Synthesis and surface engineering of iron oxide nanoparticles for biomedical applications. *Biomaterials*. 2005;26(18):3995–4021.

23. Yu P, Xia XM, Wu M, Cui C, Zhang Y, Liu L, et al. Folic acid-conjugated iron oxide porous nanorods loaded with doxorubicin for targeted drug delivery. *Colloids Surfaces B Biointerfaces*. 2014;120:142–51.
24. Hong H, Shi J, Yang Y, Zhang Y, Engle JW, Nickles RJ, et al. Cancer-targeted optical imaging with fluorescent zinc oxide nanowires. *Nano Lett*. 2011;11(9):3744–50.
25. Fujishima A, Cai RX, Otsuki J, Hashimoto K, Itoh K, Yamashita T, et al. Biochemical application of photoelectrochemistry: Photokilling of malignant cells with TiO_2 powder. *Electrochim Acta*. 1993;38(1):153–7.
26. He J, Zhou W, Zhou X, Zhong X, Zhang X, Wan P, et al. The anatase phase of nanotopography titania plays an important role on osteoblast cell morphology and proliferation. *J Mater Sci Mater Med*. 2008;19(11):3465–72.
27. Zrazhevskiy P, Gao X. Multifunctional quantum dots for personalized medicine. *Nano Today*. 2009;4(5):414–28.
28. Tripathi SK, Kaur G, Khurana RK, Kapoor S, Singh B. Quantum dots and their potential role in cancer theranostics. *Crit Rev Ther Drug Carrier Syst*. 2015;32(6):461–502.
29. Wang Q, Chao Y. Multifunctional quantum dots and liposome complexes in drug delivery. *J Biomed Res*. 2018;32(2):91–106.
30. Gillies JM. Synthesis, characterisation and bioconjugation of [109Cd]CdSe/ZnS core/shell quantum dots as "proof of principle" for the potential development of an anti-cancer theranostic. *Inorganica Chim Acta*. 2019;495(July):119001. Available from: https://doi.org/10.1016/j.ica.2019.119001.
31. Ang EH, Zeng J, Subramanian GS, Chellappan V, Sudhaharan T, Padmanabhan P, et al. Silica-coated Mn-doped ZnS nanocrystals for cancer theranostics. *ACS Appl Nano Mater*. 2020;3(3):3088.
32. Corr SA, Rakovich YP, Gun'Ko YK. Multifunctional magnetic-fluorescent nanocomposites for biomedical applications. *Nanoscale Res Lett*. 2008;3(3):87–104.
33. Pavón-Hernández AI, Rodríguez-Velázquez E, Alatorre-Meda M, Elizalde Galindo JT, Paraguay-Delgado F, Tirado-Guízar A, et al. Magnetic nanocomposite with fluorescence enhancement effect based on amino acid coated-Fe_3O_4 functionalized with quantum dots. *Mater Chem Phys*. 2020;251:123082.
34. S. Iijima. Helical microtubules of graphitic carbon. *Nature*. 1991;354:56–8.
35. Singh R, Torti SV. Carbon nanotubes in hyperthermia therapy. *Adv Drug Deliv Rev*. 2013;65(15):2045–60. Available from: https://doi.org/10.1016/j.addr.2013.08.001.
36. Garriga R, Herrero-Continente T, Palos M, Cebolla VL, Osada J, Muñoz E, et al. Toxicity of carbon nanomaterials and their potential application as drug delivery systems: In vitro studies in caco-2 and mcf-7 cell lines. *Nanomaterials*. 2020;10(8):1–21.
37. Gannon CJ, Cherukuri P, Yakobson BI, Cognet L, Kanzius JS, Kittrell C, et al. Carbon nanotube-enhanced thermal destruction of cancer cells in a noninvasive radiofrequency field. *Cancer*. 2007;110(12):2654–65.
38. Kam NWS, O'Connell M, Wisdom JA, Dai H. Carbon nanotubes as multifunctional biological transporters and near-infrared agents for selective cancer cell destruction. *Proc Natl Acad Sci USA*. 2005;102(33):11600–5.
39. Zuo X, Wu C, Zhang W, Gao W. Magnetic carbon nanotubes for self-regulating temperature hyperthermia. *RSC Adv*. 2018;8(22):11997–2003. Available from: https://doi.org/10.1039/C7RA13256E.
40. Dalal M, Greneche JM, Satpati B, Ghzaiel TB, Mazaleyrat F, Ningthoujam RS, et al. Microwave absorption and the magnetic hyperthermia applications of $Li_{0.3}Zn_{0.3}Co_{0.1}Fe_{2.3}O_4$ nanoparticles in multiwalled carbon nanotube matrix. *ACS Appl Mater Interfaces*. 2017;9(46):40831–45.

41. Huiqun C, Meifang Z, Yaogang L. Novel carbon nanotube iron oxide magnetic nanocomposites. *J Magn Magn Mater.* 2006;305(2):321–4.
42. Seal P, Alam A, Borgohain C, Paul N, Babu PD, Borah JP. Optimization of self heating properties of Fe_3O_4 using PEG and amine functionalized MWCNT. *J Alloys Compd.* 2021;882:160653. Available from: https://doi.org/10.1016/j.jallcom.2021.160653.
43. Liu Z, Yang K, Lee ST. Single-walled carbon nanotubes in biomedical imaging. *J Mater Chem.* 2011;21(3):586–98.
44. Gong H, Peng R, Liu Z. Carbon nanotubes for biomedical imaging: The recent advances. *Adv Drug Deliv Rev.* 2013;65(15):1951–63. Available from: https://doi.org/10.1016/j.addr.2013.10.002.
45. Delogu LG, Vidili G, Venturelli E, Ménard-Moyon C, Zoroddu MA, Pilo G, et al. Functionalized multiwalled carbon nanotubes as ultrasound contrast agents. *Proc Natl Acad Sci USA.* 2012;109(41):16612–7.
46. Saghatchi F, Mohseni-Dargah M, Akbari-Birgani S, Saghatchi S, Kaboudin B. Cancer therapy and imaging through functionalized carbon nanotubes decorated with magnetite and gold nanoparticles as a multimodal tool. *Appl Biochem Biotechnol.* 2020;191(3):1280–93.
47. Wang S, Zhang Q, Yang P, Yu X, Huang LY, Shen S, et al. Manganese oxide-coated carbon nanotubes as dual-modality lymph mapping agents for photothermal therapy of tumor metastasis. *ACS Appl Mater Interfaces.* 2016;8(6):3736–43.
48. Bhirde AA, Patel V, Gavard J, Zhang G, Sousa Ḱ AA, Masedunskas A, et al. Targeted killing of cancer cells in vivo nanotube-based drug delivery. *ACS Nano.* 2009;3(2):307–16.
49. Peng H, Liu X, Wang G, Li M, Bratlie KM, Cochran E, et al. Polymeric multifunctional nanomaterials for theranostics. *J Mater Chem B.* 2015;3(34):6856–70.
50. Parveen S, Sahoo SK. Polymeric nanoparticles for cancer therapy. *J Drug Target.* 2008;16(2):108–23.
51. Ray PC, Yu H, Fu PP. Toxicity and environmental risks of nanomaterials: Challenges and future needs. *J Environ Sci Health C Environ Carcinog Ecotoxicol Rev.* 2009;27:1–35.
52. Pene F, Courtine E, Cariou A, Mira JP. Toward theragnostics. *Crit Care Med.* 2009;37(SUPPL. 1):S50–8.
53. Moghimi SM, Hunter AC, Murray JC. Nanomedicine: Current status and future prospects. *FASEB J.* 2005;19(3):311–30.
54. Mahmoudi M, Sant S, Wang B, Laurent S, Sen T. Superparamagnetic iron oxide nanoparticles (SPIONs): Development, surface modification and applications in chemotherapy. *Adv Drug Deliv Rev.* 2011;63(1–2):24–46. Available from: https://doi.org/10.1016/j.addr.2010.05.006.
55. Santhamoorthy M, Thirupathi K, Krishnan S, Guganathan L, Dave S, Phan TTV, Kim SC. Preparation of magnetic iron oxide incorporated mesoporous silica hybrid composites for pH and temperature-sensitive drug delivery. *Magnetochemistry.* 2023;9(3):81.
56. Dilnawaz F, Acharya S, Sahoo SK. Recent trends of nanomedicinal approaches in clinics. *Int J Pharm.* 2018;538(1–2):263–78. Available from: https://doi.org/10.1016/j.ijpharm.2018.01.016.
57. Gaspar R. Regulatory issues surrounding nanomedicines: Setting the scene for the next generation of nanopharmaceuticals. *Nanomedicine.* 2007;2(2):143–7.

4 Functionalized Graphene Nanomaterials for Electrochemical Sensors

Manorama Singh, Vijai K. Rai, and Ankita Rai

4.1 INTRODUCTION TO GRAPHENE

Carbon has an abundant naturally occurring allotrope known as graphite. This word 'graphite' was derived from the Greek term 'graphene' having the meaning 'write'. It has a three-dimensional, dividable sheet-like structure with a layer separation of 0.337 nm. A bunch of 2-D single layers are also found which are employed in miscellaneous area as carbon brushes, lubricant, refractory and resistance materials, cathode material in batteries, writing *etc*. The study of 3-D graphite necessitates the study of its 2D single layer [1]. In the Mermin–Wagner theorem, it is stated that 2-D materials do not subsist in nature as crystal loses its long-range orderness and melts due to thermal fluctuations at any small but non-zero temperature [2]. Because of their extraordinary electronic properties, carbon sheets were the center of attention among the innumerable 2-D materials [3]. A single layer of graphite is a hexagonal arrangement of carbon atoms bonded through sp2 hybridization, and several efforts were made to isolate a single layer of graphite. In this regard, different guest molecules were inserted between the individual sheets of graphite forming graphite intercalation compound, to separate a single sheet of graphite, and removal of these intercalated molecules, unfortunately, resulted in restacking of graphite sheets. The name 'graphene' was first coined by Boehm et al. for a single layer of graphite. Since planar aromatic hydrocarbon suffix -ene is employed and graphite is in a stacked planar arrangement, the name graphene is used [4]. Geim and Novoselov isolated a single sheet of graphite, i.e., graphene, via the scotch tape mechanical exfoliation process. Using this method, single-layer and few-layer graphene with widths of 10 and 100 μM, respectively, were prepared [5]. For this revolutionary experiment on graphene, Geim and Novoselov have been awarded the Nobel Prize in Physics in 2010 by Royal Swedish Academy of Sciences. Graphene is the fundamental of other carbonaceous materials, and it can be converted from one form to another in suitable conditions, such as 0-D fullerenes (wrapping up graphene), 1-D carbon nanotubes (rolling of graphene), 2-D graphene and 3-D graphite (stacking of graphene) [6].

DOI: 10.1201/9781003316435-4

Geim et al. found that carbon-to-carbon bond length of graphene is 0.142 nm, which prevents thermal fluctuations and stabilizes it.

4.1.1 Different Derivatives of Graphene

There are different derivatives of graphene as follows: *graphene oxide* (*GO*) is the exfoliated form of graphitic oxide with sp3-hybridized C atoms. It contains carboxyls and carbonyls at the edge, and epoxy and hydroxyls at the base. The presence of oxygen functionalities on GO influences its characteristic properties: electronic (disruption of conjugation), mechanical, electrochemical, etc. [6,7] and produces structural defects, which results in some loss in electrical conductivity and thus probably restricts the direct use of GO in electrical devices. In contrast, these oxygen functionalities make GO available to various other applications due to its dispersibility in many solvents, particularly in water [8]. Besides this, the presence of the oxygen functionalities destroys its thermal stability [9,10].

Graphane is a 100% saturated, 2-D, hexagonally arranged hydrocarbon with sp^3-hybridized C–C bonds with wrinkled carbon sheet having the chemical formula CH, and it was first anticipated by Sluiter and Kawazoe in 2003 from *ab initio* calculation [11,12].

Graphyne (GY) is a one-atom-thick, 2-D hydrocarbon, in which hexagonal carbon array of graphene linked with an acetylenic (–C≡C–) bridge constructs a sp^2-sp-hybridized carbon structure. However, GY was initially suggested in 1987 [13] with one –C≡C– chain.

Graphadiyne (GDY) with one more –C≡C– chain was first synthesized in 1997 [14,15].

4.1.2 Preparation of Graphene

The unusual properties of graphene make it a special candidate in different fields, but the challenge was its synthesis in bulk amounts. On the whole, there are two main approaches to the preparation of graphene.

4.1.2.1 Top-Down Approach

The top-down approach involves breaking down of stacked graphite into a single layer. A gainful approach is applied to produce isolated graphene sheets on both microscale and nanoscale. Mechanical exfoliation (scotch tape method) [16], chemical exfoliation [17,18], chemical synthesis [19,20], and reduction of GO [4,21,22] are some of the top-down approaches to prepare graphene.

In the *micromechanical exfoliation approach*, adhesive tape was brought into play in the isolation of graphene from a graphite crystal. After peeling away the tape from the graphite crystal, multilayer graphene exists on the tape. With the repetition of the peeling process, multilayer graphene is converted into a thinner slice of few-layer graphene. Later on, the tape was affixed onto the Si/SiO_2 wafer and the tape was peeled back. Single-layer graphene can be seen through a light microscope due to the optical interference effect between oxidized silicon substrate and flakes [16]. However, high-quality, defect-free graphene is easily obtained by this method, but with some drawbacks such as less quantity, and differences in size and thickness (nm to thousands of μm), depending on the number of peelings.

Chemical exfoliation includes two steps for the complete exfoliation of graphene layers process. The first step comprises an increase in the interlayer spacing, thereby reducing the interlayer van der Waals forces, and the second step is the exfoliation of graphene layers. This is attained by inserting some species (alkali metals, halides, oxides, acids) in between graphite layers forming graphite-intercalated compounds (GICs) [17]. Ultrasonication in an organic solvent, like N-methyl-2-pyrrolidine (NMP), also results in isolation of stacked graphene layers due to solvent–graphene interaction [18].

Chemical synthesis method involves two steps: (1) oxidation of graphite, forming graphitic oxide which exhibits an almost amorphous nature with stacked layers of *GO* which exhibits a hydrophilic nature [19], and (2) reduction of graphene oxide. Oxidation of graphite was carried out by *Brodie's scheme*, *Staudenmaier's scheme*, *Hummer's scheme*, and *modified Hummer's scheme* using strong oxidizing agents such as concentrated H_2SO_4, H_3PO_4, $KClO_3$, HNO_3, and $KMnO_4$. Due to the oxidation process, oxygen functionalities such as –OH, –COOH, and epoxy are introduced which results in increase in interlayer spacing between graphene layers. To attain graphene with a superior quality, oxidation at a higher extent is required, while reduction of graphitic oxide yields graphene. The extent of oxidation is enhanced beginning with Brodie's to Staudenmaier's to Hummer's and then modified Hummer's scheme. A number of methods have been applied for reduction of GO process such as thermal [23], photochemical [24], chemical [25], and electrochemical [26] processes. However, reduced material is not recognized as graphene but is identified as reduced graphene oxide (rGO) due to partial reduction of oxygen functionalities, and of course, the resultant material differs in feature properties of graphene. If complete oxidation takes place, still graphene and rGO exhibit dissimilar properties because defects are present in higher amounts created at the stage of oxidation of graphite [22].

4.1.2.2 Bottom-Up Approach

The bottom-up approach involves the utilization of carbon at the atomic level to produce a 2-D carbon sheet. Hydrocarbons such as methane, ethane, and acetylene are used as carbon sources. Applying high temperature, high-quality graphitic materials can be obtained. Bottom-up approaches mainly involve *epitaxial growth* [27] and *chemical vapor deposition (CVD) techniques* [28].

Deposition of a single crystalline film on a single crystalline substrate produces epitaxial film, and the process is known as *epitaxial growth.* Based on the substrate and deposited film, the epitaxial growth method is of two types. As the material is the same for substrate and film, the growth is known as homo-epitaxial growth; on the other hand, when the substrate and film are different materials, it is called hetero-epitaxial growth. Graphene can be fabricated only by heating SiC crystal, which facilitates evaporation of silicon, and consequently, the remaining carbon atoms come across to fabricate the graphene sheet. The thickness and properties of produced graphene depend on the parameters applied such as temperature, time, and heating rate [27,28]. The *CVD process* involves a substrate and a suitable carbon source [29]. These compounds decompose on the surface of the substrate to facilitate the development of a thin film.

4.1.3 Salient Features (Properties) of Graphene

Graphene comprises sp^2-hybridized carbon atoms arranged in a hexagonal manner. These three sp^2-hybridized orbitals of carbons form a m σ bond with other sp2 hybridized orbital of vicinal carbon atoms and remaining pz orbital of carbon align perpendicular to the planar carbon hexagon forming a delocalized π bond with the pz orbital of a vicinal carbon atom [30]. Single-sheet graphene exhibits 97.7% optical transparency with 2.3% opacity based on its atomic thickness. Graphene shows decrease in optical transparency with increase in the number of sheets [31]. According to an atomic force spectroscopy (AFM) study, graphene is considered as the strongest material ever discovered, about 300 times stronger than the steel of equal thickness. Graphene is stretchable and has flexibility up to 20% of its original length. Single-layer graphene exhibits a surface area of 2630 m^2/g [32], Young's modulus of 1.0 TPa, and a tensile strength of 130 GPa [33]. Graphene displays a zero bandgap semiconductor nature with a minute overlap between conduction and valence bands [34]. In graphene, negatively charged electrons and positively charged holes act as charge carriers with an excellent mobility of up to 15,000 cm^2/V s with a carrier density of 10 cm^{-2} at ambient temperature [35]. Apart from the abovementioned excellent properties, graphene also exhibits a thermal conductivity of ~3,000 W/m K [36], which higher than other carbon-based materials. Adsorption and desorption of gases, like hydrogen and carbon monoxide, are also possible on graphene surface [37]. The shape, size, edges, number of layers, and additional covalent or noncovalent bonds with other atoms, which results in modifications of the electrical or chemical properties of graphene, can be determined on the basis of the arrangement of benzene rings in the entire graphene sheet.

4.1.4 Significance of Functionalized Graphene Nanomaterials

Although graphene has excellent physicochemical properties, it has the tendency of aggregation to form graphite via strong π–π and van der Waals' interactions [38], if each sheet was not well isolated from each other. Therefore, graphene sheets should be prevented from agglomeration. The prevention of aggregation is of particular importance for graphene sheets because most of their unique properties are present only when they are separated as single sheets. Therefore, the functionalization of graphene through appropriate functional group was very much required for the preparation of high-performance conducting materials and also to utilize its physicochemical properties to frame various types of sensors [39], supercapacitors [40], batteries [41], optoelectronic devices, etc. [42].

Functionalization of graphene sheets through *covalent* or *noncovalent* interactions via attachment of suitable organic or inorganic species, atoms, molecular species, etc. has attracted the interest of many researchers. Functionalization of graphene sheets with different species facilitates dispersion of graphene sheets in a variety of solvents, reduces the aggregation of graphene sheets, and generates a gap between conduction and valence bands [43,44]. Functionalization also improves the presentation of a number of electronic devices and makes it possible to produce sophisticated multifunctional appliances in different fields such as medicine, energy storage, catalysis, electronics, and sensing. [45–49].

4.2 FUNCTIONALIZATION METHODS OF GRAPHENE

Functionalization of graphene can be carried out on the surface, edges, or at a defective area. The defects are created during the synthesis of graphene, including adsorption of adatoms as well as solvent molecules, damage in sp2 carbon network, or structural defects [50,51]. The advantage of functionalization is that the properties of functionalized species include properties of both graphene and added functional species such as chromophores, supramolecules, biomolecules, and polymers [52]. Functionalization of graphene sheet can be performed in two manners as follows.

4.2.1 Covalent Functionalization

Graphene, which is entirely made up of sp^2 carbon atoms with delocalization of π electrons all over the carbon hexagon framework, exhibits chemically inertness to some extent. Covalent functionalization of 2-D carbon hexagon of graphene usually necessitates reactive species to facilitate the formation of a covalent bond with the sp2 carbon of graphene. Throughout the covalent functionalization, sp2 conjugation of graphene surface was perturbed and non-conjugated sp3 carbon was produced with a tetrahedral geometry. Covalent functionalization can enhance the properties of graphene with opening its band gap, tuning conductivity, dispersibility in various solvents such as organic and polar solvents, and stability. Graphene can be covalently functionalized in two ways: (i) the covalent attachment of C=C of graphene with free radicals and dienophiles and (ii) covalent attachment of functional group containing organic compounds with oxygen functionalities of GO. Because of the different functional groups present on GO, i.e., hydroxyl and epoxy groups at above and below the graphene surface and carboxyl at the edges, GO was used as the starting material.

4.2.1.1 The Covalent Attachment of C=C of Graphene with Free Radicals and Dienophiles

Free radicals are extremely reactive organic species that react with the C=C of graphene forming covalent bonds. Free radicals can be generated through typical schemes such as thermal decomposition (heat treatment of diazonium salt) [53] and photochemical reaction (with benzoyl peroxide) [54,55]. Besides free radicals, dienophiles also interact with C=C of graphene hexagon. A typical example of reaction of dienophiles with graphene is cycloaddition reaction. The cycloaddition reaction can be performed on the surface of the graphene. Graphene can exhibit different types of cycloaddition reaction: [2+1], [2+2], [3+2], and [4+2]. Among these, the most common cycloaddition is [3+2] cycloaddition, which is also defined as 1,3-dipolar cycloaddition reaction [56]. Carbenes and nitrenes perform [2+1] cycloadditions [57,58], resulting in cyclopropane or aziridine rings, respectively; aryne or benzyne performs [2+2] cycloaddition, resulting in a four-membered ring [59]; and [4+2] cycloaddition, which is the Diels–Alder cycloaddition, involves a diene (an electron-rich moiety) and a dienophile (an electron-deficient moiety) [60,61]. Other examples are cycloaddition reaction in graphene [62], [D] [2+2] cycloaddition reaction in graphene [63], [E] 1,3-dipolar cycloaddition reaction in graphene [64], and [F] [4+2] cycloaddition reaction in graphene [60].

4.2.1.2 Covalent Attachment of Functional Groups Containing Organic Compounds with Oxygen Functionalities of GO

4.2.1.2.1 Amidation Reaction

Amidation reaction (also called carbodiimide coupling) [65–67] occurs at the carboxylic group of GO and the amine group of organic moieties. Amidation of the carboxylic acid group of GO can be carried out in drastic or mild conditions. Numerous amidation reactions involve in the first step: activation of carboxylic group and formation of acyl chloride treating with thionyl chloride. In the second step, amine group containing species reacts to form amide [65]. Amidation reaction can also be performed via activation of carboxyl group through coupling reaction using 1-[3-[dimethylamino]propyl]-3-ethylcarbodiimide methiodide, *N,N*'-dicyclohexylcarbodiimide or 1-ethyl-3-[3-dimethylaminopropyl]carbodiimide (EDC), and hydroxybenzotriazole as coupling agents [66]. However, thionyl or oxalyl chlorides can also react with hydroxyl groups of GO performing side reactions. Therefore, it is not specific to the carboxylic acid groups.

Our group has also reported the functionalization of GO with an organic molecule 'dithiooxamide' via amidation. Furthermore, AuNPs were anchored to develop a novel tricomponent nanocomposite 'AuNPs@dithiooxamide-reduced GO'. The prepared nanocomposite offers a high active surface area, speedy electron transference, and stable physicochemical property with exceptional electrocatalytic behavior [68]. A novel, biofunctionalized, graphene-based nanocomposite was reported in which 'bovine serum albumin'-wrapped graphene was functionalized with 'Neutral Red' via amidation followed by its association with AuNPs. The prepared nanocomposite-modified glassy carbon (GC) electrode was applied for the development of a methyl parathion electrochemical sensor [69]. A voltammetric sensing proposal for bisphenol A was established using histamine-functionalized GO through amide coupling between carboxyl and amine groups of GO and histamine, respectively, and the functionalized GO was further electrochemically reduced [70]. Chitosan (CS)-incorporated rGO nanomaterial was electrophoretically deposited on an indium tin oxide glass substrate to synthesize an amide-coupled product. Amide coupling occurred between –COOH and $–NH_2$ groups of rGO and CS, respectively. This synthesized material makes availability of sites for functionalization of CS-incorporated rGO with tyrosinase enzyme for the electrochemical determination of bisphenol A. Introduction of tyrosinase enzyme results in amide coupling due to which tyrosinase enzyme spreads homogenously on CS-incorporated rGO [71]. GO was electrolytically functionalized with ethylenediamine through nucleophilic substitution and amidation reactions between amine group of ethylenediamine, and epoxy and carboxylic groups of GO, and thus nitrogen-rich GO was reduced via negative electrolysis. The synthesized nanocomposite was employed in the detection of Pb^{2+} by differential pulse anodic striping voltammetry [72]. The functionalization of graphene was done with 'sulfourea'. The *N*-terminals of sulfourea was carbodiimide coupled with carboxyls of GO. Sulfourea-functionalized graphene offers a large active surface area and a good electrocatalytic property toward the electrochemical sensing of acetaminophen. Gold-NPs@SFG acts as a more efficient electrocatalyst for the electrocatalytic oxidation of the drug 'acetaminophen' using differential pulse voltammetry with a limit of detection (LOD) of 0.09 μM in a linear range of 1.2–300 μM [73]. Silver nanoparticles (NPs) were grafted on GO forming Ag-GO which was deposited on electrode and further covalently functionalized via amide bonding with electrochemically polymerized poly L-lysine. The prepared electrode was employed for voltammetric detection of dopamine through hydrogen bonding between –COOH and –OH groups of GO and $–NH_2$ group of dopamine [74]. An electrochemical platform for the detection of Cu(II) was prepared using impedance spectroscopy, formulated by thio-Au electrode forming Au-S by thiol group of 1-octadecanethiol (ODT) and Au atom. Furthermore, carboxylated GO was interacted with Au-ODT results linking with alkyl chain of ODT via intermolecular force forming Au-ODT-CGO. It was further covalently functionalized with rhodamine B hydrazide via amide coupling [75].

Bhardiya et al. constructed an environment-friendly nanobiocomposite using SnO_2 NPs and GO. The amino acid 'L-proline' was linked with NH_2-GO via carbodiimide coupling, and furthermore, SnO_2 NPs were anchored on it. The fabricated nanocomposite was employed for the efficient determination of cadmium [II] in water samples. The synergism between proline-functionalized GO and SnO_2 NPs boosted the electrocatalytic performance of the modified electrode. The LOD was calculated to be 1×10^{-4} ppm Cd [II] in a calibration range of 0.001–0.4 ppm [76].

4.2.1.2.2 Esterification Reaction

Esterification reaction [77] occurs in the carboxyl group of GO and the hydroxyl group of organic species. As in the cases of amidation reaction, the carboxyl group of GO activated with thionyl (or oxalyl) chloride, resulting in acyl chloride and the formation of ester bond, requires application of base for deprotonation of alcohol. However, using coupling agents EDC and 4-dimethylaminopyridine (DMAP) as an alternative avoids the requirement of base. The Steglich esterification agent EDC/DMAP was first used on graphene by Mei et al. [78]. Electrochemical detections of di-[2-ethylhexyl] phthalate was made possible by ferrocene poly[amine] ester dendrimer (Fc-AED)-functionalized GO via an esterification reaction between the carboxylic terminal of Fc-AED and the hydroxyl group of GO [79].

4.2.1.2.3 Nucleophilic Epoxy Ring Opening

Epoxy ring present on the graphene surface can be open with the reaction of amine-containing species and GO, introducing hydroxyl and amine groups on graphene surface, where amine behaves as nucleophile [80]. GO was functionalized with an amine group having the ionic liquid (IL) 1-aminopropyl-3-methylimidazolium tetrafluoroborate via epoxy ring opening of GO. This IL-functionalized GO was applied for voltammetric detection of Cu [II] and antimony [III] by differential pulse voltammetry (DPV) [81]. Our group functionalized the graphene with the biomolecule 'Threonine' using a nucleophilic epoxide-ring opening. Further, it was anchored with spinel Co_3O_4. The prepared biocomposite material was applied for the electrochemical sensing of the drug 'Metronidazole' [82].

4.2.1.2.4 1,2-Cycloaddition Reaction

GO was reduced to rGO, and it was further functionalized with ω-azidodi-ethylene glycol-α-ferrocenyl carboxylic acid ester through 1,2-cycloaddition reactions between nitrene, produced by the decomposition of alkylazido compound and double bond of rGO. This functionalized product showed good solubility in water and was applied as an enzymatic glucose sensor and a nonenzymatic H_2O_2 electrochemical sensor [83].

4.2.2 Noncovalent Functionalization

Since graphene exhibits excellent surface area, which provides platform for physical attachment of molecules through noncovalent functionalization, for instance, van der Waals, electrostatic, and π–π interactions [84]. The noncovalent communications of π-structures have significance to immobilize enzymes, proteins, supramolecules, and DNA complexes [85,86]. These noncovalent communication of π-structures is applicable in the manufacture of nanodevices, because slight variations in the electronic properties of π-structures make remarkable impacts on the structure and characteristics of nanosystem [87].

4.2.2.1 π–π Interaction

The π–π interactions include two ubiquitous necessities. The first is the presence of π systems, and the second is that interacting systems should have a planar geometry, so that overlap can take place between two species. Because graphene is prosperous in π system with a nearly planar geometry [88], graphene has a preference to strong interaction with other aromatic species. The following factors have influence on π–π interactions, electron-donating or electron-withdrawing properties, substituents, and size of aromatic species [89].

GO was non-covalently functionalized with copper terephthalate metal organic framework via π–π interaction and hydrogen bonding for electrochemical reduction of acetaminophen and dopamine by cyclic voltammetry (CV) and DPV [90]. An electrochemical sensor was developed using noncovalent functionalization of graphene with iron phthalocyanine through π–π attraction, which facilitates additional active centers for electro-oxidation of NO liberated from live cells [91]. A electrochemical sensor for nitric oxide was prepared using GO in its reduced form rGO and interaction of rGO with Fe[III] *meso*-tetra-[4-carboxyphenyl] porphyrin via π-π attraction, and the obtained product was electrophoretically deposited on indium tin oxide (ITO) microelectrode and further covalently interrelated with 3-aminophenylboronic acid [92]. Hemin-functionalized GO nanomaterial was prepared via simple sonication method through π–π interaction between them and was electrochemically applied to prepare electrode for voltammetric sensing of ascorbic acid, dopamine, and uric acid [93]. Application of metal-porphyrin compound was extended through noncovalent grafting of GO with manganese-*tetra*-phenylporphyrin (Mn-TPP) via π–π stacking attraction using an ecofriendly method. After that, electrochemical reduction of GO/Mn-TPP results in rGO/Mn-TPP nanocomposite, which was applied for voltammetric determination of dopamine [94]. A facile synthesis method for electrochemical detection of 4-nitrophenol was performed through functionalization of electrochemically reduced GO with electropolymerized 3,5-diamino 1,2,4-triazole (DAT). GO was interacted with DAT via its triazole through π–π interaction, and the synthesized nanomaterial was applied to prepare electrode for electrochemical sensing of 4-nitrophenol via electrostatic attraction and hydrogen bonding [95]. A low-temperature hydrothermal process was applied for the synthesis of electrochemically active nanomaterial for voltammetric sensing of nitric oxide. For this purpose, nitrogen-doped graphene was non-covalently functionalized with 5-, 10-, 15-, 20-tetrakis [1-methyl-4-pyridino] porphyrin tetra [p-toluenesulfonate] via π–π interaction [96]. Non-covalent functionalization of electrochemically reduced GO was done with hyroxylattopillar [5] arene AuNPs via π–π staking. This fabricated nanomaterial was used to modify glassy carbon electrode (GCE) to test its electroactivity toward methyl parathion pesticide [97]. An electrochemical platform for neonicotinoid pesticide was developed by molecularly imprinted polymer (MIP)–modified graphene using *p*-vinyl benzoic acid monomer, which has alkenyl and hydroxyl groups and interacted with graphene via π–π stacking. The prepared nanomaterial was successfully applied for the sensing of thiamethoxan that occurs in grain via linear sweep voltammetry (LSV) [98]. The presence of phenothrine, a non-cyano pyrethroid insecticide, in fruit sample was electrochemically determined by modified GC electrode. For this purpose, noncovalent modification of GO was carried out with polypyrrole via π–π interaction. The electrochemical activity of the prepared material was performed by electrochemical impedance spectroscopy and CV [99]. GO in its reduced form was non-covalently functionalized with the bifunctional molecule 1-formylpyrene via π–π stacking to facilitate incorporation of tyrosinase on rGO, and this synthesized nanomaterial was drop-casted on screen-printed electrode and this modified electrode was applied to determine the existence of phenol in an aqueous sample by the DPV technique [100]. GO was covalently functionalized with polyethylene glycol (PEG) and ethylenediamine via esterification and amide coupling, respectively. The synthesized composites was used to modify working electrode, which offer the stage for electrocatalytic oxidation of bisphenol A through π stacking [101].

A nonenzymatic, graphene-based glucose sensor was fabricated using wet chemical method through noncovalent functionalization of graphene. GO reacted with poly[vinyl pyrrole] (PVP) followed by reduction to facilitate π–π interaction between graphene and PVP, and after that nickel NPs were introduced. The fabricated nanocomposite was dispersed in CHIT to immobilize the prepared nanomaterial on GC electrode to detect glucose in blood [102]. GO suspension was pipetted on interdigitated gold microelectrode and electrochemically reduced into rGO, and this prepared electrode was modified using 1-pyrenebutyl-amino-β-CD (PyCD) via π–π stacking of pyrene portion of PyCD and rGO. The as-prepared electrode was applied for the detection of picric acid with the formation of inclusion complex between nitro group of picric acid and β-CD [103].

4.2.2.2 Van der Waals' Interaction

Pristine graphene is hydrophobic in character, and because of this property, graphene exhibits interaction with hydrophobic or partially hydrophobic species [104], for instance, surfactants, [105], ionic liquids [106], or macromolecules [107]. These interactions are usually useful to disperse graphene in aqueous as well as organic medium and assimilation in polymers. The hydrophobic interaction also occurs in rGO, although rGO has aromaticity with hydrophobicity to a lesser extent [108].

4.2.2.3 Hydrogen Bonding

GO, which is hydrophilic in nature, also shows aromatic property to a very small extent, and rGO also have a small number of ionic groups, generally carboxyl and hydroxyl, which play important roles in ionic interactions or hydrogen bonding with the corresponding ionic parts of added molecules such as diethyl-N,N-bis[2-hydroxyethyl] phosphoramide (DEPA) [109], triethylenetetramine (TETA) [110], and gelatin [111]. An electrochemical sensor for ascorbic acid was facilitated by non-covalently functionalizing GO with zinc porphyrin dye via hydrogen bond and π–π interaction and further incorporation of tetra-octyl ammonium bromide and electrochemical reduction of GO [112]. β-Cyclodextrin (β-CD] non-covalently interacted with GO via hydrogen bonding, and the prepared nanomaterial was deposited on GC electrode. The obtained β-CD/GO/GC electrode further introduced with 1,2-naphthoquinone-4-sulphonic acid sodium salt (NQS), which acts as redox indicator, via host–guest interaction. As-prepared electrode was applied to determine cholylglycine (a component of bile acid) by nucleophilic substitution reaction between amine group of cholylglycine and NQS by DPV [113].

4.2.2.4 Cation–π Interaction

A new electrochemical sensor for H_2O_2 secreted from different breast cells was fabricated via cation–π interaction between 1-butyl-3-methylimidazolium tetrafluoroborate IL and graphene, and the obtained product was decorated with gold nanoflower [114].

4.2.2.5 Electrostatic Interaction

A square-wave anodic stripping voltammetry for Hg^{2+} ion was defined by functionalization of GO with silver nanowires (AgNWs) via electrostatic interaction between negative-charged GO and positive-charged AgNWs [115]. Graphene was non-covalently functionalized via π–π and electrostatic attractions with polyaniline in water by the help of bath sonicator with a different mass ratio of polyaniline and graphene, and this prepared nanocomposite was further applied as electrochemical DNA sensor [116]. GO was functionalized with hexadecyl trimethyl ammonium bromide–capped gold nanoparticles (AuNPs) via electrostatic interaction to fabricate GO/AuNPs. This GO/AuNPs were further interacted with thio-β-cyclodextrin forming Au-S bond and applied to fabricate electrode for voltammetric sensing of tetra-bromo bisphenol A [72]. GO was modified using one-pot reaction via electrostatic attraction with 1-butyl-3-methylimidazolium IL and decorated with AuNPs via electrostatic attraction. Here, IL acts as a linker between GO and AuNPs. The synthesized nanocomposite was applied for electro-oxidation of dopamine [117].

A coordination complex–functionalized rGO nanomaterial was synthesized. For this purpose, GO was firstly reduced with environment-friendly L-cystine forming rGO. rGO was functionalized via electrostatic attraction with hexamine cobalt [III] complex to fabricate electrochemical sensor for morin (a flavonoid) in fruit sample [118]. Functionalization of graphene with 1-[3-aminopropyl]-3-methyl-imidazolium bromide IL makes graphene surface positively charged and to interact electrostatically with negatively charged sulfonated polyaniline, which results in multilayer film deposited on ITO electrode to fabricate nonenzymatic H_2O_2 electrochemical sensor [119]. Noncovalent functionalization of GO was carried out via electrostatic interaction using polyethyleneimine (PEI), which acts as a functionalizing agent for GO and a stabilizing agent for AuNPs. Reduction of GO and $HAuCl_4$ also takes place simultaneously in one step. The nanocomposite was deposited on electrode and further grafted with polyaciflavin (PAF). PAF was bonded with GO via amide bond formation between residual carboxylic group of rGO and amine group of PAF. This prepared electrode was applied for sensing of iodate [120]. Due to the presence of abundant oxygen-containing functional groups, GO facilitates attraction of β-cyclodextrin via electrostatic interaction resulting in synthesis of β-CD/GO. B-CD/GO was drop-casted on electropolymerized acid yellow modifying glassy carbon electrode and resulting in β-CD/GO/PAY/GC electrode for voltammetric detection of isoprenaline [121]. Layer-by-layer functionalized graphene nanomaterials were assembled by adsorption of positively charged polyallylamine hydrochloride

(PAH) on negatively charged GCE. After that, adsorption of GO on PAH was taken place via electrostatic interaction. Then, reduction of GO was carried out by the mild reducing agent $NaBH_4$. The prepared nanomaterial was used in electrochemical sensing of Cu [II] ion through DPASV [122].

Singh et al. utilized a noncovalent way to functionalize the graphene with polyaniline using starch as a bridge. Furthermore, the embellishment of ZnO on prepared graphene was utilized for the electrochemical sensing of a toxic dye '*p*-phenylene diamine'. ZnO NPs were associated via electrostatic interactions [123].

Electrochemical sensors are extensively applied in miscellaneous areas, for instance, medical diagnostics, food testing and pharmaceutical laboratories, industrial safety, and environmental monitoring. Functionalized graphene-based materials have been extensively utilized to fabricate electrochemical sensors because of their exceptional physicochemical property, tremendous catalytic activity, and low manufacturing cost. Functionalization of graphene or GO with organic moieties, polymers, metal oxides, biomolecules, etc. can modulate the sensing signal and can enhance their selectivity, adsorption of analyte, and sensitivity [124–131]. Commonly preferred voltammetric techniques for the determination of biomolecules [132], ions [133], and organic species [134] are CV, DPV, square-wave voltammetry (SWV), etc. The monitoring of the resultant current of electrochemically active species is recorded against applied scanning potential that results from CV, DPV, or SWV voltammogram. Basically, these techniques require a three-electrode system consisting of working, counter-, and reference electrodes. Several studies have been done based on the functionalization of GO and its application as an electrochemical sensor [68–79, 81–83, 90–104, 112–123, 135–228].

4.3 SOME APPLICATIONS OF GRAPHENE-BASED NANOMATERIAL IN ELECTROCHEMICAL SENSORS

4.3.1 Functionalized Graphene Nanomaterials for Electrochemical Sensing of Metronidazole (MNZ)

A GC electrode was prepared for electrochemical sensing of MNZ by functionalizing and reducing GO by polydialkyldimethylammonium chloride (PDDA) via microwave assistance. The prepared PDDA-graphene was drop cast on GC electrode and further interacted with L-cystine to fabricate cysteic acid-PDDA-graphene-GC electrode as working electrode for MNZ detection in urine and lake water sample by CV and LSV in Britton-Robinson (BR) buffer [143]. Sulfonated graphene with silver NPs was used as working electrode material to examine MNZ in an aquatic product by CV and LSV in citric acid–trisodium citrate dehydrate. For this purpose, first GO was reduced, after that sulfonated using sulfanilic acid, and deposited on GC electrode which was further modified with silver NPs [144]. A zeolite-modified carbon paste (CP) electrode was fabricated for MNZ determination. For this purpose, Cu [II]-exchanged clinoptile NPs were used to modify CP electrode, and the modified electrode were employed for square wave

(SW) voltammetric detection technique of MNZ [145]. A sensitive electrode for detection of MNZ was fabricated by Cu [II] polycysteine nanostructure. First, Cu [II]-cysteine nanostructure was prepared and deposited on GC electrode, and afterward electroreduction of Cu [II]-cysteine and electropolymerization of cysteine was carried out via CV in phosphate-buffered saline (PBS). The prepared electrode was successfully applied for MNZ sensing by LSV technique in BR buffer [146]. An electrochemical stage for MNZ was prepared by magnetic molecularly imprinted polymer-grafted magnetic GC electrode using Fe_3O_4@SiO_2 NPs, 3-aminopropyltriethoxysilane, and tetraethyl orthosilicate. The electrochemical activity of electrode toward MNZ in milk and honey samples was performed in BR buffer by differential pulse stripping voltammetry (DPSV) [147].

A CP electrode was prepared to detect MNZ by gold nanotubes which were synthesized via electrodeposition within the polycarbonate hole. The prepared electrode was successfully applied to examine MNZ via SWV in PBS [148]. To facilitate MNZ detection in injection solution via linear sweep striping voltammetry in BR buffer, electropolymerization of L-cysteine was carried out on a GC electrode, and after that, the prepared electrode was modified by deposition of gold NPs which were functionalized with β-CD [149]. A GC electrode was formulated by electropolymerization of thionine (TH) by CV resulting in PTH-GC electrode, and after that, 3-D graphene like carbon structure was deposited on PTH-GC electrode surface. The as-fabricated electrode exhibited its electroactivity toward reduction of MNZ in real sample by CV and DPV in PBS buffer [150]. Graphite powder and paraffin oil were used in the ratio of 72:28 to prepare CP electrode for the determination of MNZ in tablet sample by SWV using BR buffer as the supporting electrolyte [151]. An electrode was prepared by growing poly-[p-aminobenzene sulfonic acid] on GC electrode by CV and was applied to sensitive determination of MNZ in tablet form by the DPV method using PBS as the supporting electrolyte [152]. To fabricate a sensitive electrode for MNZ in real drug sample, carboxyl multiwalled carbon nanotubes (CMWCNTs) were deposited on GC electrode surface. Furthermore, electropolymerization of dopamine was carried out on CMWCNT-modified GC electrode by CV. The modified electrode was successfully applied for MNZ detection by DPV in PBS electrolyte [153]. Hydrothermally synthesized, strontium-doped molybdenum di-selenide was deposited on GC electrode surface to electrochemical detection of MNZ in real sample by DPV using PBS as the supporting electrolyte [154]. A modified GC electrode was prepared by deposition of multiwalled carbon nanotubes on GC electrode surface; thereafter, CS was self-assembled on MWCNT-GC electrode followed by self-assembly of Ni^{2+}, and the prepared electrode was applied for MNZ detection by DPV in PBS [155]. DPV technique was used to determine MNZ in human blood serum and urine specimen by applying graphene-TiO_2 nanocomposite as GC electrode modifier in BR buffer. Here, CS is also used to enhance the performance by increasing current peak [156].

MNZ was amperometrically determined in drug and urine specimen by depositing CS-guarded, tetra-sulfonated, copper phthalocyanine on GC electrode used in DPV technique in PBS electrolyte [157]. An anionic surfactant sodium dodecyl sulfate was used for modification of graphene to prepare electrode material for voltammetric technique. The prepared electrode was applied for sensing of MNZ in tablet and biological specimen via DPSV technique in acetate buffer electrolyte solution [158]. A voltammetry electrode material was prepared by doping nitrogen, sulfur, and phosphorus atoms on porous carbon applying pyrolysis and carbonization procedure, which was performed at a high temperature. The prepared electrode was applied in LSV technique for the detection of MNZ in milk and pharmaceutical (tablet and injection) specimen in PBS electrolyte [159]. Our group prepared a functionalized graphene with 'Threonine' amino acid via nucleophilic epoxide-ring opening. The prepared biofunctionalized graphene was anchored with spinel Co_3O_4 for the determination of the drug 'Metronidazole' via nitro group reduction with LOD 3.9×10^{-9}M in the calibration range of 2.5–240 μM [82].

4.3.2 Functionalized Graphene Nanomaterials for the Sensing of Ascorbic Acid

Starting from a stable base material graphene, several types of nanocomposite-based sensors have been reported using various underlying electrode substrates (such as Au, glassy carbon, and quartz glass). Keeley et al. first reported graphene nanosheets immobilized on pyrolyzed photoresist film (PPF) electrodes (PPF/GNS) as a novel ascorbic acid (vitamin C) sensor, and it has a very low LOD of 0.12 mM with a very effective linear range of 0.4–6.0 mM [160]. Tig et al. modified glassy carbon electrode with silver nanoparticles (AgNPs), GO, and poly[L-arginine] (P[Arg]) and presented a hybrid composite GCE/AgNPs/P[Arg]-GO electrode with high electrocatalytic activity for ascorbic acid (AA), dopamine (DA), uric acid (UA), and L-tryptophan (L-Trp). In the case of AA, the modified electrode eradicated the interference effects of Na+, K+, L-lysine, glucose, L-cysteine, urea, and citric acid and have an LOD (S/N = 3) of 0.984 μM with linear relationships between the peak currents and the concentrations in the range of 4.0–2,400.0 μM [161]. Tian et al. reported carbon ceramic electrodes with a poly[acridine orange] film containing reduced graphene oxide–modified electrode for the selective detection of AA and UA in a mixture at working potentials of 170 and 400 mV, respectively. This electroactive material improved the electrochemical catalytic oxidation of AA and UA with resolved overlapping of anodic peaks. AA and UA exhibit concentration ranges of 0.8–5,000 and 0.6–900 μM with LODs of 0.3 and 0.2 μM, respectively [162]. Zhao et al. prepared MgO nanobelts on a graphene-modified tantalum wire (denoted as MgO/Gr/Ta) electrode. In the threefold co-existence system, the modified electrode demonstrated attractive features such as excellent sensitivity, outstanding selectivity, and good stability as a sensor for simultaneous detection of AA, dopamine (DA), and UA [163]. The most promising conducting polymer-based electrode materials, such as polyaniline (PANI) and polypyrrole (PPy), offer high conductivity, good redox reversibility, and stability and were applied as an ideal material for the construction of sensitive transducer in amperometric, voltammetric, and conductimetric/impedimetric sensors [164–171].

A number of electrochemical sensors based on PANI and PPy nanostructures have been investigated [172]. For example, Li et al. introduced a sensing strategy prepared by feasible one-pot hydrothermal process based on the self-assembly of MoS_2 nanospheres and polyaniline (PANI) loaded on reduced graphene oxide (3D MoS_2-PANI/rGO). The prepared sensing platform exhibited high sensitivity for the detection of AA. The present 3D, nanostructured sensing strategy exhibits a wide linear range from 8 to 50 mM with an LOD of 22.2 mM and offers high bioaffinity, strong catalytic effect, and good reliability in the trace determination of electroactive biomolecules [173]. Recently, a different approach was opted by Salahandish et al. to construct a novel AA electrochemical sensor NFG/AgNPs/PANI by a three-layer sandwich arrangement of nitrogen-doped functionalized graphene (NFG), AgNPs, and nanostructured polyaniline (PANI) nanocomposite. The significant alteration of the AgNPs-grafted NFG-PANI coated on very low-cost fluorine doped tin oxide electrode (FTOE) effectively enhanced the charge transfer conductivity of the electrode. The nano-biosensor exhibits high selectivity for AA in the presence of interferences as glucose, dopamine, UA, and other similar oxidizable compounds and demonstrated a linear detection range of [10–11], 460 μM with a very low LOD of 8 μM [174]. Wu et al. fabricated an electrochemical AA sensor using PdNPs-GO-modified GCE [175]. The PdNPs-GO sensor offered detection within a good linear correlation to AA concentration from 20 μM to 2.28 mM with an excellent sensitivity and exhibited a rapid response to AA within 5 s.

Similarly, the noble metal NPs (Pt, Au, and Pd) are prone to undergo impermanent agglomeration through van der Waals' interactions, which reduces the surface area [176]. Lui et al. have established a method for synthesis of AuCo alloy nanoparticles (AuCo NPs) on a thiol group functional graphene (HS-GR) modified electrode for selective determination of dopamine, AA and UA [177]. The AuCo NPs/HS-GR sensor showed high electrocatalytic activity in citrate-phosphate buffer solutions (MBS) with pH 4.5 with outstanding catalytic properties for the oxidation of these analytes and also compatible for individual determination from their mixture with a wide linear range, superior sensitivity, selectivity, good repeatability, and stability. Song et al. studied the detailed mechanism of AA oxidation on the glassy carbon electrode modified with GO sheet and AuNPs [178]. According to this study, the electrode that has the best performance presents attractive analytical features with a low LOD of 100 nM and a fast response time. Later, Jiang et al. developed reduced graphene oxide-supported Au@Pd (Au@Pd-RGO) nanocomposites by one-step synthesis for individual and modified GCE for the simultaneous determination of AA, dopamine, and UA with excellent specificity and a low LOD [179]. A novel method using a bimetallic system for the detection of glucose and AA was introduced by Darabdhara et al. The prepared bimetallic Cu-Ag/rGO nanocomposite has greater advantages over a monometallic system like it follows Michaelis–Menten kinetics with a good affinity toward TMB [180]. Llobregat et al. modified a gold-interdigitated microelectrodes array (Au-IDA) using graphene oxide doped with gold nanoparticles (AuNPs-GO/Au-IDA) and fabricated simultaneously a sensor for AA, dopamine, and UA. The fabricated sensor demonstrated resistance from commonly superior interfering biomolecules. The sensor has been utilized for the selective detection of AA in the presence of dopamine and UA and the synchronized determination of individual analytes in their mixtures with satisfactory results [181].

4.3.3 Functionalized Graphene Nanomaterials for the Electrochemical Sensing of H_2O_2

The development of proficient electrochemical hydrogen peroxide (H_2O_2) sensors for rapid and reliable determination has enormous importance due to the significance of H_2O_2 in biological systems and its various practical applications, for example, in food, pharmaceutical, and environmental analyses [182].

The electrochemical detection of H_2O_2 is mainly classified into two major groups, namely, *enzymatic* and *nonenzymatic.* Till now, a number of research works have been reported regarding this. During a biochemical reaction of enzymatic H_2O_2 sensors, enzymes must have a redox group that fascinates the electron transportation, resulting in variation in an H_2O_2 oxidation state. Enzymatic horseradish peroxidase (HRP)-based sensors that contain heme proteins are quite famous for decades due to their effective sensitivity, handiness, and very high selectivity. In the field of enzymatic H_2O_2 sensing, a quaternary nanocomposite material was synthesized and reported by Kumar et al., and they evaluated its effectiveness as a new-fangled peroxidase mimetic. The fabrication of hemin and silver-coated gold nanostars on a GO hexagonal sheet frame of carbon inflicted a nanoscale imprisonment and efficiently enhanced the catalytic performance of the nanocomposite. Under physiological conditions, the nanocomposite exhibits a nanomolar range sensitivity toward H_2O_2 with a low LOD of 1.26 nM [183]. Mercante et al. synthesized a graphene-based ternary conducting polymer nanocomposite (PEDOT:PSS-rGO-AuNPs) using poly[3,4-ethylenedioxythiophene]-poly[styrenesulfonate], rGO, and gold NPs, which was obtained via a superficial one-step approach and has a congregation with HRP. The basic phenomenon revealed that the HRP was captured on top of the film-modified electrode and functional as an H_2O_2 biosensor.

On the other hand, the development of an enzymatic hydrogen peroxide electrochemical sensor is of less interest because of low storage stability of enzymes. The developed nonenzymatic electrochemical sensor exhibited acceptable reproducibility, high accuracy, and great anti-interference ability and well-defined amperometric response toward H_2O_2 in a wide linear range of 5–400 μM, and an LOD of 0.08 μM (S/N=3) could be obtained [184]. Ju et al. introduced surfactant-free AuNPs that can provide naked catalytic surface with highly electrocatalytic activity. They prepared hybrid nanocomposite using gold NPs on nitrogen-doped graphene quantum dots (AuNPs–N-GQDs), which exhibited high sensitivity and selectivity for nonenzymatic electrochemical detection of hydrogen peroxide (H_2O_2) with a linear chronoamperometric concentration range of 0.25–13,327 μM, a sensitivity of 186.22 μA/mM cm^2, and a low LOD of 0.12 μM [185]. Yang et al. modified the gold electrode by controllable construction of AuNPs based on graphene sheets @cerium oxide (GS@CeO_2) nanocomposites via a facile solvothermal process. The prepared electrochemical sensor demonstrated an excellent performance for the electrocatalytic reduction of H_2O_2. Under the optimized conditions, detection of H_2O_2 was in a relative wide range from 1.0×10^{-3} to 10.0 mM ($R^2 = 0.9990$) with a lower LOD of 2.6×10^{-4} mM (S/N = 3) [186]. Sun et al. prepared CeO_2-montmorillonite (MMT) hybrid nanocomposites which was in agreement with classic Michaelis–Menten kinetics and demonstrated an advanced affinity to H_2O_2 [187]. Due to the stable chemical and physical character, good biocompatibility, high surface activity, and fast electron transport features, nano-sized ZnO is considered as a material for electrochemical sensors [188]. Also, AuNPs exhibit a large specific surface area, strong adsorption ability, good suitability, and good conductivity, and they can strongly interact with biomaterials and have been utilized to enhance current response in the construction of a sensitive amperometric immunosensor. Because of these properties, Xie et al. constructed AuNPs and flower-like zinc oxide through layer-by-layer method onto graphene/GCE (AuNPs/ZnO/Gr/GCE) electrochemical sensor for highly sensitive determination of H_2O_2 based on immobilization of hemoglobin (Hb). The developed sensor allows the detection of H_2O_2, with a linear response from 6.0 to 1130 M of H_2O_2, and the LOD was estimated to be 0.8 M (S/N = 3) [189]. An electrochemical sensor based on Au@TiO_2/graphene (GR) nanocomposite was introduced by Fan et al. through deposition of AuNPs on TiO_2/GR substrates, which revealed their high sensitivity toward H_2O_2 [190]. Lu et al. synthesized an excellent electrocatalytic H_2O_2 sensor via Pt-Au bimetallic NPs on graphene sheets–multiwalled carbon nanotubes (G-CNTs) hybrid nanomaterials for modification of GCE. This sensor was linear within the range from 2.0 to 8,561 μM H_2O_2 and a relatively low LOD of 0.6 μM (S/N = 3) [191]. Liu et al. [192] reported a nonenzymatic amperometric sensor for the detection of glucose and H_2O_2 on the basis of Cu_2O nanocubes wrapped by graphene nanosheets (Cu_2O/GNs) as electrocatalysts.

Under physiological conditions, the oxidation current of H_2O_2 varies linearly with respect to its concentration from 0.3 to 7.8 mM at 0.4 V and a low LOD of 20.8 mM [192]. By the use of chemical reduction of GO, Lui et al. prepared a noncovalent functionalized rGO by aniline that leads to a GO dispersion which is extremely stable without any floating or precipitated particles for several months. Furthermore, they decorated it with AgNPs by *in situ* chemical reduction of silver salts. The prepared enzyme-less AgNP/rGO sensor demonstrated good catalytic activity toward the reduction of H_2O_2 leading to the linear detection range, and the LOD is estimated to be from 100 μM to 80 mM (r = 0.9991) and 7.1 μM respectively [193]. Golsheikh et al. developed a silver NPs–decorated rGO on ITO by electrodeposition method, leading to an enzyme-less electrochemical sensor that exhibited extraordinary electrocatalytic activity for the reduction of H_2O_2 with calibration range of concentration about 0.1–100 mM ($R^2 = 0.9992$), while the LOD was 5 μM and fast amperometric response time was less than 2 s [194]. A 3D sandwich was reported by Li et al. by the association of MnO_2/graphene (GP), carbon nanotubes (CNTs), and AuNPs. An accelerated electron transfer was observed due to the good distribution of MnO_2 NPs on 3D scaffold. The prepared material exhibited a good sensitivity of 452 μA /mM cm^2 toward the reduction of H_2O_2, and the LOD was calculated to be 0.1 μM [195]. The covalently functionalized nanocomposite 'new methylene blue-GO' was prepared through cross-linking to fabricate an electrochemical sensor for the determination of H_2O_2. The prepared composite showed good electrocatalytic properties toward the reduction of H_2O_2. The calibration range for the sensing purpose was recorded from 3.3×10^{-4} to 2.28 mM with an LOD of 1.35 μM [196].

4.3.4 Functionalized Graphene Nanomaterials for the Electrochemical Sensing of Methyl Parathion (Organophosphate)

Recently, electrochemical sensors based on nanomaterial catalysis have attracted tremendous attention, which are more robust, stable, easy to handle, rapid, and sensitive in contrast to sensors [197]. Yang et al. applied a simple and cost-effective electrodeposition method for the construction of graphene–chitosan (GR–CS) hybrid composite onto glassy carbon electrode under controlled potential. The electrochemical studies revealed a significant redox response of methyl parathion (MP) on the GR–CS/GCE with a wide linear concentration range from 4.0 to 400 ng/mL and a low LOD of 0.8 ng/mL [198]. Rodrigues et al. proposed an interesting fabrication and exploration of layer-by-layer films constructed by rGO stabilized in polyelectrolytes in the existence or nonexistence of AuNPs for MP determination. They performed an organized investigation on the influence of MP allocation on the LOD and linear range of the sensor. In the absence of AuNPs, LOD and a linear range of 0.2–26 and 0.25–40 ppm were obtained, whereas in their presence, a wider linear range of 0.5–60 ppm was accomplished with an LOD of 0.770 ppm [199]. Xu et al. modified glassy carbon electrode sensor using poly[malachite green]/graphene nanosheets–nafion (PMG/GNs–NF) composite film which indirectly detected MP. Improved stability of PMG and the enhanced electron transfer rate were due to the presence of GNs in the composite film [200]. Balasubramanian et al. modified glassy carbon electrode with tannic acid–stabilized colloidal AuNPs to achieve the desired functionality. They introduced tannic acid as a bifunctional reducing cum stabilizing agent under ambient temperature (25°C). The colloidal TA@AuNPs/GCE has a better electrocatalytic activity in the determination of MP with a wide dynamic concentration range and a lower LOD. Experimental results confirm that there was no obvious change to the response current toward MP reduction in the presence of interfering ionic species [201]. Another nonenzymatic approach has been made by Li et al. involving a glassy carbon electrode modified by the combination of the individual properties of graphene nanosheets (high conductivity and adsorption affinity) and gadolinium hexacyanoferrate (high surface area and special catalytic activity) for sensitive detection of MP. Under optimum conditions, results indicated that reduction current increased with increase in MP concentration over the range from 0.008 to 10 mM. The electrochemical sensor displayed high sensitivity, acceptable stability, and a very attractive LOD 1 nM. Selectivity analysis of the GdHCF/GNs/GCE revealed that the 1000-fold of PO4-3, SO4-2, NO3-, and CO3-2 didn't interfere with the detection of MP [202].

The progress in nanotechnology, mutually with the valuable properties of nanomaterials, has unbolted a fresh perspective for the advancement of pesticide sensors. With the accomplishment of nanomaterials counting CNTs, AuNPs, ZrO_2NPs, CdS NPs, and CdS as immobilization templates, remarkable improvements in the electrocatalytic activity with extremely high sensitivity toward organophosphate pesticide (OP) detection was recognized. Fu et al. prepared graphene nanosheets (GS) through liquid-phase exfoliation of graphite powder in *N*, *N*-dimethylformamide (DMF) solvent system with the support of sodium citrate. Using *in situ* electrodeposition method, the surface of glassy carbon electrode was apparently covered with a porous reticulated nanosilica film. The prepared composite improved effectively the redox peak currents of MP. The external structure of nanocomposites has nano-cavities that significantly enhanced the rebinding rate of MP. Experimental results showed the linear concentration range of MP from 0.0005 to 5.6 μM, and LOD was calculated to be 0.07 nM (S/N=3) [203]. Song et al. developed a graphene-based, nano-TiO_2-modified glassy carbon electrode sensor for electrochemical investigation of MP behavior. At the optimal experimental condition of pH 5.2 acetate buffer solution, the modified electrode sensor showed good catalytic effects that can be concluded by improvised redox peak currents of MP. The sensor exhibited high sensitivity and good reproducibility as well as a very lower detection value of 1.0 nM (S/N=3) [204]. In addition, metal-fabricated ionic surfactant has also been used for the determination of OP. Li et al. reported a glassy carbon electrode modified by gold/sodium dodecyl benzene sulfonate NPs (nanoAu/SDBS/GCE) and utilized it for the determination of the organophosphorus pesticide MP under optimal conditions. The peak current analogous to the oxidation of the hydroxylamine group with outstanding linearity was obtained in the concentration range from 5.0×10^{-7} to 1.0×10^{-4} M and a predictable LOD of 8.6×10^{-8} M (S/N=3) [205]. Xue et al. reported a very simple approach for glassy carbon electrode modification by graphene–nafion matrix (graphene–nafion/GCE). The prepared electrochemical sensor reveals that the graphene–nafion matrix not only enhanced the adsorption to organophosphorus pesticide MP but also enhanced the sensitivity of its recognition. Experimental data showed that the peak current evidently amplified the reduction peak potential which was positively shifted for modified electrode. The response current was linearly interconnected to the concentration of MP from 0.02 to 20 μg/mL with a lower LOD of 1.6 ng/mL [206].

Gong et al. proposed a facile electrochemical one-step co-electrodeposition approach to the synthesis of high-quality graphene nanosheets decorated with zirconia nanoparticles (ZrO_2NPs-GNs) with no contamination onto a cathodic substrate. ZrO_2NPs have a high recognition and enrichment capability for phosphoric moieties and GNs with a large surface area and a high conductivity, and exhibit excellent efficiency to capture MP. The prepared sensor determined an LOD of 0.6 ng/mL (S/N=3) for MP [207]. In another study on graphene-based MP sensor, Govindasamy et al. described a low-cost electrode for the responsive amperometric detection of MP. In their work, they constructed a hybrid nanocomposite based on molybdenum disulfide nanosheets (MoS_2) and graphene via hydrothermal technique. Furthermore, using this nanocomposite, they modified glassy carbon electrode, and the modified electrode demonstrated an exceptional electrocatalytic ability toward MP. The linear concentration range is 10 nM to 1.9 mM with a LOD of 3.2 nM and a reduction in peak current measured typically at –0.60 V (*vs.* Ag/AgCl) for the pesticide MP [208].

For the first time, Zhao et al. introduced a glassy carbon electrode coated with molecularly imprinted polymer–ionic liquid–graphene composite film (MIP–IL–EGN/GCE) by free radical polymerization using MP as template. The electrochemical synthesis of sensor involved 2,2-azobis[iso-butyronitrile] as initiator and a functional monomer methacrylic acid with a cross-linking reagent ethylene glycol di-methacrylate. The proposed sensor could detect MP in the range from 0.010 to 7.0 M with a sensitivity of 12.5 A/M and an LOD of 6 nM (S/N=3) [209]. MIP offers a novel sensitive and selective electrochemical sensor constructed by electropolymerization method. MIP demonstrates high selectivity and sensitivity toward MP. Synthesis of MIP involves phenol as a functional monomer with an Au electrode in PBS using CV in the presence of MP. Determination of MP under the optimum operating conditions found to have a linear concentration range of 0.1–10 g/mL with an LOD of 0.01 g/mL [210]. Shi et al. prepared a photoelectrochemical (PEC) sensor by solvothermal method and electrochemical deposition technique successively for the determination of OPs that are based on rGO/TiO_2/CdS photoactive nanomaterials. It has a low LOD of 0.02 nM (S/N=3) and a linear response range of 0.05–10 nM for MP. The modified ITO electrode with nanocomposite rGO/TiO_2/CdS NPs exhibited enhanced photocurrent intensity with increase of the concentration of the hydrolysate of MP [211].

In the case of OPs like MP, nonenzymatic electrochemical biosensor became trendy nowadays due to their rapid, selective, and sensitive determination. Govindasamy et al. introduced an effective biosensor with an excellent capacity as an alternative to enzyme inhibition–based sensor for the detection of MP. The obtained data suggested that the proposed biosensor has an excellent capacity as an alternative to enzyme inhibition–based biosensor for the determination of MP. They constructed a BSA template Au-Ag bimetallic nanoclusters (AuAg@BSA/GCE) for modification of GCE. Experimental observation reveals that Au-Ag@BSA/GCE significantly catalyzed the redox reaction of MP through electrochemical determination. It was found that the improved electrode had high detection sensitivity to MP, with a linear concentration range from 0.02 to 8.0 and 8.0 to 200 μM with an LOD of 8.2 nM [212]. Recently, Tan et al. constructed two different MP electrochemical sensors via a wet chemistry approach and compared the works together. They synthesized a hybrid composite based on pillar [5] arene

(CP5), β-cyclodextrin (β-CD), and rGO. The pillar arene (CP5)/rGO nano hybrid modified glassy carbon electrode (CP5-rGO/GCE) was applied for the determination of MP by DPV. This sensor showed outstanding electrochemical catalytic activity, quick response, high sensitivity, excellent reproducibility, and anti-interference ability toward MP in comparison to β-cyclodextrin (β-CD)-functionalized reduced graphene (rGO) modified GCE (β-CD-rGO/GCE). The experimental observations displayed a higher supramolecular recognition capability between CP5 and MP in comparison to β-CD and MP. The sensitivity for CP5-rGO/GCE sensor was found to be directly proportional to the amount of MP molecules in solution with an LOD of 0.0003 mM (S/N=3) and a linear response concentration range of 0.001–150 mM [213].

A novel AuNPs@biofunctionalized graphene–based nanocomposite was prepared by Singh et al. in 2019 for the electrochemical sensing of MP. The responses were recorded using a DPV in the calibration range of 0.02–0.153 μM and 0.153–1.36 μM with an LOD of 6 nM [69]. One biocomposite was reported by Kaur et al. in which hemoglobin was immobilized on electrochemically rGO in the presence of chitosan. The prepared composite material exhibited a good surface coverage area and better charge transfer properties. Furthermore, it was employed for the electrochemical sensing of MP in vegetable samples with an LOD of 79.77 nM [214]. A new MP sensor was reported which has been prepared by the association of SnS_2 nanosheets and N, S-codoped drGO in one-pot hydrothermal synthesis. Using SnS_2 with NS–RGO accelerates electron movement. The SnS_2/NS–RGO exhibited a good performance with an LOD of 0.17 nM. The real-sample analysis was performed in black grape and river water samples [215].

4.3.5 Functionalized Graphene Nanomaterials for the Electrochemical Sensing of *p*-Aminophenol

Several works have been reported for the sensing of *p*-AP due to its harmful effects on environment. Graphene and hydroxyapatite nanocomposite synthesized by precipitation method employed as electrochemical sensing material for detection of *p*-AP in tap water by SWV technique in PBS via drop casting of nanocomposite on GC electrode [216]. GO-encapsulated SnO_2 hollow sphere was used for the preparation of electrode material for voltammetric determination of *p*-AP. The prepared material was deposited on a GC electrode using DPV technique in acetate buffer medium [217]. Carboxylated carbon nanotube was coupled with tetra-aminophenyl porphyrin and further incorporated with AuNPs. The as-prepared material was drop-casted on a GC electrode to fabricate voltammetric sensor for *p*-AP in real sample [218]. Carbon nanotube coupled with graphene nanoribbon was deposited on GC electrode surface. After that, β-CD and L-arginine were electropolymerized on modified GC electrode, and the prepared electrode was applied in the determination of *p*-AP via DPV in river water [219]. Palladium NPs–decorated rGO was prepared, and it was deposited on GC electrode. Furthermore, AuNPs were electrodeposited on modified GC electrode and then CS solution was added to the modified surface for voltammetric detection of *p*-AP by DPV in PBS [220]. An electrode was prepared for *p*-AP in pharmaceutical sample via electropolymerization of chromium [III] Schiff base complex in CV. The prepared electrode was applied for nanomolar concentration level detection by DPV technique in PBS [221]. Strontium mixed with 1, 10-phenanthroline-5, 6-dione [phendione] was used as a modifier to modify graphite paste electrode. The prepared electrode was used for voltammetric determination of *p*-AP in human urine and serum samples by DPV in PBS [222]. A 2-D spherical-shaped MoS_2-containing nafion modified GC electrode was prepared for voltammetric detection of *p*-AP at nanomolar concentration range in waste water sample by LSV in PBS [223]. An electrode material was synthesized based on hemin-mixed graphene. The as-prepared material was deposited on GC electrode surface on which MIP was further immobilized to detect *p*-AP by DPV in PBS [224]. Titanium dioxide was used to prepare CP electrode for *p*-AP in pharmaceutical samples by SWV in PBS [225]. A stainless steel voltammetric electrode was prepared by 3-D printing and electroplating of gold metal for the determination of *p*-AP in PBS electrolyte via CV and DPV techniques [226]. A RGO-tinnitride (TiN)–based electrode was prepared for sensing *p*-AP. For this, TiN NPs were further incorporated in the GO solution, and glucose was used to reduce GO. TiN NPs act as a spacer between graphene sheets. The synthesized composite was used to modify the GC electrode for *p*-AP detection by DPV in ammonia buffer in a real sample [227–229]. A detailed review has been published as application of metal organic frameworks (MOF) in sensing applications [230].

Functionalization of graphene was performed with polyvinyl alcohol-tungsten oxide for the electrochemical detection of *p*-AP in the calibration range of 0.003–70 μM with an LOD of 0.51 nM. The real-sample analysis was performed in pharmaceutical and some water samples [228]. Our group has also reported the tricomponent nanocomposite dithiooxamide-functionalized GO anchored with gold NPs for the electrochemical sensing of p-amino phenol. The prepared nanocomposite offers a high active surface area and stable physicochemical property with speedy electron transference. Under optimized conditions, electrochemical sensing of *p*-AP was performed in a calibration linear range of 0.1–130 mM with a LOD of 0.11×10^{-7} M. The successful sensing of *p*-AP in a real sample was also performed [68].

4.4 CONCLUDING REMARKS

The above review focused on the functionalization of graphene materials for the electrochemical sensing of various analytes such as MP, hydrogen peroxide, metronidazole, *p*-amino phenol, and AA. The covalent as well as noncovalent ways may be utilized for the preparation of functionalized graphene which can be employed for the highly sensitive sensing of analytes. We have tried to summarize the different functionalized graphene composite materials reported in the last decade for utilization in electrochemical sensors development. Certainly, it was found that 'functionalized graphene'–based composite materials offer an economical and efficient approach to fabrication of electrochemical sensors/biosensors.

ACKNOWLEDGEMENT

M. Singh is grateful to CSIR, New Delhi for financial assistance.

CONFLICTS OF INTEREST

None.

REFERENCES

1. Wallace PR. The band theory of graphite. *Phys Rev* 1947, 71: 622–34.
2. Mermin ND, Wagner H. Absence of ferromagnetism or anti-ferromagnetism in one- or two-dimensional isotropic heisenberg models. *Phys Rev Lett* 1966, 17: 1133–36.
3. Hancock Y. The 2010 Nobel Prize in physics-ground-breaking experiments on graphene. *J Phys D Appl Phys* 2011, 44: 473001–12.
4. Boehm HP, Setton R, Stumpp E. Nomenclature and terminology of graphite intercalation compounds [IUPAC Recommendations 1994], *Pure Appl Chem* 1994, 66: 1893–901.
5. Novoselov KS, Geim AK, Morozov SV, Jiang D, Zhang Y, Dubonos SV, Grigorieva IV, Firsov AA. Electric field effect in atomically thin carbon films. *Science* 2004, 306: 666–69.
6. Geim AK, Novoselov KS. The rise of graphene. *Nature Mater* 2007, 6: 183–91.
7. Allahbakhsh A, Sharif F, Mazinani S. The influence of oxygen-containing functional groups on the surface behavior and roughness characteristics of graphene oxide. *Nano* 2013, 8: 1350045–8.
8. Smith AT, La Chance AM, Zeng S, Liu B, Sun L. Synthesis, properties, and applications of graphene oxide/reduced graphene oxide and their nanocomposites. *Nano Mater Sci* 2019, 1: 31–47.
9. Konios D, Stylianakis MM, Stratakis E, Kymakis E. Dispersion behaviour of graphene oxide and reduced graphene oxide. *J Coll Interf Sci* 2014, 430: 108–12.
10. Pham TA, Kim JS, Kim JS, Jeong YT. One-step reduction of graphene oxide with L-glutathione. *Colloids Surf A Physicochem Eng Asp* 2011, 384: 543–48.
11. Sluiter MHM, Kawazoe Y. Cluster expansion method for adsorption: Application to hydrogen chemisorption on graphene. *Phys Rev B Condens Matter* 2003, 68: 085410.
12. Sofo JO, Chaudhari AS, Barber GD. Graphane: A two-dimensional hydrocarbon. *Phys Rev B Condens Matter Mater Phys* 2007, 75: 153401.
13. Baughman RH, Eckhardt H, Kertesz MJ. Structure-property predictions for new planar forms of carbon: Layered phases containing sp2 and sp atoms. *Chem Phys* 1987, 87: 6687–99.
14. Haley MM, Brand SC, Pak JJ. Stepwise assembly of site specifically functionalized dehydrobenzo[18]annulenes. *Angew Chem Int Ed Engl* 1997, 36: 836–38.
15. Lu N, Li Z, Yang J. Half-metallicity in edge-modified zigzag graphene nanoribbons. *Phys Chem C* 2009, 113: 16741.
16. Inagaki M, Kang F. Graphene derivatives: Graphane, fluorographene, graphene oxide, graphyne and graphdiyne. *J Mater Chem A* 2014, 2: 13193.

17. Casiraghi C, Hartschuh A, Lidorikis E, Qian H, Harutyunyan H, et al. Rayleigh imaging of graphene and graphene layers. *Nano Lett* 2007, 7: 2711–17.
18. Valles C, Drummond C, Saadaoui H, Furtado CA, He M, et al. Solutions of negatively charged graphene sheets and ribbons. *J Am Chem Soc* 2008, 130: 15802–04.
19. Hernandez Y, Nicolosi V, Lotya M, Blighe FM, Sun Z, De S, Mc Govern IT, Holland B, Byrne B, Gun'Ko YK, et al. High-yield production of graphene by liquid-phase exfoliation of graphite. *Nat Nano* 2008, 3: 563–68.
20. Park S, Ruoff RS. Chemical methods for the production of graphenes. *Nat Nanotechnol* 2009, 4: 217–24.
21. Dreyer DR, Park S, Bielawski CW, Ruoff RS. The chemistry of graphene oxide. *Chem Soc Rev* 2010, 39: 228.
22. Paredes JI, Villar-Rodil S, Martinez-Alonso A, Tascon JMD. Graphene oxide dispersions in organic solvents. *Langmuir* 2008, 24: 10560–64.
23. Edwards RS, Coleman KS. Graphene synthesis: Relationship to applications. *Nanoscale* 2013, 5: 38–51.
24. Sofer Z, Jankovsky O, Simek P, Sedmidubsky D, Sturala J, Kosina J, Miksova R, Mackova A, Mikulics M, Pumera M. Insight into the mechanism of the thermal reduction of graphite oxide: Deuterium-labeled graphite oxide is the key. *ACS Nano* 2015, 9: 5478–85.
25. Stroyuk L, Andryushina NS, Shcherban ND, Il'in VG, Efanov VS, Yanchuk IB, Kuchmii SY. Pokhodenko VD. *Theor Exp Chem* 2012, 48: 1–12.
26. Stankovich S, Dikin DA, Piner RD, Kohlhaas KA, Kleinhammes A, Jia Y, Wu Y, Nguyen ST, Ruoff RS. Synthesis of graphene-based nanosheets via chemical reduction of exfoliated graphite oxide. *Carbon* 2007, 45: 1558–65.
27. Toh SY, Loh KS, Kamarudin SK, Daud WRW. Graphene production via electrochemical reduction of graphene oxide: Synthesis and characterisation. *Chem Eng J* 2014, 251: 422–34.
28. Berger C, Song ZM, Li TB, Li XB, Ogbazghi AY, Feng R, Dai ZT, Marchenkov AN, et al. Ultrathin epitaxial graphite: 2D electron gas properties and a route toward graphene-based nanoelectronics. *J Phys Chem B* 2004, 108: 19912–16.
29. Lahiri J, Miller TS, Ross AJ, Adamska L, Oleynik II, Batzill M. Graphene growth and stability at nickel surfaces. *New J Phys* 2011, 13: 025001–19.
30. Plutnar J, Pumera M, Sofer Z. The chemistry of CVD graphene. *J Mater Chem C* 2018, 6: 6082–101.
31. Yang G, Li L, Lee WB, Ng MC. Structure of graphene and its disorders: A review. *Sci Technol Adv Mater* 2018, 19: 613–48.
32. Nair RR, Blake P, Grigorenko AN, Novoselov KS, Booth TJ, Stauber T, Peres NMR, Geim AK. Fine structure constant defines visual transparency of graphene. *Science* 2008, 320: 1308.
33. Dai JF, Wang GJ, Ma L, Wu CK. Surface properties of graphene: Relationship to graphene-polymer composites. *Rev Adv Mater Sci* 2015, 40: 60–71.
34. Lee C, Wei X, Kysar JW, Hone J. Measurement of the elastic properties and intrinsic strength of monolayer graphene. *Science* 2008, 321: 385–88.
35. Zhu Y, Murali S, Cai W, Li X, Suk JW, Potts JR, Ruoff RS. Graphene and graphene oxide: Synthesis, properties, and applications. *Adv Mater* 2010, 22: 3906–24.
36. Shahil KMF, Balandin AA. Thermal properties of graphene and multilayer graphene: Applications in thermal interface materials. *Solid State Commun* 2012, 152, 1331–40.
37. Gadipelli S, Guo ZX. Graphene-based materials: Synthesis and gas sorption, storage and separation. *Progress Mate Sci* 2015, 69: 1–60.

38. Farquhar K, Brooksby PA, Downard AJ. Controlled spacing of few-layer graphene sheets using molecular spacers: Capacitance that scales with sheet number. *ACS Appl Nano Mater* 2018, 1: 1420–29.
39. Viswanathan P, Ramraj R. *Graphene-Based Electrochemical Sensor for Biomolecules*. 2019, Chapter 2, pp. 43–65. doi: 10.1016/C2017-0-02915-4.
40. Ke Q, Wang J. Graphene-based materials for supercapacitor electrodes - A review. *J Materiomics* 2016, 2: 37–54.
41. Li G, Huang B, Pan Z, Su X, Shao Z, An L. Advances in three-dimensional graphene-based materials: Configurations, preparation and application in secondary metal [Li, Na, K, Mg, Al]-ion batteries. *Energy Environ Sci* 2019, 12: 2030–53.
42. Bonaccorso F, Sun Z, Hasan T, Ferrari AC. Graphene photonics and optoelectronics. *Nature Photon* 2010, 4: 611–22.
43. Rani P, Jindal VK. Stability and electronic properties of isomers of B/N co-doped graphene. *Appl Nanosci* 2014, 4: 989–96.
44. Wagner P, Ewels CP, Adjizian JJ, Magaud L, Pochet P, Roche S, Lopez- Bezanilla A, Ivanovskaya VV, Yaya A, Rayson M, Briddon P, Humbert B. Band gap engineering via edge-functionalization of graphene nanoribbons. *J Phys Chem C* 2013, 117: 26790–96.
45. Shareena TPD, Dasari S, Danielle MS, Dasmahapatra AK, Paul BT. A review on graphene-based nanomaterials in biomedical applications and risks in environment and health. *Nano-Micro Lett* 2018, 10: 53–86.
46. Xu C, Xu B, Gu Y, Xiong Z, Sun J, Zhao XS. Graphene-based electrodes for electrochemical energy storage. *Energy Environ Sci* 2013, 6: 1388–14.
47. Adeel M, Bilal M, Rasheed T, Sharma A, Iqbal HMN. Graphene and graphene oxide: Functionalization and nano-bio-catalytic system for enzyme immobilization and biotechnological perspective. *Int J Biological Macromole* 2018, 120: 1430–40.
48. Torrisi F, Carey T. Graphene, related two-dimensional crystals and hybrid systems for printed and wearable electronics. *Nano Today* 2018, 23: 73–96.
49. Nag A, Mitra A, Mukhopadhyay SC. Graphene and its sensor-based applications: A review. *Sens Actuators A* 2018, 270: 177–94.
50. Quintana M, Tapia JI, Prato M. Liquid-phase exfoliated graphene: Functionalization, characterization, and applications. *Beilstein J Nanotechnol* 2014, 5: 2328–38.
51. Banhart F, Kotakoski J, Krasheninnikov AV. Structural defects in graphene. *ACS Nano* 2011, 5: 26–41.
52. Georgakilas V, Otyepka M, Bourlinos AB, Chandra V, Kim N, Kemp KC, Hobza P, Zboril R, Kim KS. Functionalization of graphene: Covalent and non-covalent approaches, derivatives and applications. *Chem Rev* 2012, 112: 6156–214.
53. Sarkar S, Bekyarova, E, Haddon RC. Covalent chemistry in graphene electronics. *Materials Today* 2012, 15: 276–85.
54. Liu H, Ryu S, Chen Z, Steigerwald ML, Nuckolls C, Brus LE. Photochemical reactivity of graphene. *J Am Chem Soc* 2009, 131: 17099–101.
55. Hamilton CE, Lomeda JR, Sun Z, Tour JM, Barron AR. High-yield organic dispersions of unfunctionalized graphene. *Nano Lett* 2009, 9: 3460–62.
56. Georgakilas V, Bourlinos AB, Zboril R, Steriotis TA, Dallas P, Stubos AK, Trapalis C. Organic functionalisation of graphene. *Chem Commun* 2010, 46: 1766–68.
57. Petrushenko IK. [2+1] Cycloaddition of dichlorocarbene to finite-size graphene sheets: DFT study. *Monatsh Chem* 2014, 145: 891–96.
58. Strom TA, Dillon EP, Hamilton CE, Barron AR. Nitrene addition to exfoliated graphene: A one-step route to highly functionalized graphene. *Chem Commun* 2010, 46: 4097–99.

59. Denis PA, Iribarne F. [2+2] Cycloadditions onto graphene. *J Mater Chem* 2012, 22: 5470–77.
60. Sarkar S, Bekyarova E, Niyogi S, Haddon RC. Diels–alder chemistry of graphite and graphene: Graphene as diene and dienophile. *J Am Chem Soc* 2011, 133: 3324–27.
61. Faghani A, Donskyi IS, Gholami MF, Ziem B, Lippitz A, Unger WES, Bçttcher C, Rabe JP, Haag R, Adeli M. Controlled covalent functionalization of thermally reduced graphene oxide to generate defined bifunctional 2D nanomaterials. *Angew Chem Int Ed* 2017, 56: 2675–79.
62. Sulleiro MV, Quiroga S, Pena D, Pérez D, Guitián E, Criado A, Prato M. Microwave-induced covalent functionalization of few-layer graphene with arynes under solvent-free condition. *Chem Commun* 2018, 54: 2086–89.
63. Zhang N, Cong X. Enhanced nonlinear absorption performance of reduced graphene oxide nanohybrid covalently functionalized by porphyrin via 1,3-dipolar cycloaddition. *Mater Sci Appl* 2018, 9: 972–84.
64. Tang XZ, Li W, Yu ZZ, Rafiee MM, Rafiee J, Yavari F, Koratkar N. Enhanced thermal stability in graphene oxide covalently functionalized with 2-amino-4,6-didodecylamino-1,3,5–triazine. *Carbon* 2011, 49: 1258–65.
65. Emadi F, Amini A, Gholami A, Ghasemi Y. Functionalized graphene oxide with chitosan for protein nanocarriers to protect against enzymatic cleavage and retain collagenase activity. *Sci Rep* 2017, 7: 42258–13.
66. Fonseca LC, de Araujo MM, de Moraes ACM, da Silva DS, Ferreira AG, Franqui LS, Martinez DST, Alves OL. Nanocomposites based on graphene oxide and mesoporous silica nanoparticles: Preparation, characterization and nanobiointeractions with red blood cells and human plasma proteins. *Appl Surf Sci* 2018, 437: 110–21.
67. Yu D, Yang Y, Durstock M, Baekand JB, Dai L. Nitrogen doped holey graphene as an efficient metal-free multifunctional electrochemical catalyst for hydrazineoxidation and oxygen reduction. *ACS Nano* 2010, 4: 5633–40.
68. Singh M, Sahu A, Mahata S, Singh PK, Rai VK, Rai A. Efficient electrochemical determination of p-aminophenol using a novel tricomponent graphene-based nanocomposite. *New J Chem* 2019, 43: 14972.
69. Singh M, Kashyap H, Singh PK, Mahata S, Rai VK, Rai A. AuNPs/Neutral red-biofunctionalized graphene nanocomposite for nonenzymatic electrochemical detection of organophosphate via NO_2 reduction. *Sens Actuators B Chem* 2019, 290: 195–202.
70. Tian X, Tan Z, Zhang Z, Zhan T, Liu X. An electrochemical sensor based on an ionic liquid covalently functionalized graphene oxide for simultaneous determination of copper [II] and antimony [III]. *Chem Select* 2018, 3: 8252–58.
71. Luo S, Wu Y, Mou Q, Li J, Luo X. A thio-β-cyclodextrin functionalized graphene/gold nanoparticle electrochemical sensor: A study of the size effect of the gold nanoparticles and the determination of tetrabromobisphenol A. *RSC Adv* 2019, 9: 17897–17904.
72. Li M, Li Z, Liu C, Chang Y, Wen J, Zhao H, et al. Amino-modification and successive electrochemical reduction of graphene oxide for highly sensitive electrochemical detection of trace Pb^{2+}. *Carbon* 2016, 109: 479–86.
73. Singh M, Sahu A, Singh PK, Verma F, Rai A, Rai VK. A novel ternary graphene-based nanocomposite modified electrode for acetaminophen detection. *Electroanal* 2020, 32: 1516–23.
74. Palakollu VN, Chiwunze TE, Gill AAS, Thapliyal N, Maru SM, Karpoormath R. Electrochemical sensitive determination of acetaminophen in pharmaceutical formulations at iron oxide/graphene composite modified electrode. *J Molecular Liq* 2017 248: 953–62.

75. Rooyanian S, Bagherzadeh M, Akrami Z, Golikand AN. A simple route to surface functionalization of graphene nanosheets by benzoic acid and its application toward Pb[II] sensing. *New J Chem* 2018, 42: 17371–78.
76. Bhardiya SR, Asati A, Sheshma H, Rai A, Rai VK. A novel bioconjugated reduced graphene oxide-based nanocomposite for sensitive electrochemical detection of cadmium in water. *Sens Actuators B Chem* 2021, 328: 129019.
77. Mei KC, Rubio N, Costa PM, Kafa H, Abbate V, Festy F, Bansal SS, Hider RC, Al-Jamal KT. Synthesis of double-clickable functionalised graphene oxide for biological applications. *Chem Commun* 2015, 51: 14981–84.
78. Yang H, Shan C, Li F, Han D, Zhang Q, Niu L. Covalent functionalization of polydisperse chemically-converted graphene sheets with amine-terminated ionic liquid. *Chem Commun* 2009, 2009: 3880–82.
79. Zou HL, Li BL, Luo HQ, Li NB. A novel electrochemical biosensor based on hemin functionalized graphene oxide sheets for simultaneous determination of ascorbic acid, dopamine and uric acid. *Sens Actuat B*. 2015, 207: 535–41.
80. Kuila T, Bose S, Mishra AK, Khanra P, Kim NH, Lee JH. Chemical functionalization of graphene and its applications. *Prog Mater Sci* 2012, 57: 1061–105.
81. Zhang Y, Xiao J, Lv QY, Wang L, Dong X, Asif M, Ren J, He W, Sun Y, Xiao F, Wang S. In situ electrochemical sensing and real-time monitoring live cells based on freestanding nanohybrid paper electrode assembled from 3D functionalized graphene framework. *ACS Appl Mater Interfaces* 2017, 9: 38201–210.
82. Sahu A, Shukla P, Mahata S, Rai VK, Rai A, Singh M. First bio-covalent functionalization of graphene with threonine towards drug sensing via electrocatalytic transfer hydrogenation. *Sens Actuators B Chem* 2019, 281: 1045–53.
83. Xu H, Liao C, Liu Y, Ye BC, Liu B. Iron phthalocyanine decorated nitrogen-doped graphene biosensing platform for real-time detection of nitric oxide released from living cells. *Anal Chem* 2018, 90: 4438–44.
84. Li D, Zhang W, Yu X, Wang Z, Suand G, Wei G. When biomolecules meet graphene: From molecular level interactions to material design and applications. *Nanoscale* 2016, 8: 19491–509.
85. Ciesielski A, Samori P. Supramolecular approaches to graphene: From self-assembly to molecule-assisted liquid-phase exfoliation. *Adv Mater* 2016, 28: 6030–51.
86. Singh NJ, Lee HM, Suh SB, Kim KS. De novo design approach based on nanorecognition toward development of functional molecules/materials and nanosensors/nanodevices. *Pure Appl Chem* 2007, 79: 1057.
87. Gray D, McCaughan A, Mookerji B. Crystal structure of graphite, graphene and silicon. *Phys Solid State Appl* 2009, 6: 1–3.
88. Zhang XF, Liu SP, Shao XN. Silver nanoparticles: Synthesis, characterization, properties, applications, and therapeutic approaches. *Spectrochim Acta Part A* 2013, 113: 92–9.
89. Upadhyay RK, Soin N, Roy SS. Role of graphene/metal oxide composites as photocatalysts, adsorbents and disinfectants in water treatment: A review. *RSC Adv* 2014, 4: 3823–51.
90. Qiao W, Wang L, Ye B, Li G, Li J. Electrochemical behavior of palmatine and its sensitive determination based on an electrochemically reduced L-methionine functionalized graphene oxide modified electrode. *Analyst* 2015, 140: 7974–83.
91. Reza KK, Ali MA, Srivastava S, Agrawal VV, Biradar AM. Tyrosinase conjugated reduced graphene oxide based biointerface for bisphenol A. *Biosens Bioelectron* 2015, 74: 644–51.

92. Li J, Wang Y, Sun Y, Ding C, Lin Y, Sun W, Luo C. A novel ionic liquid functionalized graphene oxide supported gold nanoparticle composite film for sensitive electrochemical detection of dopamine. *RSC Adv* 2017, 7: 2315–22.
93. Kokulnathan T, Sakthinathan S, Chen SM, Karthik R, Chiu TW. Hexammine cobalt[III] coordination complex grafted reduced graphene oxide composite for sensitive and selective electrochemical determination of morin in fruit samples. *Inorg Chem Front* 2018, 5: 1145–55.
94. Azadbakht A, Abbasi AR, Derikvand Z, Karimi Z. Fabrication of an ultrasensitive impedimetric electrochemical sensor based on graphene nanosheet/polyethyleneimine/gold nanoparticle composite. *J Electroanal Chem* 2015, 757: 277–87.
95. Liu H, Li S, Sun D, Chen Y, Zhou Y, Lu T. Layered graphene nanostructures functionalized with NH_2-rich polyelectrolytes through self-assembly: Construction and their application in trace Cu[II] detection. *J Mater Chem B* 2014, 2: 2212–19.
96. Kang M, Peng D, Zhang Y, Yang Y, He L, Yan F, Sun S, Fang S, Wang P, Zhang Z. An electrochemical sensor based on rhodamine B hydrazide-immobilized graphene oxide for highly sensitive and selective detection of Cu[II]. *New J Chem* 2015, 39: 3137–44.
97. Xie T, Zhang M, Chen P, Zhao H, Yang X, Yao L, Zhang H, Dong A, Wang J, Wang Z. A facile molecularly imprinted electrochemical sensor based on graphene: Application to the selective determination of thiamethoxam in grain. *RSC Adv* 2017, 7: 38884–94.
98. Tefera M, Tessema M, Admassie S, Iwuoha EI, Waryo TT, Baker PG. Electrochemical determination of phenothrin in fruit juices at graphene oxide-polypyrrole modified glassy carbon electrode. *Sens Bio-Sens Res* 2018, 21: 27–34.
99. Hua Z, Qin Q, Bai X, Huang X, Zhang Q. An electrochemical biosensing platform based on 1-formylpyrene functionalized reduced graphene oxide for sensitive determination of phenol. *RSC Adv* 2016, 6: 25427–34.
100. Zhang P, Wang Y, Zhang D, Liu C, Wang D, He S, Hu G, Tang X. Calixarene-functionalized graphene oxide composites fixed on glassy carbon electrodes for electrochemical detection. *RSC Adv* 2016, 6: 91910–20.
101. Seenivasan R, Chang WJ, Gunasekaran S. Highly sensitive detection and removal of lead ions in water using cysteine-functionalized graphene oxide/polypyrrole nanocomposite film electrode. *ACS Appl Mater Interfaces* 2015, 7: 15935–43.
102. Huang J, Wang L, Shi C, Dai Y, Gu C, Liu J. Selective detection of picric acid using functionalized reduced graphene oxide sensor device. *Sens Actuat B* 2014, 196: 567–73.
103. Liu Y, Liang Y, Yang R, Li J, Qu L. A highly sensitive and selective electrochemical sensor based on polydopamine functionalized graphene and molecularly imprinted polymer for the 2, 4-dichlorophenol recognition and detection. *Talanta* 2019, 195: 691–98.
104. Crescenzo AD, Profio PD, Siani G, Zappacosta R, Fontana A. Optimizing the interactions of surfactants with graphitic surfaces and clathrate hydrates. *Langmuir* 2016, 32: 6559–70.
105. Dong D, Vatamanu JP, Wei X, Bedrov D. The 1-ethyl-3-methylimidazolium bis[trifluoro-methylsulfonyl]-imide ionic liquid nanodroplets on solid surfaces and in electric field: A molecular dynamics simulation study. *J Chem Phys* 2018, 148: 193833–9.
106. SimsiSkova M, Sikola T. Interaction of graphene oxide with proteins and applications of their conjugates. *J Nanomed Res* 2017, 5: 00109.

107. Xiao M, Li N, Ma Z, Song H, Lu K, Li A, Meng Y, Wang D, Yan X. The effect of doping graphene oxide on the structure and property of polyimide-based graphite fibre. *RSC Adv* 2017, 7: 56602–10.
108. Zhao B, Liu PW, Liu DY, Kolibaba TJ, Zhang CY, Liu YT, Liu YQ. Functionalized graphene oxide based on hydrogen-bonding interaction in water: Preparation and flame-retardation on epoxy resin. *Macromol Mater Eng* 2019, 304: 1900164.
109. Jin T, Easton CD, Yin H, de Vries N, Hao X. Triethylenetetramine/hydroxyethyl cellulosefunctionalized graphene oxide monoliths for the removal of copper and arsenate ions. *Sci Technol Adv Mater* 2018, 19: 381–95.
110. Piao Y, Chen B. One-pot synthesis and characterization of reduced graphene oxide-gelatin nanocomposite hydrogels. *RSC Adv* 2016, 6: 6171–81.
111. Perreault F, de Faria AF, Elimelech M. Environmental applications of graphene-based nanomaterials. *Chem Soc Rev* 2015, 44: 5861–96.
112. Liu M, Wang L, Meng Y, Chen Q, Li H, Zhang Y, Yao S. [4-Ferrocenylethyne] phenylamine functionalized graphene oxide modified electrode for sensitive nitrite sensing. *Electrochim Acta* 2014, 116: 504–11.
113. Yokus OA, Kardas F, Akyıldırım O, Eren T, Atar N, Yola ML. Efficient removal and trace determination of chlorophenols from water by mixed hemi/ad-micelle ionic liquid-coated magnetic graphene oxide and adsorption mechanism. *Sens Actuat B* 2016, 233: 47–54.
114. Rahman MT, Kabir MF, Gurung A, Reza KM, Pathak R, Ghimire N, Baride A, Wang Z, Kumar M, Qiao Q. Graphene oxide-silver nanowire nanocomposites for enhanced sensing of Hg^{2+}. *ACS Appl Nano Mater* 2019, 2: 4842–51.
115. Zheng Q, Wu H, Shen Z, Gao W, Yu Y, Ma Y, Guang W, Guo Q, Yan R, Wang J, Ding K. An electrochemical DNA sensor based on polyaniline/graphene: High sensitivity to DNA sequences in a wide range. *Analyst* 2015, 140: 6660–70.
116. Rabti A, Martinez CCM, Pires LB, Raouafi N, Merkoçi A. Ferrocene-functionalized graphene electrode for biosensing applications. *Anal Chim Acta* 2016, 926: 28–35.
117. Wu H, Li X, Chen M, Wang C, Wei T, Zhang H, Fan S. A nanohybrid based on porphyrin dye functionalized graphene oxide for the application in non-enzymatic electrochemical sensor. *Electrochim Acta* 2018, 259: 355–64.
118. Luo J, Chen Y, Ma Q, Liu R, Liu X. Layer-by-layer assembled ionic-liquid functionalized graphene-polyaniline nanocomposite with enhanced electrochemical sensing properties. *J Mater Chem C* 2014, 2: 4818–27.
119. Sakthinathan S, Lee HF, Chen SM, Tamizhdurai P. Reduced graphene oxidegold tetraphenyl. *J Colloid and Interface Sci* 2016, 468: 120–27.
120. Guo Z, Huang G, Li J, Wang Z, Xu X. Gold nanoparticle and poly arginine modified GCE for simultaneous determination of hydroquinone and catechol. *J Electroanal Chem* 2015, 759: 113–21.
121. Kumar DR, Kesavan S, Baynosa ML, Shim JJ. 3,5-Diamino-1,2,4-triazole@electrochemically reduced graphene oxide film modified electrode for the electrochemical determination of 4-nitrophenol. *Electrochim Acta* 2017, 246: 1131–40.
122. Suhag D, Sharma AK, Patni P, Garg SK, Rajput SK, Chakrabarti S, Mukherjee M. Hydrothermally functionalized biocompatible nitrogen doped graphene nanosheet based biomimetic platforms for nitric oxide detection. *J Mater Chem B* 2016, 4: 4780–89.
123. Singh M, Sahu A, Mahata S, Shukla P, Rai A, Rai VK. Efficient electrocatalytic oxidation of *p*-phenylenediamine using a novel PANI/ZnO anchored bio-reduced graphene oxide nanocomposite. *New J Chem* 2019, 43: 6500.

124. Hu C, Song L, Zhang Z, Chen N, Feng Z, Qu L. Tailored graphene systems for unconventional applications in energy conversion and storage devices. *Energy Environ Sci* 2015, 8: 31–54.
125. Adil SF, Khan M, Kalpana D. *Multifunctional Photocatalytic Materials for Energy*, Woodhead Publishing in Materials. 2018, pp 127–52. doi: 10.1016/C2016-0-01653-4.
126. Lin YK, Hong YT, Shyue JJ, Hsueh CH. Construction of Schottky junction solar cell using silicon nanowires and multi-layered graphene. *Superlattices Microstruct* 2019, 126: 42–8.
127. Han TH, Kim H, Kwon SJ, Lee TW. Graphene-based flexible electronic devices. *Mater Sci Eng R* 2017, 118: 1–43.
128. Yadav SK, Chandra P, Goyal RN, Shim YB. A review on determination of steroids in biological samples exploiting nanobio-electroanalytical methods. *Anal Chimic Acta* 2013, 762: 14–24.
129. Gan T, Hu S. Electrochemical sensors based on graphene materials. *Microchim Acta* 2011, 175: 1–19.
130. Devi PN, Sathiyabama J, Rajendran S, Rathish RJ, Prabha SS. Influence of malic acid-Zn2+ system on inhibition of corrosion of mild steel insimulated concrete pore solution prepared in well water *J Chem Pharm Res* 2015, 7: 133–40.
131. Sinha DA, Lu X, Wu L, Tan D, Li Y, Chen J, Jain R. Voltammetric sensing of biomolecules at carbon based electrode interfaces: A review. *Trends Anal Chem* 2018, 98: 174–89.
132. Lu Y, Liang X, Niyungeko C, Zhou J, Xu J, Tian G. A review of the identification and detection of heavy metal ions in the environment by voltammetry. *Talanta* 2018, 178: 324–38.
133. Slepchenko GB, Gindullina TM, Deryabina VI, Akeneev YA, Otmakhov VI. Voltammetric determination of organic ecotoxicants on modified electrodes. *Procedia Chem* 2015, 15: 350–54.
134. Muralikrishna S, Sureshkumar K, Thomas SV, Nagaraju DH, Ramakrishnappa T. *In situ* reduction and functionalization of graphene oxide with l-cysteine for simultaneous electrochemical determination of cadmium(II), lead(II), copper(II), and mercury(II) ions. *Anal Methods* 2014, 6: 8698–705.
135. Manna B. Rational functionalization of reduced graphene oxide with an imidazole group for the electrochemical sensing of bisphenol A-an endocrine disruptor. *Analyst* 2018, 143: 3451–57.
136. Dave S, Kirubavathy SJ. Biosensors based on metal-organic framework (MOF): Paving the way to point-of-care diagnosis. In *Electrochemical Applications of Metal-Organic Frameworks*. 2022 (pp. 255–267). Elsevier.
137. Xiao F, Guo M, Wang J, Yan X, Li H, Qian C, Yu Y, Dai D. Ferrocene-terminated dendrimer functionalized graphene oxide layered sensor toward highly sensitive evaluation of Di [2-ethylhexyl] phthalate in liquor samples. *Anal Chimic Acta* 2018, 1043: 35–44.
138. Palakollu VN, Chiwunze TE, Gill AAS, Thapliyal N, Maru SM, Karpoormath R. Electrochemical sensitive determination of isoprenaline at β-cyclodextrin functionalized graphene oxide and electrochemically generated acid yellow 9 polymer modified electrode. *J Molecular Liq* 2017, 248: 953–62.
139. Hou X, Liu X, Li Z, Zhang J, Du G, Ran X, Yang L. Electrochemical determination of methyl parathion based on pillar [5] arene@ AuNPs@ reduced graphene oxide hybrid nanomaterials. *New J Chem* 2019, 43: 13048–57.
140. Baruah U, Chowdhury D. Functionalized graphene oxide as an electrochemical sensing platform for detection of Bisphenol A. *Adv Mater Lett* 2018, 9: 516–25.

141. Dave S, Das J. Technological model on advanced stages of oxidation of wastewater effluent from food industry. In *Advanced Oxidation Processes for Effluent Treatment Plants*. 2021 (pp. 33–49). Elsevier.
142. Liu W, Zhang J, Li C, Tang L, Zhang Z, Yang M. A novel composite film derived from cysteic acid and PDDA-functionalized graphene: Enhanced sensing material for electrochemical determination of metronidazole. *Talanta* 2013, 104: 204–11.
143. Dave S. Electrochemical and spectral characterization of silver nanoparticles synthesized employing root extract of Curculigo orchioides. *Indian J Chem Technol (IJCT)* 2018, 25(2): 201–207.
144. Shahrezaieab ES, Ejhieh AN. A zeolite modified carbon paste electrode based on copper exchanged clinoptilolite nanoparticles for voltammetric determination of metronidazole. *RSC Adv* 2017, 7: 14247–53.
145. Gu Y, Yan X, Liu W, Li C, Chen R, Tang L, Zhang Z, Yang M. Biomimetic sensor based on copper-poly [cysteine] film for the determination of metronidazole. *Electrochim Acta* 2015, 152: 108–16.
146. Chen D, Deng J, Liang J, Xie J, Hu C, Huang K. A core-shell molecularly imprinted polymer grafted onto a magnetic glassy carbon electrode as a selective sensor for the determination of metronidazole. *Sens Actuat B* 2013, 183: 594–600.
147. Mollamahale YB, Ghorbani M, Ghalkhani M, Vossoughi M, Dolati A. Highly sensitive 3D gold nanotube ensembles: Application to electrochemical determination of metronidazole. *Electrochim Acta* 2013, 106: 288–92.
148. Gu Y, Liu W, Chen R, Zhang L, Zhang Z. β-cyclodextrin-functionalized gold nanoparticles/Poly[L-cysteine] modified glassy carbon electrode for sensitive determination of metronidazole. *Electroanalysis* 2013, 25: 1209–16.
149. Yang M, Guo M, Feng Y, Lei Y, Cao Y, Zhu D, Yu Y, Ding, L. Sensitive voltammetric detection of metronidazole based on three-dimensional graphene-like carbon architecture/polythionine modified glassy carbon electrode. *J Electrochem Soc* 2018, 165: B530–5.
150. Nikodimos Y, Amare M. Electrochemical determination of metronidazole in tablet samples using carbon paste electrode. *J Anal Methods Chem* 2016, Article ID 3612943. doi: 10.1155/2016/3612943.
151. Saglikogluand G, Yilmaz S. Voltammetric sensitive determination of metronidazole at poly[p-aminobenzene sulfonic acid]-modified glassy carbon electrode. *Russian J Electrochem* 2015, 51: 862–6.
152. Tursynbolat S, Bakytkarim Y, Huang J, Wang L. Ultrasensitive electrochemical determination of metronidazole based on polydopamine/carboxylic multi-walled carbon nanotubes nanocomposites modified GCE. *J Pharmaceut Anal* 2018, 8: 124–30.
153. Sakthivel M, Sukanya R, Chen SM, Dinesh B. Synthesis of two-dimensional Sr-doped $MoSe_2$ nanosheets and their application for efficient electrochemical reduction of metronidazole. *J Phys Chem C* 2018, 122: 12474–84.
154. Mao A, Li H, Yu L, Hu X. Electrochemical sensor based on multi-walled carbon nanotubes and chitosan-nickel complex for sensitive determination of metronidazole. *J Electroanal Chem* 2017, 799: 257–62.
155. Sehatnia B, Sabzi RE, Kheiri F, Nikoo A. Sensitive determination of metronidazole based on Graphene-TiO_2 modified glassy carbon electrode in human serum and urine samples. *Euro J Chem* 2015, 6: 31–6.
156. Meenakshi S, Pandian K, Jayakumari LS, Inbasekaran S. Enhanced amperometric detection of metronidazole in drug formulations and urine samples based on chitosan protected tetrasulfonated copper phthalocyanine thin-film modified glassy carbon electrode. *Mater Sci Eng C* 2016, 59: 136–44.

157. Zhu M, Ye H, Lai M, Ye J, Kuang J, Chen Y, Wang J, Mei Q. Differential pulse stripping voltammetric determination of metronidazole with graphene-sodium dodecyl sulfate modified carbon paste electrode. *Int J Electrochem Sci* 2018. 13: 4100–14.
158. Yalikun N, Mamat X, Li Y, Hu X, Wang P, Hu G. N, S, P-triple doped porous carbon as an improved electrochemical sensor for metronidazole determination. *J Electrochem Soc* 2019. 166:B1131–7.
159. Hudari FF, Almeida LC, Silva BF, Zanoni MVB. Voltammetric sensor for simultaneous determination of *p*-phenylenediamine and resorcinol in permanent hair dyeing and tap water by composite carbon nanotubes/chitosan modified electrode. *Microchem J* 2014. 116: 261–8.
160. Keeley GP, O'Neill A, McEvoy N, Peltekis N, Coleman JN, Duesberg GS. Electrochemical ascorbic acid sensor based on DMF-exfoliated graphene. *J Mater Chem* 2010, 20: 7864–9.
161. Tığ GA. Development of electrochemical sensor for detection of ascorbic acid, dopamine, uric acid and L-tryptophan based on Ag nanoparticles and poly[L-arginine]-graphene oxide composite. *J Electroanal Chem* 2017, 807: 19–28.
162. Tian L, Zhang B, Sun D, Chen R, Wang B, Li T. A thin poly [acridine orange] film containing reduced graphene oxide for voltammetric simultaneous sensing of ascorbic acid and uric acid. *Microchim Acta* 2014, 181: 589–95.
163. Zhao L, Li H, Gao S, Li M, Xu S, Li C, Yang B. MgO nanobelt-modified graphene-tantalum wire electrode for the simultaneous determination of ascorbic acid, dopamine and uric acid. *Electrochim Acta* 2015, 168: 191–8.
164. O'Connell PJ, Gormally C, Pravda M. Guilbault GG. Development of an amperometric L-ascorbic acid [Vitamin C] sensor based on electropolymerised aniline for pharmaceutical and food analysis. *Anal Chim Acta* 2001, 431: 239–47.
165. Hosseini M, Momeni MM, Faraji M. Electrochemical fabrication of polyaniline films containing gold nanoparticles deposited on titanium electrode for electro-oxidation of ascorbic acid. *J Mater Sci* 2010, 45: 2365–71.
166. Pei L, Cai Z, Xie Y, Pei Y, Fan C, Fu D. Electrochemical behaviors of ascorbic acid at $CuGeO_3$/polyaniline nanowire modified glassy carbon electrode. *J Electrochem Soc* 2012, 159: 107–11.
167. Zhang X, Lai G, Yu A, Zhang H. A glassy carbon electrode modified with a polyaniline doped with silicotungstic acid and carbon nanotubes for the sensitive amperometric determination of ascorbic acid. *Microchim Acta* 2013, 180: 437–43.
168. Liu Y, Su Z, Zhang Y, Chen L, Gu T, Huang S, Liu Y, Sun L, Xie Q, Yao S. Amperometric determination of ascorbic acid using multiwalled carbon nanotube-thiolated polyaniline composite modified glassy carbon electrode. *J Electroanal Chem* 2013, 709: 19–25.
169. Zhang H, Huang F, Xu S, Xia Y, Huang W, Li Z. Fabrication of nanoflower-like dendritic Au and polyaniline composite nanosheets at gas/liquid interface for electrocatalytic oxidation and sensing of ascorbic acid. *Electrochem Commun* 2013, 30: 46–50.
170. Moharana M, Pattanayak SK, Khan F, Dave S. Biosensors for Infectious Diseases-Fundamentals. In Sushma Dave and Jayashankar Das (eds.) *Point-of-Care Biosensors for Infectious Diseases* 2023, pp.1–14. Wiley.
171. Shao L, Wang X, Yang B, Wang Q, Tian Q, Ji Z, Zhang J. A highly sensitive ascorbic acid sensor based on hierarchical polyaniline coated halloysite nanotubes prepared by electrophoretic deposition. *Electrochim Acta* 2017, 255: 286–97.
172. Pakapongpan S, Mensing JP, Phokharatkul D, Lomas T, Tuantranont A. Highly selective electrochemical sensor for ascorbic acid based on a novel hybrid graphene-copper phthalocyanine-polyaniline nanocomposites. *Electrochim Acta* 2014, 133: 294–301.

173. Li Y, Ma Y, Liu Y, Xin G, Wang M, Zhang, Z, Liu Z. Electrochemical sensor based on a three dimensional nanostructured MoS_2 nanosphere-PANI/reduced graphene oxide composite for simultaneous detection of ascorbic acid, dopamine, and uric acid. *RSC Adv* 2019, 9: 2997–3003.
174. Salahandish R, Ghaffarinejad A, Naghib SM, Niyazi A, Majidzadeh AK, Janmaleki M, Nezhad AS. Sandwich-structured nanoparticles-grafted functionalized graphene based 3D nanocomposites for high-performance biosensors to detect ascorbic acid biomolecule. *Sci Rep* 2019, 9: 1226.
175. Wu GH, Wu YF, Liu XW, Rong MC, Chen XM, Chen X. An electrochemical ascorbic acid sensor based on palladium nanoparticles supported on graphene oxide. *Anal Chim Acta* 2012, 745: 33–7.
176. Daniel MC, Astruc, D. Gold nanoparticles: Assembly, supramolecular chemistry, quantum-size-related properties, and applications toward biology, catalysis, and nanotechnology. *Chem Rev* 2004, 104: 293–346.
177. Liu Z, Wang X, Sun L, Yu Z. Using AuCo alloy nanoparticles/HS-graphene modified electrode for the selective determination of dopamine, ascorbic acid and uric acid. *Anal Methods* 2014, 6: 9059–65.
178. Song J, Xu L, Xing R, Li Q, Zhou C, Liu D, Song H. Synthesis of Au/graphene oxide composites for selective and sensitive electrochemical detection of ascorbic acid. *Sci Rep* 2014, 4: 7515.
179. Jiang J, Du X. Sensitive electrochemical sensors for simultaneous determination of ascorbic acid, dopamine, and uric acid based on Au@Pd-reduced graphene oxide nanocomposites. *Nanoscale* 2014, 6: 11303–9.
180. Venkadesh A, Mathiyarasu J, Dave S, Radhakrishnan S. Amine mediated synthesis of nickel oxide nanoparticles and their superior electrochemical sensing performance for glucose detection. *Inorg Chem Commun* 2021, 131: 108779.
181. Llobregat AA, Vidal L, Amaro RR, Murcia AB, Canals A, Morallón E. Au-IDA microelectrodes modified with Au-doped graphene oxide for the simultaneous determination of uric acid and ascorbic acid in urine samples. *Electrochim Acta* 2017, 227: 275–84.
182. Niethammer P, Clemensr G, Thomas LA, Timothy JM, Look TA, Mitchison JT. A tissue-scale gradient of hydrogen peroxide mediates rapid wound detection in zebrafish. *Nature* 2009, 459: 996–99.
183. Kumar S, Bhushan P, Bhattacharya S. Facile synthesis of Au@Ag-hemin decorated reduced graphene oxide sheets: A novel peroxidase mimetic for ultrasensitive colorimetric detection of hydrogen peroxide and glucose. *RSC Adv* 2017, 7: 37568–77.
184. Mercante LA, Facure MHM, Sanfelice RC, Migliorini FL, Mattoso LHC, Correa DS. One-pot preparation of PEDOT: PSS-reduced graphene decorated with Au nanoparticles for enzymatic electrochemical sensing of H_2O_2. *Appl Surf Sci* 2017, 407: 162–70.
185. Ju J, Chen W. In situ growth of surfactant-free gold nanoparticles on nitrogen-doped graphene quantum dots for electrochemical detection of hydrogen peroxide in biological environments. *Anal Chem* 2015, 87: 1903–10.
186. Yang X, Ouyang Y, Wu F, Hu Y, Ji Y, Wu Z. Size controllable preparation of gold nanoparticles loading on graphene sheets@cerium oxide nanocomposites modified gold electrode for nonenzymatic hydrogen peroxide detection. *Sens Actuators B Chem* 2017, 238: 40–7.
187. Sun L, Ding Y, Jiang Y, Liu Q. Montmorillonite-loaded ceria nanocomposites with superior peroxidase-like activity for rapid colorimetric detection of H_2O_2. *Sens Actuators B Chem* 2017, 239: 848–56.

188. Palanisamy S, Chen SM, Sarawathi R. A novel nonenzymatic hydrogen peroxide sensor based on reduced graphene oxide/ZnO composite modified electrode. *Sens Actuators B Chem* 2012, 166–167: 372–77.
189. Xie L, Xu Y, Cao X. Hydrogen peroxide biosensor based on hemoglobin immobilized at graphene, flower-like zinc oxide, and gold nanoparticles nanocomposite modified glassy carbon electrode. *Colloids Surf B Biointerfaces* 2013, 107: 245–50.
190. Fan Y, Yang X, Yang C, Liu J. Au-TiO_2/graphene nanocomposite film for electrochemical sensing of hydrogen peroxide and NADH. *Electroanalysis* 2012, 24: 1334–39.
191. Lu Y, Zhang S, Lin L, Wang L, Wang C. Synthesis of PtAu bimetallic nanoparticles on graphene-carbon nanotube hybrid nanomaterials for nonenzymatic hydrogen peroxide sensor. *Talanta* 2013, 112: 111–16.
192. Liu M, Liu R, Chen W. Graphene wrapped Cu2O nanocubes: Non-enzymatic electrochemical sensors for the detection of glucose and hydrogen peroxide with enhanced stability *Biosens Bioelectron* 2013, 45: 206–12.
193. Liu S, Wang L, Tian J, Luo Y, Zhang X, Sun X. Aniline as a dispersing and stabilizing agent for reduced graphene oxide and its subsequent decoration with Ag nanoparticles for enzymeless hydrogen peroxide detection. *J Colloid Interface Sci* 2011, 363: 615–19.
194. Golsheikh AM, Huang NM, Lim HN, Zakaria R, Yin CY. One-step electrodeposition synthesis of silver-nanoparticle-decorated graphene on indium-tin-oxide for enzymeless hydrogen peroxide detection. *Carbon* 2013, 62: 405–12.
195. Li SJ, Zhang JC, Li J, Yang H, Meng JJ, Zhang B. A 3D sandwich structured hybrid of gold nanoparticles decorated MnO_2/graphene-carbon nanotubes as high performance H_2O_2 sensors. *Sens Actuators B Chem* 2018, 260: 1–11.
196. Chen J, Gao Z, Yang R, Jiang H, Bai L, Shao A, Wu H. New methylene blue covalently functionalized graphene oxide nanocomposite as interfacial material for the electroanalysis of hydrogen peroxide. *Front Chem* 2021, 9: 788804.
197. Musameh M, Notivoli MR, Hickey M, Huynh CP, Hawkins SC, Yousef JM, Kyratzis IL. Carbon nanotube-Web modified electrodes for ultrasensitive detection of organophosphate pesticides. *Electrochim Acta* 2013, 101: 209–15.
198. Yang S, Luo S, Liu C, Wei W. Direct synthesis of graphene-chitosan composite and its application as an enzymeless methyl parathion sensor. *Colloids Surf B* 2012, 96: 75–9.
199. Rodrigues G, Miyazaki CM, Rubira RJG, Constantino CJL, Ferreira M. Layer-by-layer films of graphene nanoplatelets and gold nanoparticles for methyl parathion sensing. *ACS Appl Nano Mater* 2019, 2: 1082–91.
200. Xu M, Zhu J, Su H, Dong J, Ai S, Li R. Electrochemical determination of methyl parathion using poly [malachite green]/graphene nanosheets-nafion composite film-modified glassy carbon electrode. *J Appl Electrochem* 2012, 42: 509–16.
201. Balasubramanian P, Balamurugan TST, Chen SM, Chen TW, Sharmila G, Yu MC. One-step green synthesis of colloidal gold nano particles: A potential electrocatalyst towards high sensitive electrochemical detection of methyl parathion in food samples. *J Taiwan Inst Chem Eng* 2018, 87: 83–90.
202. Li Y, Xu M, Li P, Dong J, Ai S. Nonenzymatic sensing of methyl parathion based on graphene/gadolinium Prussian Blue analogue nanocomposite modified glassy carbon electrode. *Anal Methods* 2014, 6: 2157–62.
203. Fu J, Tan XH, Li YH, Song XJ. A nanosilica/exfoliated graphene composite film-modified electrode for sensitive detection of methyl parathion. *Chinese Chem Lett* 2016, 27: 1541–46.

204. Song B, Cao W, Wang Y. A methyl parathion electrochemical sensor based on Nano-TiO_2, graphene composite film modified electrode. *Fuller Nanotubes Carbon Nanostruct* 2016, 24: 435–40.
205. Li C, Wang Z, Zhan G. Electrochemical investigation of methyl parathion at gold-sodium dodecylbenzene sulfonate nanoparticles modified glassy carbon electrode. *Colloids Surf B Biointerfaces* 2011, 82: 40–5.
206. Xue R, Kang TF, Lu LP, Cheng SY. Electrochemical sensor based on the graphene-nafion matrix for sensitive determination of organophosphorus pesticides. *Anal Lett* 2013, 46: 131–41.
207. Gong J, Miao X, Wan H, Song D. Facile synthesis of zirconia nanoparticles-decorated graphene hybrid nanosheets for an enzymeless methyl parathion sensor. *Sens Actuators B Chem* 2012, 162: 341–47.
208. Govindasamy M, Chen SM, Mani V, Akilarasan M, Kogularasu S, Subramani B. Nanocomposites composed of layered molybdenum disulfide and graphene for highly sensitive amperometric determination of methyl parathion. *Microchim Acta* 2016, 184: 725–33.
209. Zhao L, Zhao F, Zeng B. Electrochemical determination of methyl parathion using a molecularly imprinted polymer-ionic liquid-graphene composite film coated electrode. *Sens Actuators B Chem* 2013, 176: 818–24.
210. Xue X, Wei Q, Wu D, Li H, Zhang Y, Feng R, Du B. Determination of methyl parathion by a molecularly imprinted sensor based on nitrogen doped graphene sheets. *Electrochim Acta* 2014, 116: 366–71.
211. Shi JJ, Wang Y, Meng LR, Zhu JC, Shu RW, He J. Synthesis of rGO/TiO_2/CdS nanocomposites and its enhanced photoelectrochemical performance in determination of parathion-methyl. *Nano* 2018, 13: 1850054.
212. Govindasamy M, Umamaheswari R, Chen SM, Su S. Graphene oxide nanoribbons film modified screen-printed carbon electrode for real-time detection of methyl parathion in food samples. *J Electrochem Soc* 2017, 164: 403–8.
213. Tan X, Liu Y, Zhang T, Luo S, Liu X, Tian H, Chen C. Ultrasensitive electrochemical detection of methyl parathion pesticide based on cationic water-soluble pillar [5] arene and reduced graphene nanocomposite. *RSC Adv* 2019, 9: 345–53.
214. Kaur R, Rana S, Lalit K, Singh P, Kaur K. Electrochemical detection of methyl parathion via a novel biosensor tailored on highly biocompatible electrochemically reduced graphene oxide-chitosan-hemoglobin coatings. *Biosens Bioelectron* 2020, 167: 112486.
215. Shunmugum R, Manavalan S, Chen SM, Keerthi M, Lin LH. Methyl parathion detection using SnS_2/N, S-Co-doped reduced graphene oxide nanocomposite. *ACS Sustain Chem Eng* 2020, 30: 11194–203.
216. Lavanya N, Sudhan N, Kanchana P, Radhakrishnan S, Sekar C. A new strategy for simultaneous determination of 4-aminophenol, uric acid and nitrite based on a graphene/hydroxyapatite composite modified glassy carbon electrode. *RSC Adv* 2015, 5: 52703–709.
217. Gan T, Wang Z, Wang Y, Li X, Sun J, Liu Y. Flexible graphene oxide–wrapped SnO_2 hollow spheres with high electrochemical sensing performance in simultaneous determination of 4–aminophenol and 4–chlorophenol. *Electrochim Acta* 2017, 250: 1–9.
218. Shi P, Xue R, Wei Y, Lei X, Ai J, Wang T, Shi Z, Wang X, Wang Q, Soliman FM, Guo H, Yang W. Gold nanoparticles/tetraaminophenyl porphyrin functionalized multiwalled carbon nanotubes nanocomposites modified glassy carbon electrode for the simultaneous determination of p-acetaminophen and p-aminophenol. *Arabian J Chem* 2020, 13: 1040–51.

219. Yi Y, Zhu G, Wu X, Wang K. Highly sensitive and simultaneous electrochemical determination of 2-aminophenol and 4-aminophenol based on poly[L-arginine]-β-cyclodextrin/carbon nanotubes@graphene nanoribbons modified electrode. *Biosens Bioelectron* 2016, 77: 353–58.
220. Wang H, Zhang S, Li S, Qu J. Electrochemical sensor based on palladium-reduced graphene oxide modified with gold nanoparticles for simultaneous determination of acetaminophen and 4-aminophenol. *Talanta* 2018, 178: 188–94.
221. Kumar SP, Giribabu K, Manigandan R, Munusamy S, Muthamizh S, Padmanaban A, Dhanasekaran T, Suresh R, Narayanan V. Simultaneous determination of paracetamol and 4-aminophenol based on poly[chromium Schiff base complex] modified electrode at nanomolar levels. *Electrochim Acta* 2016, 194: 116–26.
222. Narouie S, Shahbakhsh M, Hashemzaei Z, Nouri A, Saravani H, Noroozifar M. Modified graphite paste electrode with strontium phen-dione complex for simultaneous determination of a ternary mixture of 4-aminophenol, uric acid and Tryptophan [Part I]. *Int J Electrochem Sci* 2017, 12: 10911–32.
223. Ramasubramanian PA, Thangavel S, Nallamuthu G, Kirabakaran K, Vasudevan V, Ravichandran K, Venugopal G. A novel MoS_2 structures for electrochemical detection of 4-aminophenol. *J Mater Sci Mater Electron* 2018, 29: 5696.
224. Liu Y, Yan K, Wang B, Yang C, Zhang J. An electrochemical sensor for selective detection of p-aminophenol using hemin-graphene composites and molecularly imprinted polymer. *J Electrochem Soc* 2017, 164: B776–80.
225. Dave S, Khan AM, Purohit SD, Suthar DL. Application of green synthesized metal nanoparticles in the photocatalytic degradation of dyes and its mathematical modelling using the Caputo–Fabrizio fractional derivative without the singular kernel. *J Math* 2021: 1–8.
226. Cheng TS, Nasir MJM, Ambrosi A, Pumera M. 3D-printed metal electrodes for electrochemical detection of phenols. *Appl Mater Today* 2017, 9: 212–19.
227. Kong FY, Gu SX, Wang JY, Fang HL, Wang W. Facile green synthesis of graphene-titanium nitride hybrid nanostructure for the simultaneous determination of acetaminophen and 4-aminophenol. *Sens Actuators B* 2015, 213: 397–403.
228. Buledi JJA, Solangi AR, Hyder A, Batool M, Mahar N, Mallah A, Maleh HK, Karaman O, Karaman C, Ghalkhani M. Fabrication of sensor based on polyvinyl alcohol functionalized tungsten oxide/reduced graphene oxide nanocomposite for electrochemical monitoring of 4-aminophenol. *Environ Res* 2022, 212: 113372.
229. Manna B, Rational functionalization of reduced graphene oxide with an imidazole group for the electrochemical sensing of bisphenol A-an endocrine disruptor. *Analyst* 2018, 143: 3451–57.
230. Dave S, Sahu R, Tripathy BC, *Electrochemical Applications of Metal-Organic Frameworks: Advances and Future Potential*. Elsevier, 2022.

5 DNA Nanotechnology for Point of Care Diagnosis

Dipak Maity, Urvashi Gupta, and Ganeshlenin Kandasamy

5.1 INTRODUCTION

Medical diagnostics are critical for the discovery, monitoring, and treatment of many illnesses; hence, creating effective diagnostic instruments is very crucial. While clinical lab tests have made significant progress, there is still a need for the development of novel diagnostic methods with high specificity and sensitivity as well as broad application in point of care (POC) conditions. As a result, significant advancements in the health sector and analytical process have focused on producing portable, reusable, and efficient miniature platforms or POC technologies. POC devices are designed with the assumption that all tests may be performed at or close to the point of treating patients. POC testing is a fundamental shift from conventional diagnostic procedures in the lab to near-patient locations, allowing physicians to make more informed decisions about diagnosis and treatment by presenting them with diagnostic data in real time. Recently, DNA nanotechnology has demonstrated considerable promise for developing such POC platforms [1–4].

Numerous benefits of nanoscale size are exploited by the science of nanotechnology, which has found applications in many disciplines such as agriculture, storage devices, and biomedical technologies. Controlling material nanoscale properties can result in novel physicochemical characteristics and behaviours. Nanomaterials may be prepared by top-down methods by using a bulk material and deconstructing it into nanometer scale sizes or by bottom-up methods by using smaller building blocks and arranging them into nanostructures. DNA is one such substance that could be utilised to build nanostructures from the bottom-up approach. Because of the programmability of Watson–Crick base pairing, DNA has become a frequently utilised building component to produce nanoscale addressable materials and dynamic molecular structures with predefined geometries. These biomimetic molecular devices, which come in a variety of sizes and functions, are distinguished by characteristics such as sequence programmability, obvious biocompatibility, chemical addressability and excellent biostability. These nanoplatforms can transport or process information independently and,

DOI: 10.1201/9781003316435-5

when combined with other functional elements, can be used for smart tasks such as sensing, computing, signal amplification, or biological activity modification [5–7].

Because of the inherent characteristics of DNA, such as predictable intermolecular interactions (Watson–Crick base pairing), easily automated chemistry formation, handy modifying enzymes, externally comprehensible code, high functional group density, and prototype for many derivatives, numerous DNA or DNA-based nanostructures, ranging from simple to complex and small to large, have been self-assembled with carefully controlled size and shape in one, two, or three dimensions by a technique known as self-assembly. Furthermore, when specific base pairs are formed, DNA strands hybridise with each other, allowing them to be conveniently designed and built into a functional nanostructure with strongly spatial programmability. Moreover, DNA strands mixed with other nanomaterials, such as nanosheets, polymers, gold nanoparticles (AuNPs), quantum dots, and iron oxides, showed significant promise for early and POC diagnosis [8,9].

In this chapter, we highlight some of the most noteworthy advances in the design and deployment of DNA nanotechnology in recent years for the development of easy point of care diagnostic platforms. First, we give a brief background about structural DNA nanotechnology by discussing three fundamental processes of preparation, i.e., DNA hybridisation, branched-DNA molecules and desired sequence synthesis. Further self-assembly of structural DNA nanotechnology is discussed via a detailed description of rigid motifs, and modular and origami methods. Finally, we give a comprehensive study of various recent DNA nanoplatforms that have shown immense potential for their application in POC diagnosis. For this section, we mainly focus on DNA tetrahedrons, DNA hydrogels and DNA-integrated fluorescent/inorganic nanoparticles (NPs) and 2D nanomaterials. Moreover, we discuss about the principles of various signal amplification strategies and summarise the most recent developed DNA nanoplatforms based on the abovementioned technologies in the form of tables.

5.2 STRUCTURAL DNA NANOTECHNOLOGY (SDNAT)

Structural DNA nanotechnology (SDNAT) mainly deals with the formation of matter via DNA with/having control on spatiotemporal structures in any dimension – e.g., one dimension (1D), two dimensions (2D) and three dimensions (3D). SDNAT is generally shaped via three fundamental processes, namely, (i) DNA hybridisation (DNAH), (ii) branched-DNA molecules (BDNAM), and (iii) desired sequence synthesis (DSS).

DNAH

DNAH is a process that involves the hydrogen bonding of two different but linear double-stranded DNA through their cohesive sticky ends. This is based on the complementing nature of adenine (A)-thymine (T) (with two hydrogen bonds) and guanine (G)-cytosine (C) (with three hydrogen bonds) – which is proposed as a double-helix model by Watson and Crick for DNA formation. This process can be effectively used in the formation of a single or an individual motif.

BDNAM

Both (i) intermediaries occurring during natural DNA metabolism and (ii) Holliday junction with four arms form the basis for the formation of BDNAM. Herein, a single four-arm-based branched-DNA having sticky ends will cohesively bond with the counterparts of three other four-arm-based branched-DNA to form the BDNAM via the complementary mechanism. The formation of the four arms along with the sticky ends involves different mechanisms that include cutting and assembling via respective enzymes – i.e., restriction and ligase. This BDNAM can further join/bond with other four-arm branched-DNA and can form 2D-lattice or 3D structures.

DSS

Usually, in a four-arm-based branched-DNA/Holliday junction (that is available in nature), sequences will be the same in at least two pairs of DNA strands and can display symmetry. This symmetry could lead to instability, if 2D/3D structures are further formed in real time, due to the relocation/migration process within the symmetric structures. Hence, it is essential to lessen the symmetry. This can be done via a combination of different phenomena that include breaking, prevention of flanking branch points, usage of free energy dissimilarities, and/or inhibition of homo-polymer tracts, and this can lead to the DSS.

5.3 SELF-ASSEMBLY OF STRUCTURAL DNA NANOTECHNOLOGY

In nature, DNA self-assembles individually or in combination with other biological structures, for example, to form junctions and chromosomes (as mentioned above), respectively. Scientists have observed this nature and modulated them to form different DNA structures via different methods, which are explained in the following.

5.3.1 Rigid Motifs

In the early 1980s, the presence of SDNAT in nature had been observed in the form of motifs (a design/pattern/shape) – for instance, three-way/Holliday junctions. Then, Seeman et al. developed a novel motif – e.g., a four-way junction (also called a crossover (Xo) junction). Later, Seeman and his group performed many investigations and prepared/formed different rigid SDNAT-based motifs – e.g., reciprocal-/double-/triple-Xo junction, and junction Xo. These motifs are essential in the formation of 1D and 2D structures. For instance, Seeman et al. have used double Xo motifs and formed a 4×4 tile structure, which has been expanded to 2D lattices/tubular structures that have been further extended to 2D arrays having different shapes (triangular/hexagonal). The same authors have furthermore formed 3D-based cubical and octahedron structures. Later in the 1990s, by utilising the above concepts, the making of 3D-based polyhedra structures (i.e., tetra-/octa-/icosa-) have been facilitated [10]. However, these structures have specific disadvantages that include the following: (i) 2D/3D structures can be formed only at lower concentrations and this has resulted in low yield, and (ii) intrinsic difficulties found during the biological molecule conjugation and also cargo loading. Only in the later part of 2000, alternatives, i.e., modular self-assembly and DNA origami, have been developed, which are explained in the following sections.

5.3.2 Modular Method

Gothef et al. have developed molecular modules that can be self-assembled and then covalently bonded to form distinct structures [11] without the need for any supplementary templates. For this, in their work, they have initially formed the linear and tripoidal oligonucleotide-functionalised modules with the salicylaldehyde-based organic backbone, which have helped later in bonding, after the self-assembly, through complementary sequences, to form the complex oligomers. Later, the same authors formed macromolecular nanostructures (i.e., nanoscaffolds) by using the modules via two diverse approaches, i.e., templated multicomponent reactions (TMR) and direct multicomponent couplings (DMC) [12]. Herein, TMR and DMC, respectively, involve peptide nucleic acid (PNA) oligomers formed via a DNA template and self-assembly with the coupling of oligonucleotide-based modules. Similarly, diethylene glycol-possessing γPNA (formed via changes in γ-position of f N-(2-aminoethyl) glycine in PNA) has been utilised by Kumar et al. as a modular self-assembling base substance to form the three-helix nanofibers, where variety and stability are incorporated in these structures by using different organic solvent mixtures and anionic surfactants (e.g., sodium dodecyl sulphate) [13].

Liu et al. have utilised the modular self-assembling approach to form rhombus-like structures (from tile modules), which are further self-assembled and made into different DNA lattice structures [14]. In a recent investigation, Zhang et al. have formed DNA tessellations, especially Archimedean tiling patterns, (4.8.8) and (3.6.3.6), by using multi-arm DNA junctions [15]. Krishnan et al. have formed platonic-solid-based polyhedra – for instance, DNA icosahedra – through a modular self-assembly method [16]. This involves the systematic unification of different modules – i.e., discrete five-way junctions – via bonding of their overhangs/cohesive sticky ends. Herein, it has also been noted that the higher concentrations can be utilised to form DNA icosahedra-based nanocages/nanocapsules with a better yield, as the cooperation is higher between the as-formed pre-folded intermediate modules during the assembly. In this work, the effective loading of gold nanoparticles inside the nanocages/nanocapsules has also been verified through images of a transmission electron microscope (TEM). In a very recent investigation, an icosahedron-based DNA cage has been produced by using the modular method, where two half-icosahedron structures are initially formed (via a unique combination of three five-way junctions), and then they are combined to form a complete icosahedron structure [17]. This structure possessed a large inner cavity (0.829 – which enhanced the caging of gold nanoparticles) as compared to other formed tetrahedron (0.302) and octahedron (0.605) structures.

5.3.3 Origami Method

Origami is a form of Japanese art to create patterns and shapes by folding a flat sheet of paper. Similar to that, in 2006, Paul Rothumend has developed a series of simple to complex structures – including square, rectangle, triangle, star (with five points), disc and smiley shapes with sizes extending to 100 nm – by using a single long DNA strand (acting as a scaffold) along with the help of short oligonucleotide strands (acting as staple strands for holding the scaffold intact) [18]. Herein, basically, the M13 bacteriophage virus–based DNA strand has been utilised as the scaffold, and during the slow annealing process, the staple strands will get fixed at distinct positions to finally form a definite nanostructure. This seminal work on DNA origami, while providing a better yield with the accurate arrangement of complex structures, does not follow the precise stoichiometric ratios between the strands. This makes them advantageous over the other methods and has been the fundamentals for many other single-/multi-layered works on DNA nanotechnology in future. For instance, analogic China's map has been recreated by Lulu et al. in 2006 using DNA origami with the aid of single-strand DNA of 7 kilobase (Kb) [19]. Pound et al. have designed and made thin DNA origami nanostructures possessing shapes like branched "T", "U", "Y", and "B" and their combinations via polymerase chain reactions [20]. In a later investigation, the DNA origami method (via multi-arm junctions) has been involved to create (i) 2D nano-patterns that include star, Penrose tiling, a wavy grid, a sphere array, fishnet and a flower-and-bird, and also (ii) 3D wire-frame structures that include cuboctahedron [21]. In another work, using DNA origami, multi-layered 3D wire-frame structures like a parallelogram (two-layered), triangular cavity (three-layered) and square (nine-layered ($40\times20\,nm^2$)/15-layered ($40\times40\,nm^2$)) are designed and developed by implementing the crossover pairs to link nearby the DNA helices [22].

In a study, Andersen et al. created a 3D hollow nano-box with dimensions of $42\times36\times36\,nm^3$ via the DNA origami method by utilising M13 bacteriophage DNA as a scaffold strand and 220 staple strands [23]. The nano-box has been made to have a lid that can be dynamically opened and closed (verified by fluorescence), and this phenomenon can be useful in employing the nano-box as a drug-loading/releasing container. Kershner et al. have taken a different approach to frame DNA origami–based nanostructures, wherein initially the triangular DNA structures with a size of 127 nm on each side are initially formed in a solution and then deposited/aligned in the templates (formed via electron beam lithography) through binding sites to finally form DNA origami [24]. In a similar study, four rectangular DNA origami templates are made with DNA nano-ribbon on one side, and their other side is used to connect with linkers-attached, DNA-functionalised, single-walled carbon nanotubes (SWCNTs) through a self-assembly process [25]. Steinhauer et al. have formed similar rectangular ($100 \times 70\,nm^2$ sized) DNA origami nanostructures, which are conjugated with ATTO655-based fluorescence molecules to use in calibration of/validating the super-resolution far-field fluorescence microscopy [26]. In another study, the rectangular ($100 \times 70\,nm^2$ sized) DNA origami nanostructures are first formed and then attached with streptavidin molecules at specific positions [27]. Herein, the reaction between the conjugated streptavidin with biotin (via covalent bonding) at a single-molecule level has been effectively identified through atomic force microscopy (AFM), indicating the potential of DNA structures to be exploited as a "breadboard for chemical reactions".

Later, Douglas et al. created an origami multi-layered structure of a honeycomb-pleated based lattice model of DNA by utilising a one-pot reaction with 10 nM of M13 bacteriophage virus–based scaffold strand, 50 nM of short oligonucleotide staple strands, monovalent/divalent cation based salts (NaCl/$MgCl_2$) and buffer [28]. This mixture has been annealed to 60°C from 80°C within 80 minutes, but then slowly cooled to room temperature from 60°C for a period of 173 hours. Besides, in this work, the following 3D shapes are also formed: (i) monolith, (ii) square nut, (iii) railed bridge, (iv) genie bottle, (v) stacked cross and (vi) slotted cross by slightly altering the reaction conditions. The same authors, in another interesting work, have formed multi-layered origami-based 3D DNA nanostructures with twists with angles of 40° and –40° (in 10-by-6 helix DNA bundle made of B-form DNA) and curves of 30° increment – i.e., 0°, 30°, 60°, 90°, 120°, 150°, and 180° (in 3-by-6 helix DNA bundle made of B-form DNA) [29]. This has been achieved by the insertion and/or the deletion of specific base pairs into/from the 3D array of DNA bundles – derived from a honeycomb-pleated lattice model. In an analogous work, Han et al. have developed specific origami-based DNA nanostructures with high curvatures by using similar folding principles [30]. Herein, the crossovers are placed at specific positions of the scaffold (made via parallelly arranging the helical axes of B-form DNA) – i.e., M13 bacteriophage virus–based scaffold with 7 Kb. This includes the 2D concentric rings (with nine layers with each layer having different base pairs (200–600), crossovers (5–10) and radius (10.3–30.9 nm)). Moreover, in and out-of curvatures are also produced by altering the crossover positions to produce 3D nanostructures like 3D spherical shells (24 rings with a final diameter of 42 nm), ellipsoidal shells (29 rings with 9.8 nm of pole diameter and 34.6 nm of equator diameter), and round-bottom nano-flask (35 concentric rings with 13.2 nm of neck diameter, 70 nm of height and 40 nm of widest-point diameter). It can be noted that multi-layered DNA origami is better at making distinct designs and structures with a better rigidity than their single-layered counterparts.

Apart from the above, DNA origami can act as a mould/template to form nanomaterials/nanoparticles. For instance, Sun et al. have created a stiff DNA nano-mould through origami by combining the scaffold with staples, for growing the nanoparticles inside the mould [31]. For this, initially, a stiff DNA barrel with a specific handle (on the inner side) and connectors (on top and bottom) is made. The seed (for growing nanoparticles) with an anti-handle is then attached to the inner handle of the DNA barrel, and then the DNA-based lids having anti-connectors are attached to the connectors of the DNA barrel on top and bottom to close it. Then, the nanoparticles are grown inside the cavity of the DNA barrel. Through this process, gold and silver nanostructures with different shapes like cuboids, triangles, spheres and Y-shape are made by attaching corresponding seeds. In a recent investigation, Ye et al. also formed casting DNA nano-moulds having four distinct mould–mould interfaces (i.e., attractive and repulsive) along with metal seeds to further make the metallic nanostructures [32]. Herein, the nano-moulds are combined together to form different linear/lengthy superstructures – i.e., tri-/tetra-/penta-/octa-/nona-meric superstructures (based on specific interfacing) as shown in Figure 5.1, which have been further employed in the formation of linear metallic (i.e., gold) nanostructures for further use in nano-plasmonics.

In another investigation, conducting gold nanowires (20–30 nm diameter) are grown from their seeds that are placed inside the cavities of the assembled linear superstructures (via complementary sequences), which are primarily formed from two different DNA nano-moulds [33]. In a recent study, gold nanowires/nano-blocks possessing high anisotropic and high aspect ratio (up to 7) are similarly produced from the chain-like superstructures assembled from DNA moulds [34].

DNA origami can also be combined with other nanomaterials/nanoparticles to form hybrid nanostructures. For example, Kuzyk et al. have successfully attached approximately nine gold nanoparticles (with a size of 10 nm) in the form of helices around both right-handed and left-handed DNA origami helix bundles, which have further improved the nano-plasmonic performance in these nanostructures [35]. In another investigation, silica has been formed and combined with (i.e., deposited onto) the DNA scaffolds to finally produce different DNA-based nano-architectures in two (square/triangle/cross/diatom) and three (cube/tetrahedron/hemisphere/toroid/ellipsoid) dimensions at distinct size ranges [36]. In a similar study, the silica shell (with a specific thickness) is made around the DNA origami to improve its structural strength [37]. Herein, initially, the DNA origami (14 helix-bundle) has been made stable in a solution containing $MgCl_2$ and N-trimethoxysilylpropyl-N,N,N-trimethylammonium chloride (TMAPS), and then tetraethoxy orthosilicate (TEOS) has been introduced for further hydrolysis and condensation to coat the silica on DNA, where these molecules are added based on the number of DNA phosphate groups. In a very recent investigation, silica has been grown on two different DNA origami–based nanostructures (24 helix-bundle and 13 helix-ring) through a series of reactions involving (3-aminopropyl)triethoxysilane (APTES)/TMAPS and TEOS [38]. Lately, Meyer et al. have precisely arranged a specific number of the DNA-modified iron oxide nanoparticles onto the surface of the DNA origami rod (made of 16 helix-bundle) as shown in Figure 5.2, and have tuned the magnetic resonance imaging (MRI) contrast [39].

In the further part of this work, we explain the applications in detail based on the above discussions on the SDNAT and their self-assembly.

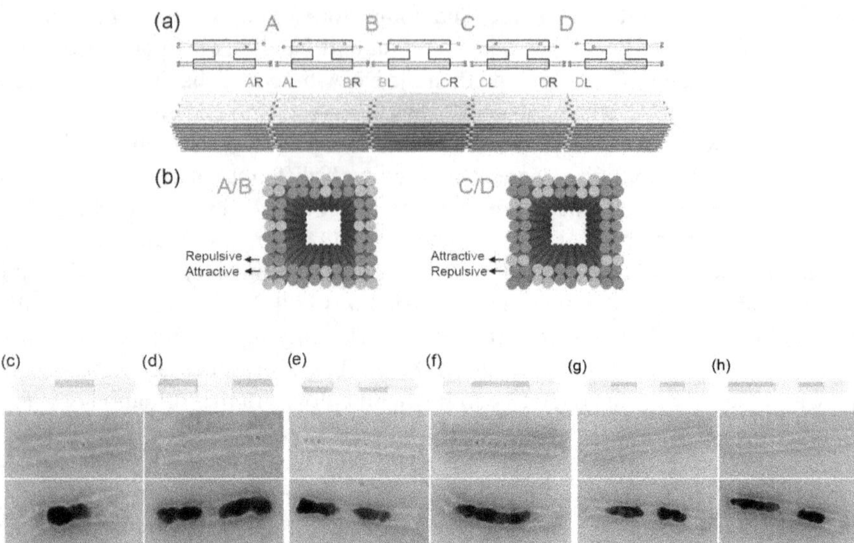

FIGURE 5.1 (a-b) Employing four perpendicular interfaces, a construction approach for DNA mould superstructures is proposed. (a) A hollow pentameric mould superstructure design approach as per the particular interfaces A, B, C, and D (as the 3D model shown at bottom). DNA ends at interfaces are either appealing or repellent. Squares and triangles indicate the 5′ and 3′ staple ends, respectively. Attractive ends have either protruding 5′-staple ends or recessed 3′-staple ends (A and C interfaces) or both protruding 3′-staple ends and recessed 5′-staple ends (B and D interfaces). Both staple ends of both ends have overhangs. A mould R-end of a certain interface must only interact with a mould L-end of the same interface, allowing monomers with varied interface combinations at their L- and R-ends to be built into a specified higher-order structure. (b) View of the interface of mould monomers A or B (left) and C or D (right). Both designs include 24 appealing and 40 repelling helix ends. (c-h) Metal deposition at particular locations inside trimeric, tetrameric, and pentameric mould superstructures. On top of the subfigures, schemes illustrate the desired lengths and locations of selective metal deposition. The acquired patterns of seeds (centre) and metal development within each structure are shown by SEM pictures. Mould trimers with a central or two terminal gold block (a,b). (c,d) Create tetramers with two distinct or two linked core gold blocks. (e,f) Make a pentamer out of two linked or three asymmetrically positioned gold bricks. All SEM pictures have scale bars of 20 nm. Reproduced with permission from Ref. [32].

5.4 DNA NANOTECHNOLOGIES FOR ESTABLISHING DIAGNOSTIC NANOPLATFORMS

As discussed in the previous sections, DNA can be strongly designed to self-assemble diverse nanoplatforms. Furthermore, constructed DNA nanoparticles could be controlled with unique shapes and functionalities at nanoscale spatial precision. Shapes, alignments and distances of DNA nanomaterials, for example, may

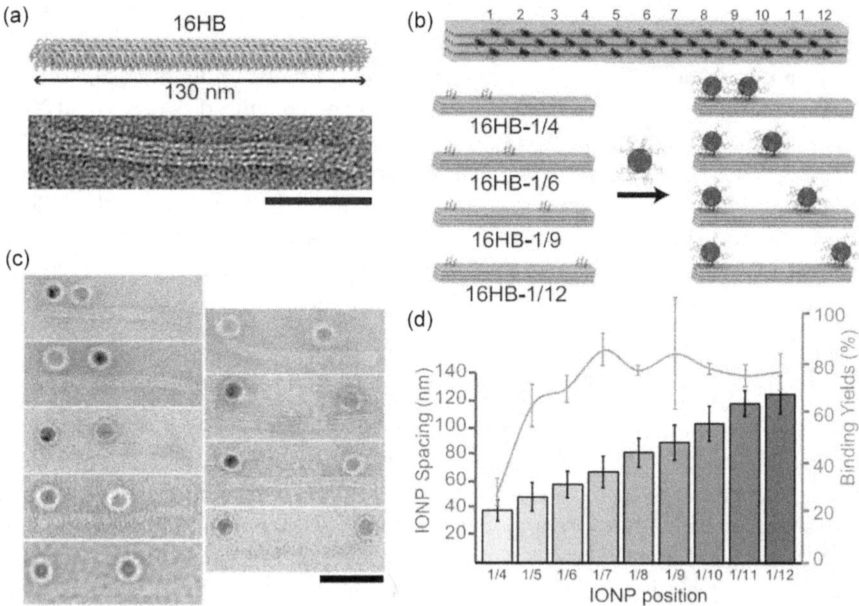

FIGURE 5.2 Schematic of 16 helix-bundle (16HB) DNA origami rod-iron oxide nanoparticles (IONP) linking and monitoring of IONP distancing. (a) 16 16HB scaffold and staple strands (top) model with typical TEM picture (bottom). (b) Schematic of 16HB demonstrating the placement of "capture" DNA extensions to provide 12 binding sites (top). The integration of staple strands with extensions only at particular locations allows for the installation of IONPs at distinct locations along 16HB (bottom). (c) Simulated TEM images of 16HB with two bound IONPs positioned at locations 1 and 412. (d) Interparticle distance as a parameter of binding site location for 16HBs with two bound IONPs and yields of 16HBs with exactly two bound particles in terms of binding site position (red line). The results are reported as the mean SD of two separate trials. N=52 (16HB-1/4), 57 (16HB-1/5), 86 (16HB-1/6), 88 (16HB-1/7), 73 (16HB-1/8), 98 (16HB-1/10), 67 (16HB-1/11), 119 (16HB-1/12). 50nm scale bars. Reproduced with permission from Ref. [39].

accurately be adjusted with varying amounts of base pairs, end to end DNA chain distance, and counts of DNA molecules. Exact modification of DNA nanoparticles offers a cost-effective technique for creating functional structures having intricate, sequential and organised constructions. Among these diverse self-assembled nanostructures, DNA tetrahedron and DNA hydrogel have lately received the greatest interest for preparing easy and simple diagnostic platforms. Hence in the following sections, we talk about these two nanotechnologies in detail. Moreover, aside from the structural qualities of self-assembly, molecules of DNA have distinct sequence-mediated functionalities. Moreover, DNA nanostructures having fascinating functionalities are aiding in the advancement of DNA-integrated nanotechnology. Several nucleic acids (NAs) have been shown in recent decades to have additional activities, for instance, recognising different molecules, catalysis, and possessing medicinal properties. These unique NAs are known as "functional NAs", and they comprise DNAzymes, ribozymes, i-motifs, aptamers, and others. Among these, aptamers and DNAzymes are largely recognised as functional NAs, and they are being extensively used as functional groups in the development of functional NA-based DNA nanostructures which have been shown to have substantial practical use in biomedical sensing and imaging. Therefore, in the following subsection, we discuss various nanoplatforms based on these functional NAs, namely, DNA-integrated fluorescent/inorganic nanoparticles (NPs)/2D nanomaterials and various signal amplification–based technologies.

5.4.1 DNA Tetrahedron–Based Nanoplatforms

DNA nanotechnology has lately attracted a lot of attention because it allows for the bottom-up fabrication of splendid 2D and 3D structures ranging in different sizes or forms, such as tetrahedron, triangular prism, octahedron, icosahedron, and sophisticated DNA origami constructions, with outstanding controllability and high accuracy. These constructed nanostructures inherit the benefits of nucleic acid, including their compact size, strong programmability, various functionalisation capacity with high addressability, and outstanding biocompatibility. Various DNA nanostructures have been described and widely used in biomedical applications throughout the last few decades. Among these concise nanostructures, the DNA tetrahedron is the most basic and fascinating three-dimensional framework, which has recently received a lot of attention for its contribution to POC diagnostics [40–43].

The DNA tetrahedron is the most basic three-dimensional DNA nanomaterial with uniform edges and acmes forming a hard nanostructure. The DNA tetrahedron has a variety of appealing qualities and functions due to its one-of-a-kind structure. Edges and acmes, for example, can give well-defined places for the construction of advanced nanomaterials and can be coupled to produce a solid structure that delivers DNA tetrahedron with great temperature stability and exceptional enzyme tolerance. The DNA tetrahedron, in general, has a stiff nanostructure having four acmes and six edges. Furthermore, covalent bonds may be used to modify the edges and acmes with various materials such as protein, medicinal compounds, and nanoparticles. Moreover, because DNA nanostructures are extremely programmable, accurate placement of functional components on the DNA tetrahedron is often possible [44–46].

In terms of living cell investigations and medication delivery, the benefits of DNA tetrahedron may be summarised as follows. First, without the need for transfection agents, it may autonomously enter negative-charged cellular membranes via receptor-mediated endocytotic internalisation. Because most internalised tetrahedrons are found in the cytoplasm, they can be employed as inexpensive and simple platforms for biological research. Third, many enzymes in live cells have the capacity to disintegrate or discard external probes, resulting in an unsustainable signal and an increased likelihood of false positives. Due to steric hindrance, the DNA tetrahedron can withstand nuclease attacks and maintain structural integrity for prolonged periods. Fourth, cytotoxicity is a common issue for a wide range of nanostructures. However, because DNA is a biologically friendly substance, the DNA tetrahedron has almost little cytotoxicity. Taking these advantages into account, the DNA tetrahedron has found widespread use in cellular bioanalysis for molecular detection and biocompatible carriers for cargo transport [47–49]. Various recently prepared nanoplatforms based on DNA tetrahedron are highlighted in Table 5.1.

5.4.2 DNA Hydrogel–Based Nanoplatform

Hydrogels are crosslinked 3D networks of hydrophilic polymer chains that, due to their hydrophilic nature, can store a large quantity of water [50,51]. As a result, the hydrogel networks can expand significantly in an aqueous medium. Given that water serves as the most prevalent component of our body, a hydrogel capable of absorbing large volumes of water is regarded to have great promise for biological applications [51,52]. Hydrogels possess better properties as compared to other biomaterials, like better biocompatibility, regulating biodegradability, plasticity, high porosity, and so on [51,53,54]. Because of these features, hydrogels are frequently employed as scaffolds for drug delivery and diagnosis [55].

Furthermore, DNA-based hydrogels have received a lot of interest due to the unique properties of NAs, which are summarised in the following. First and foremost, there is the merit of stability. DNA is more stable than antibodies, proteins and enzymes under intense heating, pressure, and chemical processing. Second, the flexibility of DNA hybridisation offers a big collection of hydrogel constructs. Moreover, DNA strand programmability, which is based on purine and pyrimidine base pairing principles and DNA secondary structures, results in accurately anticipated DNA structure. Furthermore, stimuli-responsive alterations in DNA conformation result in switchable characteristics. When exposed to external stimuli, some functional DNAs experience sudden structural changes, resulting in reversible and switchable alterations in DNA-based hydrogels. Finally, DNA-based hydrogels have simple production and modification approaches. DNA can be produced in vast numbers using an automated solid-phase approach and modified with a variety of functional groups, including acrydite, amino, carboxyl, and thiol, which can further react with other functional units. In addition, with the advancement of phosphoramidite chemistry, most DNA changes may now be easily inserted by configuring a DNA synthesiser [56–59].

DNA hydrogels can be created by either chemically linking DNA molecules or physically entangling DNA strands. The crosslinking done chemically denotes covalent connections of continuous two DNA molecules or one DNA molecule and a polymer, which often necessitates time-consuming synthesis processes indulging various reagents. Chemical crosslinking has the distinct benefit of forming permanent and irreversible bonds, resulting in physiologically stable hydrogels having excellent mechanical strength. Intermolecular bondings that are not covalent, for example, hydrogen bonding connecting complementary DNAs, coordination linkage of DNA molecules and metals, and linkage between DNA and cationic electrolytes through electrostatic forces, cause physical crosslinking.

TABLE 5.1
Potential Point of Care DNA Nanoplatforms Based on DNA Tetrahedrons and DNA Hydrogels

DNA Nanotechnology	Components/Working Mechanism	Target Disease/Pathogen/ Disease-Related Biomarkers	Detection Limit	Key Features	Ref.
Tetrahedron-based nanoplatforms	• The tetrahedron structure built using 4 distinct DNA probes • Various fluorescence signals formed by modifying substrate strand using DNAzyme and fluorophore	High sensitivity for COVID-19, Bat-SL-CoVZC45 and SARS-CoV detection	2.5, 3.1 and 2.9 fM, respectively	• High sensitivity and selectivity; robust platform; negligible interference from clinical samples • Multiple logic biocomputing capabilities "and–or", "inhibit–and", "and–and–and" and "and–inhibit" • Can also identify SARS-COV-2 delta and lambda variants • Multireadout mode	[65]
	• Created by combining DNA mtase-responsive DNA tetrahedral crosslinked hydrogel with personal glucose metre for portable and precise signal reading	DNA adenine methyltransferase (Dam) activity	0.001 U/mL	• Portable, sensitive, selective and user-friendly point of care testing device • Traps glucose-producing enzymes for target recognition and signal transduction • Can be applied to screen inhibitor and analyse dam activity in spiked serum samples • All the reactions for dam assay performed on paper; hence, simple to use at home or field	[66]

(Continued)

TABLE 5.1 (*Continued*)
Potential Point of Care DNA Nanoplatforms Based on DNA Tetrahedrons and DNA Hydrogels

DNA Nanotechnology	Components/Working Mechanism	Target Disease/Pathogen/ Disease-Related Biomarkers	Detection Limit	Key Features	Ref.
	• DNA tetrahedron nanostructures (DTNSs) self-assembled from 7 tailored single-stranded chains of NAs comprising 3 target miRNA recognition elements • Fluorophores and quenchers placed together at three edges of DTNSs, causing fluorescence quenching • In presence of target miRNAs, fluorophores and quenchers separated, and fluorescence recovered	miRNA-21, miRNA-122 and mRNA-194 (for cancer diagnosis)	0.13 nM, 0.64 nM and 0.68 nM, respectively	• Fluorescence "OFF" to "ON" mode analysis • Improved resistance to enzymatic digestion • High cellular uptake efficiency • Ability to simultaneously monitor three intracellular miRNAs • Can also identify cancer cell subtypes and act as an anti-cancer drug	[67]
	• Smart DNA logic-gated nanorobot (DLGN): a universal DNA tetrahedral scaffold (DTS) that attaches to the cell membrane and allows numerous aptamers and medicines to be loaded • DLGN – Comprises of 2 recognition robotic toes (aptamers), 3 anchor robotic arms (bulky electronegative streptavidins, SA), and 1 effector robotic head (drug-conjugated aptamer)	PTK7 antigen (for cancer diagnosis)	-	• Multimode detection and selective death of 5 different cell lines • Could distinguish between different amounts of target antigen expression in diverse comparable cell lines in 30 minutes • "Sense-then-release" technique can functionalise additional markers such as her-2 or egfr • Rapid tumour profiling, *in situ* capturing and separation, and accurate medication delivery	[68]

(*Continued*)

TABLE 5.1 (*Continued*)
Potential Point of Care DNA Nanoplatforms Based on DNA Tetrahedrons and DNA Hydrogels

DNA Nanotechnology	Components/Working Mechanism	Target Disease/Pathogen/ Disease-Related Biomarkers	Detection Limit	Key Features	Ref.
	• Sandwich cytosensor premised on the PCN-224 metal-organic framework and a DNA tetrahedron connected dual-aptamer • Tetrahedral DNA structures connected dual aptamers (AS1411 and MUC1) immobilised on Au electrode interface for identifying entrapped targeted cancer cells • Enhanced surface nanoprobe density and positioning • PCN-224 was adorned with PtNPs that had been modified by G-quadruplex/hemin DNAzyme, horseradish peroxidase (HRP) and dual-aptamer • Nanoprobes created and used to accelerate the oxidation of H_2O_2 for the purpose of enhancing electrochemical signals	MCF-7 cancer cells	6 cells/mL	• Reusable based on electrochemical desorption method • Convenient and efficient strategy for detecting cancer cells at preclinical stages • High sensitivity and selectivity	[69]

(Continued)

TABLE 5.1 (*Continued*)
Potential Point of Care DNA Nanoplatforms Based on DNA Tetrahedrons and DNA Hydrogels

DNA Nanotechnology	Components/Working Mechanism	Target Disease/Pathogen/ Disease-Related Biomarkers	Detection Limit	Key Features	Ref.
DNA hydrogel–based nanoplatforms	• A microfluidic chip integrated with a target-responsive DNA hydrogel • CK-MB aptamer with matching sDNA strand attached individually on polyacrylamide strand • Base-paired linking creates a hydrogel • Aptamer binds to CK-MB upon contact • Hydrogel disintegrated, releasing previously entrapped AuNPs • The hydrogel was then coupled with microfluidic chip, and the colour shift induced by the liberated AuNPs was used to capture a photo and calculate the average grey value	Creatine kinase MB (CK-MB)	0.027 nM	• Portable visual quantitative assay • Could be detected by cell phone • Good portability and visualisation • Simple sample handling	[70]

(*Continued*)

TABLE 5.1 (*Continued*)
Potential Point of Care DNA Nanoplatforms Based on DNA Tetrahedrons and DNA Hydrogels

DNA Nanotechnology	Components/Working Mechanism	Target Disease/Pathogen/ Disease-Related Biomarkers	Detection Limit	Key Features	Ref.
	• DNAzyme crosslinked hydrogel capillary sensor • When Pb^{2+} present, crosslinker substrate strand cleaves, causing hydrogel to partially rupture • Hydrogel film's size is altered that is sealing ends of the capillary tube • Amount of Pb^{2+} influences the activity of fluid flowing through capillary regulated by hydrogel sheet • Precise detection of Pb^{2+} by monitoring distance and duration with naked eyes	Pb^{2+} detection	10 nM	• Visual platform for in-field applications • High sensitivity and selectivity • Simple, cost-effective and rapid • Target directly detected by the naked eye • No equipment required • Detection in less than 1 hour	[71]
	• Paper-based microfluidic ruler-reading and CRISPR Cas12a-responded hydrogel-integrated quantitative tool • CRISPR Cas12a system as target identifier • DNA hydrogel linked to an enzyme pathway for signal enhancement and transmission • Microfluidic chips based on paper for naked-eye visible quantitative interpretation	8s rRNA fragments of *Candida* or *Aspergillus*	4.90 and 4.13 CFU/mL, respectively	• Visible and quantitative point of care testing • Detection by unaided eyes • High sensitivity and selectivity • Low cost • Ease of operation	[72]

(*Continued*)

TABLE 5.1 (*Continued*)
Potential Point of Care DNA Nanoplatforms Based on DNA Tetrahedrons and DNA Hydrogels

DNA Nanotechnology	Components/Working Mechanism	Target Disease/Pathogen/ Disease-Related Biomarkers	Detection Limit	Key Features	Ref.
	• Two Y-shaped DNA units and a double-stranded DNA labelled with fluorophores were self-assembled and mounted with curative siRNA • When intracellular telomerase was highly expressed, DNA nanohydrogel crashed due to prolongation of telomeric primer at terminal series of particular Y-shaped DNA units • FRET of DNA nanohydrogel restored and entrapped siRNA released, allowing for reliable sensing	Telomerase detection (for cancer diagnosis)	33 cells	• DNA nanohydrogel with specific targeting capability • Great biocompatibility and specificity • Programmable and controllable • Can be stimuli-activated for simultaneous *in vitro* telomerase detection and *in vivo* telomerase-triggered gene therapy • Minimal systemic toxicity	[73]
	• Synthesised from pH-sensitive ZnO-NH_2 and CO-Y-DNA probe assembled by three matching strands • DNA hydrogels used to detect fluorescence ratios • Under acidic circumstances, ZnO-NH_2 dissolved, releasing CO-Y-DNA probe • Target hybridised to CO-Y-DNA probe, resulting in a shift in fluorescence ratio involving TAMRA and Cy5, both of which were changed in CO-Y-DNA probe	miRNA-21 detection	83 pM	• pH-responsive DNA hydrogels with ratiometric fluorescence • Ratiometric nucleic acid probe with built-in correction used for eliminating environmental interferences • High accuracy and sensitivity • Low detection limit • Long-term stability against DNAse I and GSH	[74]

(*Continued*)

TABLE 5.1 (*Continued*)
Potential Point of Care DNA Nanoplatforms Based on DNA Tetrahedrons and DNA Hydrogels

DNA Nanotechnology	Components/Working Mechanism	Target Disease/Pathogen/ Disease-Related Biomarkers	Detection Limit	Key Features	Ref.
	• The target ctDNA causes rolling circle amplification and formation of a DNA hydrogel comprising G-quadruplex molecules, which can be seen with bare eyes • Using the DNAzyme function of G-quadruplex/heme combination, hydrogel catalyse the colourless ABTS to green oxidative product ABTS* • Quantification achieved with change in colour	Circulating tumour DNA (ctDNA) biomarker (for non-invasive access of tumour dynamics)	0.32 pM	• Visible strategy for ctDNA detection based on ctDNA-triggered and DNAzyme-functionalised hydrogel • Sensitive in a concentration from 1 pm to 10 nm • Does not require expensive equipment • Successfully applied to simulate analysis of clinical blood samples	[75]

(*Continued*)

TABLE 5.1 (*Continued*)
Potential Point of Care DNA Nanoplatforms Based on DNA Tetrahedrons and DNA Hydrogels

DNA Nanotechnology	Components/Working Mechanism	Target Disease/Pathogen/Disease-Related Biomarkers	Detection Limit	Key Features	Ref.
	• Ferrocene-tagged identification probes were crosslinked with DNAs mounted on polyacrylamide backbones to generate hybrid DNA hydrogels, which were then immobilised on a 3-(trimethoxysilyl) propyl methacrylate (KH 570)-coated ITO electrode • When the recognition probe hybridised with target miRNA-21, hydrogel disintegrated, resulting in loss of ferrocene tags and a decrease in current, as measured by cyclic and differential pulse voltammetry	Lung cancer–specific microRNA, miRNA-21 detection	5 nM	• Electrochemical biosensor based on hybrid DNA hydrogel immobilised on indium tin oxide/polyethylene terephthalate (ITO/PET) electrode • Linear read-out from 10 nm to 50 μm • Flexible sequence design of recognition probe	[76]

Non-covalent links in DNA hydrogels, which are formed via physical crosslinking, can be reversed and are weaker than covalent interactions. Physical crosslinking, as opposed to chemical crosslinking, does not need chemical reagents or chemically altered DNA molecules. Therefore, hydrogels formed via physical crosslinking have good biocompatibility and biodegradability with way less cytotoxicity [41,60,61].

DNA hydrogels are classified into two types based on their composition: hybrid and pure DNA hydrogels. Chaining functional NAs to various polymers results in the formation of hybrid hydrogels. However, because modifying hybrid hydrogels requires numerous processes, pure DNA hydrogel is proposed for overcoming the constraints posed by hybrid hydrogels. Pure DNA hydrogel is made entirely of DNAs, put together using enzymatic ligations and polymerisation, and DNA motifs' specific bonding. Furthermore, the creation of smart stimuli-responsive DNA hydrogels (SRDHs) has piqued the curiosity of many researchers. SRDHs can react to outside stimuli by changing phase properties/crosslinking density. Delivery platforms based on SRDHs enable regulated targeting, payload build-up, and controlled release, enhancing therapeutic profiles and reducing adverse impacts. There are two types of triggers that might cause a response: nonbiological triggers and biological triggers. Temperature, light, magnetism, pH, metal ions, and reducing agents are examples of nonbiological triggers. Biomolecules such as NAs, antigens, enzymes, and ATP are examples of biological stimuli. Because of the broad biomolecular identification capabilities, many additional biological triggers have been investigated. To create smart DNA hydrogels, responsive crosslinking units or preload-sensitive nanoparticles must be built. Furthermore, hydrogels that are crosslinked with DNA molecules have been gaining a lot of attention for being appropriate for signal transduction techniques for POC testing due to their stability, mobility, simplicity of storage, and cheap cost [62–64]. Various recently prepared nanoplatforms based on DNA hydrogels are given in Table 5.1.

5.4.3 DNA-Integrated Fluorescent NPs

Because of the benefits of dependability, the requirement for uncomplicated techniques, enhanced sensitivity for diagnosis, rapid response time and multimodal assays using dyes of various colours, the fluorescence-based assay has received much consideration lately and has become a compelling technique for diagnostics [77]. Fluorescence may be defined simply as the process of emitting light when a molecule absorbs light of a specific frequency [78]. Fluorescent particles, often known as fluorophores, react to light differently than ordinary compounds. As illustrated in Figure 5.3a, a photon of excited light gets absorbed by a fluorophore's electron, increasing the energy level associated with that electron to an excited state. Throughout this brief period of excitation, part of the energy is wasted by colliding molecules or taken by a nearby particle, and the rest of the energy is released in the form of photons so that the electron can be returned to its stable state. Because the emitted photon typically contains lower energy, it possesses a longer wavelength as compared to the excitation photon, and it is possible

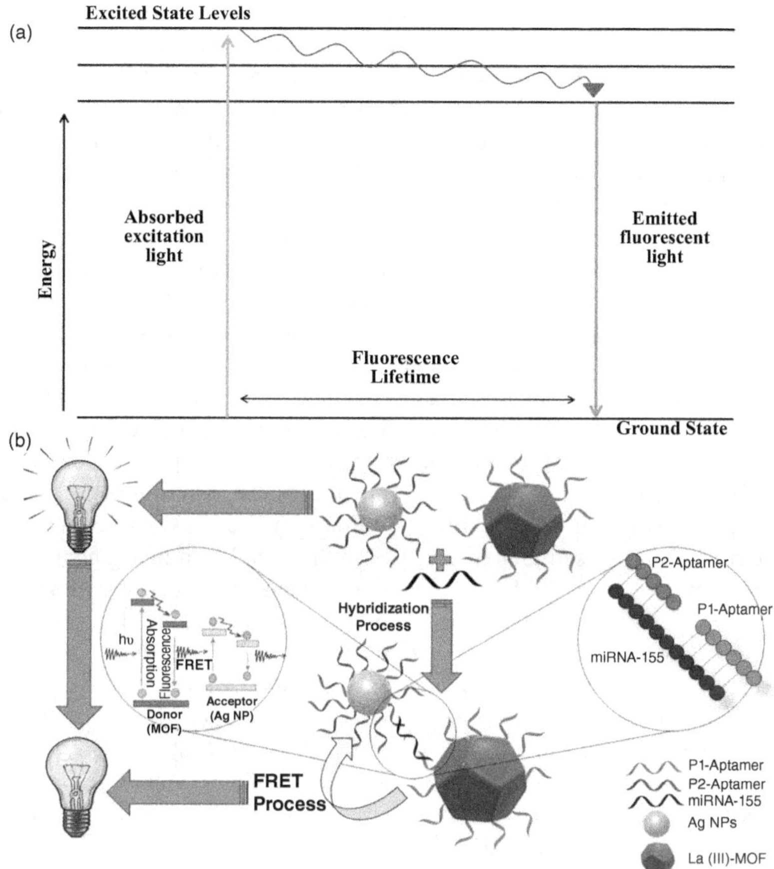

FIGURE 5.3 (a) Schematic of principle behind the phenomenon of fluorescence. (b) A schematic diagram of photoluminescence quenching–based detection of miRNA-155 as a cancer biomarker by the FRET process. Reproduced with permission from Ref. [86].

to differentiate emitted fluorescence from the excitation light. A fluorophore's excitation and photon emission are cyclic, and it can be stimulated repeatedly until it is irreparably destroyed. Fluorophores may thus produce a large number of photons as a result of the series of excitation and emission, and they are consequently utilised in various scientific applications. Furthermore, because fluorescence emission is very sensitive to a fluorophore's immediate surroundings, it has been used in the creation of various sensing applications. The fluorescence of a fluorophore is affected by any characteristic that might interact with it at the molecular level. Temperature, pressure, viscosity, pH, hydrogen bonds, polarity, ions, and other essential chemical and physical characteristics all have an impact on fluorescence [78].

Furthermore, the accessibility of NPs for imaging applications has resulted in a range of imaging approaches with characteristics such as enhanced brightness, inertness to their surroundings, and more uniform dispersion. NPs-mediated fluorescence might be caused by its intrinsic fluorescence owing to quantum confinement, as seen in semiconducting quantum dots, or by the attachment of tiny fluorescent molecules/dyes to it [79,80]. Unlike molecular probes (MPs), NPs are not always toxic and are not susceptible to unwanted binding by cellular biomacromolecules or undesired sequestration. The binding of MPs by cellular proteins can change the optical characteristics of the probe as well as the function of the protein or binding site. Inherently fluorescent NPs, on the other hand, are nearly inert and do not interact with biological proteins, nor are their optical characteristics influenced by proteins outside the cell. Notably, all known NPs possess photostability that outperforms MPs. Many NPs are easily absorbed into cells and tissues (based on charge and surface chemistry) and can even be targeted to specific sites. When compared to fluorescent proteins, NPs are easier to handle and produce more predictable outcomes. Many different types of NPs are widely accessible [81]. Even though a variety of fluorophores, for instance, organic dyes, quantum dots (QDs), and metal NPs, are being immensely used in biomedical sensing, many difficulties remain. Organic dyes, for example, have limited photostability, semiconductor QDs are huge and cytotoxic, and metal NPs have little quantum yields. Hence, DNA-templated fluorescence nanomaterials have lately gained increased attention in biomedical applications because of their exclusive fluorescent features: outstanding photophysical characteristics, stability, decreased cytotoxicity, high fluorescence emission, and excellent biocompatibility. A recent work, for example, offered a new diagnostic device based on DNA-templated fluorescent Ag nanoclusters (DNA-AgNCs) coupled with magnetic NPs. MNP-DNAzyme-acetylcholinesterase (MDA) complex is used for the diagnosis of harmful bacteria utilising *Escherichia coli* as a target organism. The MDA complex is made up of three components: MNP functions as a separator, DNAzyme functions as a bacteria-specific identifier, and AChE functions as an enzyme unit. This technology combines an enzyme-responsive fluorescent signal element based on DNA-AgNCs with a DNAzyme recognition element [82,83].

Furthermore, DNA nanostructures with better stability and permeability have emerged as interesting possibilities for improving the delivery effectiveness and stability of nucleic acid probes. These nanostructures might be easily created via molecular self-assembly. For additional bio-recognition, the placements and quantities of DNA ligands on the surface may be carefully regulated. DNA nanostructures have shown improved stability over nuclease cleavage when used as nano-carriers to transfer NAs into cells [84]. Tetrahedral DNA nanostructure (TDN) has received a lot of interest as a scaffolded biosensor since it is one of the most regularly utilised DNA nanostructures. A functionalised tetrahedral DNA nanoprobe (TDNp) with fluorescence resonance energy transfer (FRET)-ON capacity for accurate probing of intracellular telomerase (up-regulated in more than 90% of tumour cells for uncontrolled proliferation) was produced in a recent work, for example. Förster or FRET is a non-radiative energy transfer phenomenon involving dipole–dipole pairing amid two fluorophores in which the transferred emission energy from the donor causes fluorescence emission from the acceptor, which is characteristically located between 1 and 10 nm of the donor [85]. Another study presented a highly sensitive and selective fluorescent biosensor based on the "sandwich-type" oligonucleotide hybridisation FRET approach. It detects and quantifies the expression levels of miRNA-155 (cancer biomarker). In this study, a modified La(III)-metal-organic framework (MOF) and AgNPs were employed as energy donor–acceptor pairs in the FRET technique to quench fluorescence. La(III)-MOF was produced and subsequently crosslinked with glutaraldehyde. The AgNPs were also produced, and their surfaces were coupled with various 5′-amino-conjugated aptamers [86] Figure 5.3b depicts a schematic picture of the FRET method for detecting miRNA-155 as a cancer biomarker via photoluminescence quenching.

5.4.4 Signal Amplification–Based DNA Nanotechnologies

Because all living species include DNA, methods for detecting particular DNA sequences allow the creation of a plethora of biomedical applications [87]. Furthermore, these approaches are often adaptable to identify particular sequences of concern [88]. Polymerase chain reaction (PCR) amplification is the most popular way of identifying the presence of a given DNA sequence in a specimen, followed by an affirmation of DNA existence by gel electrophoresis or fluorescence-based approaches [89]. However, PCR necessitates skilled employees and costly resources, which renders it unsuitable for POC diagnostics [90]. In recent years, a variety of simple and effective alternative DNA amplification techniques have been discovered (as discussed below).

5.4.4.1 Rolling Circle Amplification

The isothermal enzymatic DNA replication method has recently been developed known as rolling circle amplification (RCA). A short DNA is amplified for generating a long, single-stranded DNA (ssDNA) when a circular DNA template is present and a specific isothermal DNA polymerase with strand displacement activity to stretch a single primer which is annealed to a round DNA template in the RCA reaction [91,92]. The strand displacement activity will help newly synthesised DNA to displace previously created DNA, resulting in the release of ssDNA. This enzymatic process of primer extension and strand displacement results in a lengthy ssDNA with a repetitive sequence complementing the circular template. When combined with molecular beacons (MBs), the RCA product with repetitive DNA domains opens and restores the fluorescence of multiple MBs [92]. Furthermore, a schematic demonstrating the fundamental principle of RCA is given in Figure 5.4.

5.4.4.2 Catalytic Hairpin Assembly

Catalytic hairpin assembly (CHA) is a method of nonenzymatic amplification. In this strategy, two complementary DNA hairpins are engineered to inactivate the process. Then, either of the hairpins might be opened by toehold-regulated strand displacement only in the presence of the initiator strand, allowing the assembly

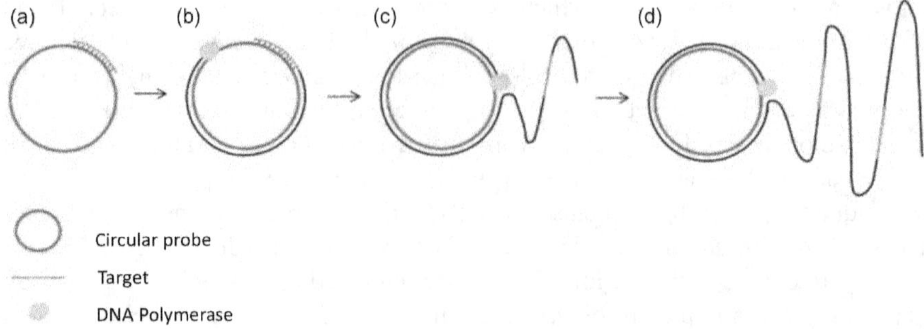

FIGURE 5.4 Schematic of rolling circle amplification (RCA). **(a)** The circular template is annealed by a primer that is complementary to an area of a circular probe. **(b)** DNA polymerase starts the DNA synthesis. **(c)** Strand displacement permits DNA synthesis to continue along the circular template. **(d)** The synthesis of DNA continues to produce a lengthy ssDNA product. Reproduced with permission from Ref. [91].

of both hairpins [93,94]. Ultimately, as a catalyst, the target strand can be autonomously shifted and recycled to induce additional hairpin assembly processes. As a result, in recent years, CHA has been used for the detection of different NAs having great sensitivity and specificity [95–97]. Moreover, CHA is being designed for providing hundreds-fold catalytic amplification having a minimal background and can transduce analyte interaction to several diagnostic modalities, including fluorescent and electrochemical signals [98,99]. However, developing real-time CHA monitoring has historically presented some obstacles. Many isothermal amplification operations are performed at temperatures of 60°C or more, which may enhance the background owing to hairpin breathing [100–103]. Yu et al. created a thermally stable CHA platform which functions at temperatures as high as 60°C without compromising efficiency (as demonstrated in Figure 5.5) [102].

5.4.4.3 Hybridisation Chain Reaction

The hybridisation chain reaction (HCR) is an enzyme-free, toehold-mediated strand displacement reaction (SDR)–mediated approach for biomedical sensing. HCR is a kinetically regulated method that involves a succession of hybridisation procedures among thermodynamically stable DNA probes [93]. The result is often a prolonged double-stranded DNA (dsDNA) with highly efficient signal amplification. Unlike conventional PCR, HCR is carried out without the use of enzymes and at a steady temperature, making it ideal for the investigation of thermally sensitive moieties such as proteins and exosomes. With moderate circumstances, the reaction procedure is made utterly simple, confirming strong practical use [104,105]. Furthermore, the target is not reproduced in an HCR process. The created lengthy DNA product is the source of the output signal. As a result, false positives may be effectively managed with great sensitivity and selectivity. Hence, HCR has widely been considered as an excellent solution for NAs amplification in biomedical sensing and imaging. Moreover, a standard linear

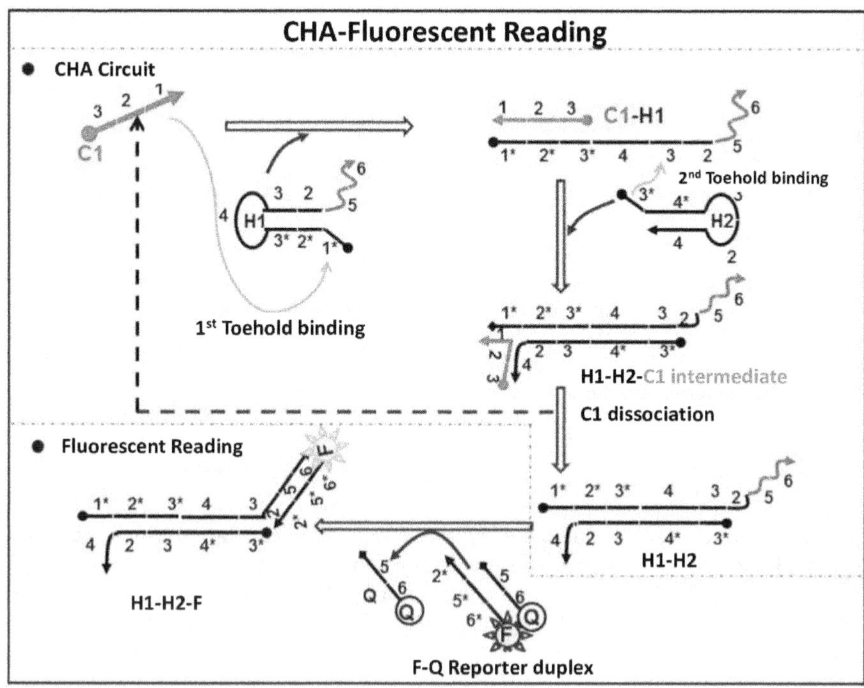

FIGURE 5.5 Schematic outline of catalytic hairpin assembly. Domain 1 (8-base, Table S1) on strand C1 (here referred to as $C1_{LT}$, where "LT" signifies "low temperature") acts as a toehold for domain 1* on $H1_{LT}$, triggering a branch migration response that opens the $H1_{LT}$ stem (16-base). The $H1_{LT}$ domain 3 (8-base) subsequently acts as a second toehold to begin another strand displacement reaction that opens the $H2_{LT}$ stem (11-base), resulting in the $C1_{LT}$-$H1_{LT}$-$H2_{LT}$ intermediate. $C1_{LT}$ can detach from $H1_{LT}$ and stimulate further hairpin assembly processes. $H1_{LT}$-$H2_{LT}$ starts strand displacement (through a 7-base toehold) of a Black(R) fluorescence quencher (Q_{LT}) from a fluorescein amidite (FAM)-labelled oligonucleotide (F_{LT}), permitting the amplification approach to be tracked. Reproduced with permission from Ref. [102].

HCR system necessitates a minimum of two hairpin-shaped DNA probes as fuel strands enabling serial hybridisation (typically called H1 and H2). H1 and H2 include the stem, loop, and toehold sections near the hairpin's terminus. The loop section stores potential energy [106,107]. Figure 5.6 explains the reaction principle of a typical HCR.

5.4.4.4 DNA Walker

Although biomolecule-based amplifications for electrochemical analysis have been established, these techniques still have several disadvantages, such as sluggish electron transfer of amplified DNA sequences and poor catalytic cycle turnover. The recent discovery of the DNA walker technique (originally found by Seeman et al. in 2004) may give a novel way to solve the challenge [108].

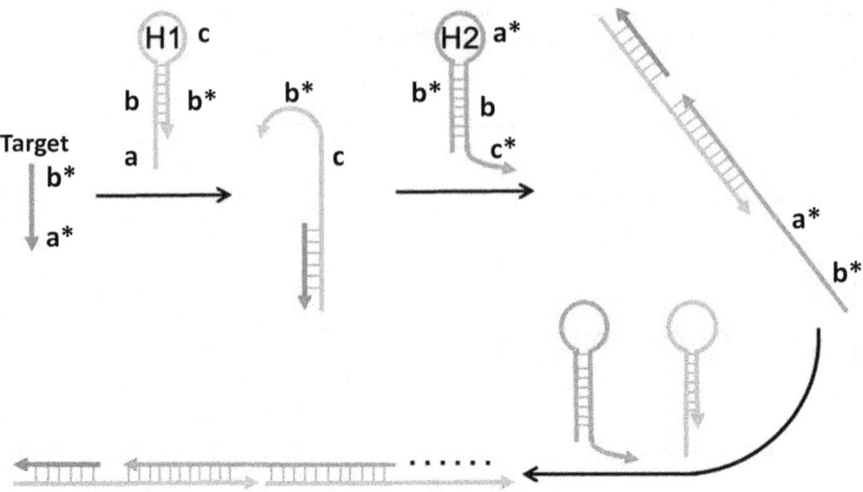

FIGURE 5.6 Schematic outline of hybridisation chain reaction. When the target is absent, H1 and H2 exist together unmodified having metastable configurations at first. Rapid interactions are prevented by the kinetic traps. Following the introduction of target, H1 (a, b) first partly hybridises with target (b*, a*), and entropy-driven SDR ensues, progressively opening the hairpin configuration of H1. The unrestricted single-stranded portion (c, b*) hybridises with the H2 toehold, and another SDR results in H2 hairpin opening. The resulting hybridisation reactions between alternating new H1 and H2 strands are triggered by the free single-stranded portion of H2 (b*, a*). Finally, alternatingly supplied H1 and H2 can be used to build a long and nicked dsDNA polymer. Reproduced with permission from Ref. [106].

The DNA walker is made up of a walker, an efficiently formulated path, and an energy source. It has been demonstrated as a form of the molecular machine that manipulates particular DNA (walking strand) to travel autonomously over predefined oligonucleotide tracks including double-stranded DNA, DNA origami and DNA monolayer [109–111]. Outside stimuli, featuring strand exchange events, nicking enzymes, DNAzyme-based DNA hydrolysis, and light can modify the DNA walker, resulting in cascade signal augmentation and target identification. Moreover, walker movements can demolish tracks and create single-stranded products for signal amplification. Thus, it has a high potential for widely applicable applications such as biological sensing, nanomedicine, logic gates units, controlled formulation, and nano-transporters, as well as cargo sorting [112–114] (Table 5.2).

5.4.5 DNA-Integrated Inorganic Nanoparticles

Functional DNA (fDNA) particles, such as aptamers (links to targets selectively), DNAzymes (similar to enzymes, provide catalysis), and aptazymes (integration of both) have many advantageous properties for the biomedical industry, including nanoscale, little immunogenicity, the comfort of formation and alteration, and

TABLE 5.2
Potential Point of Care DNA Nanoplatforms Based on DNA-Signal Amplifications and DNA-Integrated Fluorescent NPs

DNA Nanotechnology	Components/Working Mechanism	Target Disease/ Pathogen/ Disease-Related Biomarkers	Detection Limit	Key Features	Ref.
DNA-signal amplification–based nanoplatforms	• POCKET (point of care kit for the entire test) • Constructed with an embedded chip (i-chip) and a foldable box (f-box) • Sample preparation using i-chip with 3-times signal amplification • f-box for a smartphone as a heater, a signal detector and a result reader	Multiple types of DNA	$<10^3$ copies/mL	• Versatile sample-to-answer platform • Less than 100 g and smaller than 25 cm in length • Sensitive and specific (single-base differentiation) • Speedy (<2 hours) • Stable (>10 weeks shelf life) • Inexpensive and ultraportable	[115]

	• Incorporated rotary microfluidic system proficient for performing:
	  • glass microbead–mediated DNA extraction
	  • loop-based isothermal amplification
	  • colorimetric lateral flow strip–mediated detection
	  • with optimised microfluidic design and a rotational speed control
		DNA diagnosis of *Salmonella typhimurium* and *Vibrio parahaemolyticus*	50 CFU in 80 minutes	• Three multiple samples simultaneously analysed on a single device
				• Rapid, automatic and cost-effective sample-to-result genetic analysis
					[116]

(*Continued*)

TABLE 5.2 (*Continued*)
Potential Point of Care DNA Nanoplatforms Based on DNA-Signal Amplifications and DNA-Integrated Fluorescent NPs

DNA Nanotechnology	Components/Working Mechanism	Target Disease/ Pathogen/ Disease-Related Biomarkers	Detection Limit	Key Features	Ref.
	• Components: polystyrene electrospun nanofibrous membrane as sensing interface material • H2 strand as a target-triggered catalytic hairpin assembly moiety • G-quadruplex/hemin as the plasmonic reporter • Distinct colour change from red to blue enabled detection	HIV DNA biomarker	10–17 M in whole serum	• Facile and portable visualisation sensor • Ultrasensitive and selective detection • Naked-eye detection	[117]

(*Continued*)

TABLE 5.2 (*Continued*)
Potential Point of Care DNA Nanoplatforms Based on DNA-Signal Amplifications and DNA-Integrated Fluorescent NPs

DNA Nanotechnology	Components/Working Mechanism	Target Disease/ Pathogen/ Disease-Related Biomarkers	Detection Limit	Key Features	Ref.
	• A magnetic 3D DNA walker/AuNPs-based colorimetric platform • Magnetic 3D DNA walker for signal amplification • Hundreds of substrate single-stranded DNA (DNA tracks) and dozens of blocked walking strands attached on an Au-Fe_3O_4 nanocomposite and applied as a magnetic 3D DNA walker • Target-activated DNA walker by DNAzyme cleavage mechanism • Many single-stranded product (displaced ssDNA) generated • After magnetic separation displaced ssDNA incubated with AuNPs • Colour change from greyish black to purple • Quantitative detection by UV–vis spectroscopy	miRNA-155 in human serum	16.7 fM	• For POC nucleic acids diagnostics • Sensitive and specific • No complicated sample pretreatment required	[118]

(*Continued*)

TABLE 5.2 (*Continued*)
Potential Point of Care DNA Nanoplatforms Based on DNA-Signal Amplifications and DNA-Integrated Fluorescent NPs

DNA Nanotechnology	Components/Working Mechanism	Target Disease/ Pathogen/ Disease-Related Biomarkers	Detection Limit	Key Features	Ref.
	• Combining a Ru-SiO2@polydopamine (Ru-SiO2@PDA) nanoplatform with a DNA strand displacement signal amplification strategy based on near-infrared light (NIR) • When fuel DNA and carboxyfluorescein (FAM)-labelled signal DNA co-assembled on their external side, the green fluorescence of FAM was suppressed, resulting in a low ratiometric signal • When MiRNA present, target displaced signal DNA from encaptured DNA, signal DNA released (at a distance from the Ru-sio2@PDA) • Green fluorescence restored resulting in improved I_{green}/I_{red} • When exposed to NIR light, Ru-sio2@PDA elevated the surface temperature around the probe, causing the emission of fuel DNA • Target miRNA restored; ratiometric signal efficiently amplified	miRNA let-7a and its *in vivo* up- and down-regulation expressions	-	• Highly sensitive ratiometric fluorescence imaging • Simplistic tool for extremely sensitive and precise intracellular miRNA diagnosis • Single-step incubation	[119]

(*Continued*)

TABLE 5.2 (*Continued*)
Potential Point of Care DNA Nanoplatforms Based on DNA-Signal Amplifications and DNA-Integrated Fluorescent NPs

DNA Nanotechnology	Components/Working Mechanism	Target Disease/ Pathogen/ Disease-Related Biomarkers	Detection Limit	Key Features	Ref.
	• Superparamagnetic combinations and molecular beacons provide a dual functional framework • Mediated by aptamer immunoaffinity, with ultrasensitive diagnosis efficiency and repairable isolation capability, which benefit from nonenzymatic amplification techniques, magnetic separation and restriction cleavage, respectively	Prostate cancer	100 particles/µL in urine	• To analyse prostate cancer cell–derived exosomes in urine • Exosomes quantification can be exactly amplified and transformed into single-strand DNA detection • Linear relationship between the logarithmic concentration of exosomes and fluorescence intensity of the molecular beacon • Prostate-specific membrane antigen aptamers employed to detect and capture PMSA-positive exosomes from urine samples	[120]
	• Ultraviolet-induced *in situ* AuNPs united with loop-based isothermal amplification (LAMP)	Coronavirus (COVID-19)	42 fg/µL^{-}	• Handy sample delivery and multiple diagnosis • Elevated sensitivity and uncomplicated design • Quick colorimetric detection (10 minutes)	[121]

(*Continued*)

TABLE 5.2 (*Continued*)
Potential Point of Care DNA Nanoplatforms Based on DNA-Signal Amplifications and DNA-Integrated Fluorescent NPs

DNA Nanotechnology	Components/Working Mechanism	Target Disease/ Pathogen/ Disease-Related Biomarkers	Detection Limit	Key Features	Ref.
	• FRET-mediated localised hairpin-DNA pathway amplifier • System: 2 metastable hairpin DNAs (H1 and H2) localised on a DNA nanocube	Intracellular tumour-related miRNA	-	• Rapid, efficient and reliable imaging • Significantly accelerated (7 times faster) speed of detection • Improved cell permeability and better nuclease resistance • Ability to avoid false-positive signals	[122]

(Continued)

TABLE 5.2 (*Continued*)
Potential Point of Care DNA Nanoplatforms Based on DNA-Signal Amplifications and DNA-Integrated Fluorescent NPs

DNA Nanotechnology	Components/Working Mechanism	Target Disease/ Pathogen/ Disease-Related Biomarkers	Detection Limit	Key Features	Ref.
DNA-integrated fluorescent NPs	• A DNA tetrahedral nanostructure (DTN) containing 3 adapter oligos on each of its edges • TOTO-1, as a fluorescent contributor, may bind to DTN's natural NAs framework • Three organic dye-functionalised strands (FRET oligos) are used as fluorescence receptors • When target miRNAs are present, they hybridise with FRET oligos and adaptor oligos on the corners of DTN, resulting in the formation of stable DNA tetrahedron nanotags • As an outcome of TOTO-1 confinement being close to three fluorescence dyes, the FRET between TOTO-1 and three fluorescence dyes was efficiently formed	miRNA-21, miRNA-122 and miRNA-223 for liver cancer diagnosis	-	• Detection of multiple miRNAs based on FRET • Sensitive multiplexed quantification in 10% human serum samples	[123]

(*Continued*)

TABLE 5.2 (*Continued*)
Potential Point of Care DNA Nanoplatforms Based on DNA-Signal Amplifications and DNA-Integrated Fluorescent NPs

DNA Nanotechnology	Components/Working Mechanism	Target Disease/ Pathogen/ Disease-Related Biomarkers	Detection Limit	Key Features	Ref.
	• Portable device integrating reverse transcription, fast thermocycling (via plasmonic heating through magneto-plasmonic nanoparticles) and *in situ* fluorescence detection following magnetic clearance of the nanoparticles	Acute respiratory syndrome 2 (SARS-CoV-2) RNA	3.2 gene copies per μL	• Fast one-pot PCR with reverse transcription (RT-PCR) technology for COVID-19 diagnostics • Fast, portable and automated nucleic acid detection • Concurrently measures three samples within 17 minutes • Excellent diagnostic accuracy (>99%)	[124]

easy surface immobilisation. The incorporation of fDNA into NPs provides NPs with specialised recognition capabilities toward various targets, including small compounds, biomacromolecules, and even viruses and pathogens [125–128]. fDNA may be turned into highly efficient and sensitive sensing probes by making use of the unique optical and magnetic features of inorganic NPs. AuNPs are one of the most potential NPs. Because of their low cytotoxicity and specific optical features, AuNPs are recurrently engaged in biomedical research applications such as biosensors and biomedical imaging. Flora et al. recently created a colorimetric lateral flow biosensor (LFB: a paper-mediated detection unit which provides a quick examination in a single and simple step) in order to visually detect RNA of dengue-1 utilising dextrin-capped AuNPs as a tag. The diagnosis was mediated by NAs sandwich hybridisation between an AuNPs-tagged DNA reporter probe, target RNA, and a DNA capturing probe specific to dengue-1 mounted on a nitrocellulose membrane. The detection mechanism is illustrated in Figure 5.7(a and b). A positive test resulted in a red test line on the LFB strip, allowing for detection with naked eyes (Figure 5.7(c)) [129]. Similarly, Li et al. created a fluorescence sensing approach for miRNA by combining duplex-specific nuclease (DSN)-based amplification and a dumbbell DNA switch. AuNPs, which offer a three-dimensional response surface, were used. They were good fluorescence quenchers too. Figure 5.7(d) depicts the functioning mechanism. First, gold-sulphur chemistry is used to functionalise naked AuNPs with Probe A. DSN recognises a DNA/

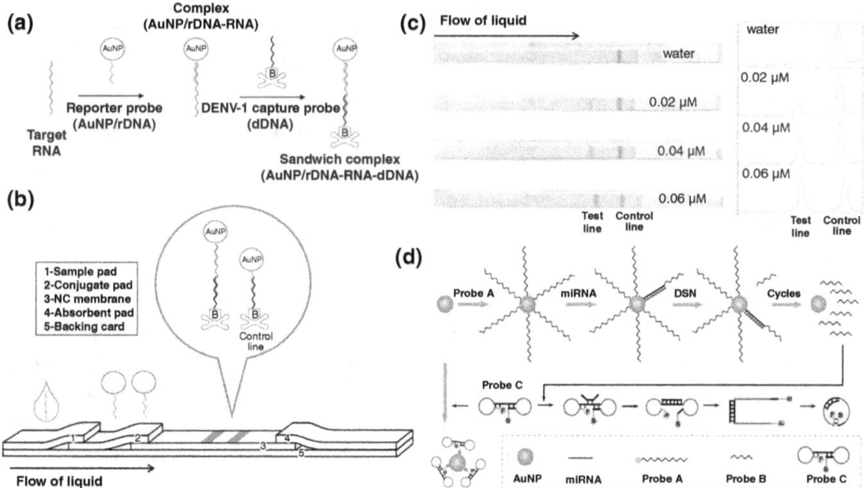

FIGURE 5.7 (a-c) A diagram of the detecting method. (a) The assembly of an AuNP/rDNA-RNA-dDNA sandwich complex. (b) Visual diagnosis diagram. (c) ImageJ analysis produced photo pictures showing genuine lateral flow biosensor (LFB) results at the stated T-1 concentrations, as well as the accompanying profile plots. Reproduced with permission from Ref. [129]. (d) Diagram of the sensing technique for miRNA detection (DSN: duplex-specific nuclease; AuNP: gold nanoparticle; F: Alexa Fluor 488; S: thiol group). Reproduced with permission from Ref. [129].

RNA duplex produced by hybridisation between Probe A and miRNA. The other single-stranded segment (Probe B) and miRNA were released when the DNA strand was digested. Target miRNA was recycled to make more Probe B strands. Second, the dumbbell-shaped Probe C has 30 terminal Alexa Fluor 488 and 50 terminal thiol groups. Probe C's stem interacts with the Probe B sequence, releasing the two loops. Furthermore, self-hybridisation occurs between the 50 and 30 terminals. As a result, the thiol group is concealed in the new stem segment, limiting Probe C adsorption on AuNPs FRET. Alexa Fluor 488 displayed high emission intensity, which could be used to determine the original concentration of miRNA [130].

Another recent research by Z. Sun et al. created a colorimetric sensor array by combining a zirconium metal-organic framework (Zr-MOF) with single-strand DNA–conjugated AuNPs (ssDNA-AuNPs) for speedy and reliable semen detection in male infertility diagnosis [131]. As illustrated in Figure 5.8(a&b), on the surface of AuNPs, six randomly chosen single-strand DNA sequences are changed to produce unique sensor components for array sensing. UiO-66, a standard Zr-based porphyrinic MOF NP, may effectively connect with oligonucleotides due to correlations between both the Zr6 complexes and DNA phosphate backbone. Furthermore, aromatic electron-rich ligands in the MOFs' structure may be coupled with ssDNA through hydrogen bonding and stacking. Consequently, Zr-MOF may bind and precipitate ssDNA-AuNPs, dimming the colouration of the precipitate. Upon mixing of various semen samples, a few components, for instance, proteins, would be adsorbed to ssDNA-AuNPs surface by nonspecific bonds, influencing the succeeding co-precipitation of Zr-MOF and ssDNA-AuNPs. Diverse colorimetric patterns will emerge as a result of the different interactions of different chemicals in semen and ssDNA-AuNPs, along with MOF. As a result, various sperm samples may be easily distinguished by monitoring the absorbance values of the precipitate before and after the samples of semen were added (Figure 5.8c–e). Apparently, the colour-based output reading requires no specialised instrumentation, and the manufactured biosensing unit employs biostable and inexpensive chemicals. Hence, this method is especially well suited for POC diagnostics.

Furthermore, fluorescent QDs (having a 5 nm radius) have been the foundational notion of nanotechnology from their conception. QDs have several distinct structural, electrochemical, and photochemical features, making them appealing biosensing nanoplatforms. These nanostructures have the potential to significantly improve the analytical capabilities of biosensors, namely, detection limit, sensitivity, and selectivity. Scientists are formulating QDs not just for their potential to amplify signals, but also for their great capacity for functionalisation with bioreceptors. A recent study created biocompatible functional nanocomposites by mixing painstakingly tailored unimolecular DNA and fine-sized graphene QDs [132]. When these nanocomposites were used as diagnostic probes, a huge build-up of fluorescence signals in live cells was generated by a modest quantity of cellular APE1 (a cancer diagnostic and predictive biomarker) via repetitive enzymatic catalysis.

Magnetic nanoparticles (MNPs) are another major class of NPs that are often made from pure metals (Fe, Co, Ni, and other rare earth metals) or a metal–polymer combination. The ability of MNPs to be magnetically modulated by an

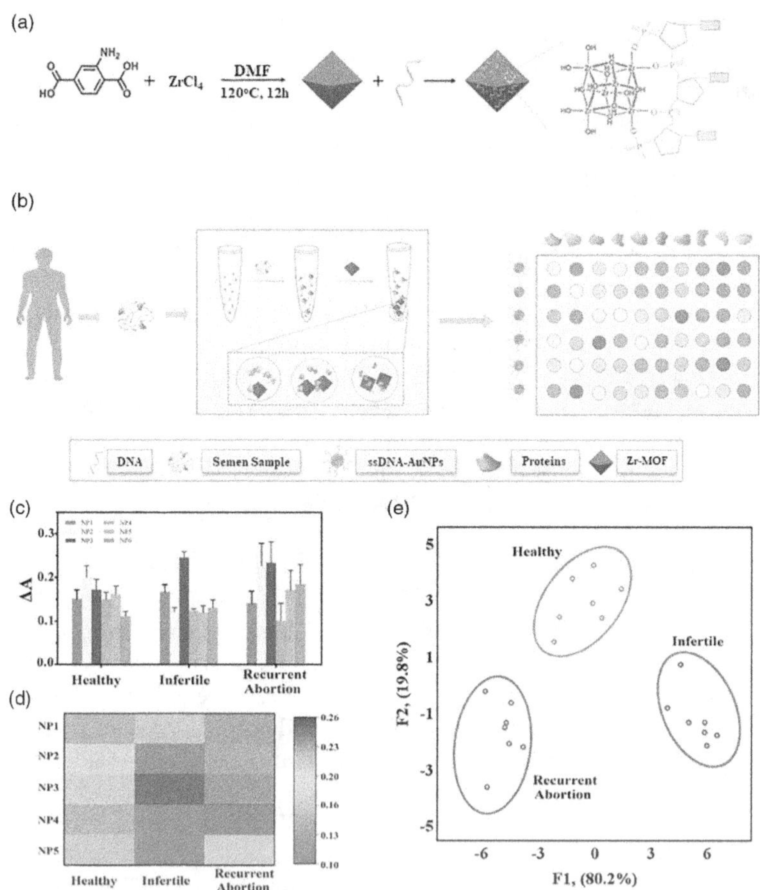

FIGURE 5.8 (a) Manufacturing of UiO-66-NH2 NPs and their association with DNA; (b) working of a colorimetric sensor array technique in order to detect semen samples. (c) Absorbance response pattern (A, A0-A) produced from distinct components of sensing unit (NP1-NP6) in opposition to three distinct semen sample scenarios. The standard deviations of six parallel readings are represented by the error bars. (d) Absorbance response pattern heat map for three independent examples of sperm samples. (e) Canonical score plot based on the first two absorbance response pattern components. Each point reflects reaction pattern of a particular semen species. Reproduced with permission from Ref. [131].

external magnetic field permits them to be widely studied for biological applications. Fuji et al. have devised a technique for detecting microRNAs utilising MNPs [133]. MicroRNAs have critical functions in various severe disorders, resulting in them being sought after as possible medical detection markers. MicroRNAs can be easily extracted from blood and urine, and quantified using q-RTPCR or microarray. Biosensing tools using nanopores have recently gained attention for single-molecule analysis of microRNAs. Ongoing approaches, on the other hand, are technically demanding, involving numerous instruments, and decontamination and tagging of microRNA samples before use. This newly designed platform uses a simple process that does not need purification or labelling. Magnetic beads attached with DNA/nanopores over a liposomal film are used for this method. It creates a duplex with complementary DNA while target microRNAs are there, and that's further split by a nuclease specific to the duplex. The divided DNA, with attached liposome, is then freed from the magnetic bead, fuses to the lipid bilayer of the chip, and generates an electrical signal caused by the development of a nanopore. The signals emitted by microRNAs can be predicted to increase in an isothermal reaction due to a feature of the DSN. Zhi Li et al. announced DNA-templated MNP QD-aptamer copolymers (MQAPs) for highly sensitive separation and monitoring of circulating tumour cells (CTCs) with great capture efficiency and purity [134]. Using DNA as a template allows for regulated assembly of magnetic, fluorescent, and biomarkers into a single compressed configuration, allowing each functionality's performance to be rationally designed and amplified. Furthermore, many recently developed nanoplatforms based on DNA-integrated inorganic NPs for POC diagnosis are listed in Table 5.3.

5.4.6 DNA-Integrated 2D Nanomaterials

Two-dimensional (2D) nanomaterials are considered a tremendous accomplishment in the technology of nanoscience and nanomaterials, where stacked atomic sheets with amazing physiochemical characteristics were discovered, sparking a huge interest in a variety of applications and industries. The dual large surface of 2D nanomaterials not just increases surface area but also provides a consistent platform for biomolecule integration. The remarkable electrical, mechanical, electrochemical, and optical properties of 2D nanomaterials have attracted considerable interest over the last decade because of their broad application in a variety of sectors, including disease diagnostics and therapies. There are different types of 2D materials that have been studied for diverse biosensing applications, including graphitic carbon nitride, transition metal dichalcogenides, graphene, metal halides, metal oxides, and MOFs. Among these, 2D nanosheet structures based on graphene or graphene oxide are typically modified with DNA and are being extensively researched for the preparation of POC diagnosis platforms, due to graphene's efficient DNA adhesion, ease of bioconjugation, surface-enhanced Raman scattering (SERS) and good fluorescence quenching [135,136].

Moreover, 2D molybdenum disulphide (MoS_2) nanomaterials from transition metal dichalcogenides have also received a lot of interest recently. This is due to great biocompatibility, strong electrochemical catalytic activity, ease of modification, high specific surface area, large electrode/electrolyte junction area, and sensitive surface states (high surface-to-volume ratio) of MoS_2. By stacking covalently bonded S-Mo-S via weak van der Waals' contacts, each Mo is coordinated to six S atoms, increasing the planar electric transportation capabilities. MoS_2 nanosheets (MoS_2 NSs) may adsorb single-stranded DNA due to the van der Waals interaction between nucleobases and the MoS_2 NSs basal plane. These benefits, together with the presence of an appropriate band gap as

TABLE 5.3
Potential Point of Care DNA Nanoplatforms Based on DNA-Integrated Organic/Inorganic and 2D Nanomaterials

DNA Nanotechnology	Components/Working Mechanism	Target Disease/ Pathogen/ Disease-Related Biomarkers	Detection Limit	Key Features	Ref.
DNA-integrated inorganic NPs–based nanoplatforms	• Fluorescent sensing strategy by combining duplex-specific nuclease (DSN)–mediated amplification and dumbbell DNA structural switch • AuNPs are employed, which provide a 3D reaction interface. They also act as effective fluorescence quenchers	miRNA detection; cancer diagnosis	0.1 fM	• Highly sensitive detection • Could load multiple probe • Good reproducibility • Differentiate interfering miRNAs with excellent selectivity	[130]
	• Gold NPs–based multipedal DNA walker • AuNPs used to load multiple "legs" for DNA walking and electrochemical amplification by tris(2-carboxyethyl) phosphine hydrochloride employed to enhance the signal • UV–vis absorption response incorporated contributing to ratiometric analysis	Circulating tumour cell (CTC) (for cancer diagnosis)	1 cell/mL	• High sensitivity and anti-interference ability • Good selectivity • Resolution of single-cell level • Excellent ability of distinguishing CTC in blood samples	[139]

(Continued)

TABLE 5.3 (*Continued*)
Potential Point of Care DNA Nanoplatforms Based on DNA-Integrated Organic/Inorganic and 2D Nanomaterials

DNA Nanotechnology	Components/Working Mechanism	Target Disease/ Pathogen/ Disease-Related Biomarkers	Detection Limit	Key Features	Ref.
	• DNA-linked gold nanoprobes (DNA-AuNPs) • Liquid-phased miRNA quantification assay followed by receiver operating characteristic (ROC) curve–based correlation analysis	miR-21/miR-141/ miR-375 detection (prostate cancer diagnosis)	-	• Integrated nano-biosensing technology for the PCR-free, non-invasive liquid biopsies of multiple miRNA • Simple, rapid and ultrasensitive quantification of serum miRNA • Direct and target-specific detection • Single-step quantification • Multimodal liquid-phase essay	[140]
	• A DNA biosensor relying on silsesquioxane-functionalised AuNPs that use an oxidised glassy carbon electrode (ox-GCE) customised with silsesquioxane-functionalised AuNPs • Positively charged polyelectrolyte immobilised on ox-GCE for coupling with thiolated DNA probe • Univariate and multivariate optimisation • Target identification mediated by distinction of charge transfer resistance of redox marker ($[Fe(CN)_6]^{3-/4-}$) and roughness of electrode interface	Zika virus	0.82 pmol L^{-1}	• Sensitive label-free impedimetric DNA biosensor • Showed suitable stability and selectivity to quantify ZIKV in human serum samples	[141]

(*Continued*)

TABLE 5.3 (*Continued*)
Potential Point of Care DNA Nanoplatforms Based on DNA-Integrated Organic/Inorganic and 2D Nanomaterials

DNA Nanotechnology	Components/Working Mechanism	Target Disease/ Pathogen/ Disease-Related Biomarkers	Detection Limit	Key Features	Ref.
	• Aptamer-integrated magnetic nanoparticles • Iron oxide-magnetised nanoparticles bifunctional with l-cysteine and bonded to streptavidic • Magnetic nanoparticles bound with biotin carrying an epitope precise to a breast cancer biomarker protein	Breast cancer biomarker protein	15.63 µg/mL	• Used to separate MUC 1 proteins from MCF-7 cell lysates • Proteins isolated measured using a Qubit fluorimeter and verified using MALDI-TOF-MS • Can provide amplified sensitivity	[142]

(*Continued*)

TABLE 5.3 (*Continued*)
Potential Point of Care DNA Nanoplatforms Based on DNA-Integrated Organic/Inorganic and 2D Nanomaterials

DNA Nanotechnology	Components/Working Mechanism	Target Disease/ Pathogen/ Disease-Related Biomarkers	Detection Limit	Key Features	Ref.
	• Magnetic nanoparticles (MNPs) with atomic transfer radical polymeric techniques to improve for fluorescent detection • Helix DNA probe (pDNA) marked by 5′ thio and 3′ azide groups was immobilised on the interface of amino group–modified magnetic NPs using sulfo-N-succinimidyl-4-maleimidobutyrate sodium salt (sulfo-GMBS) cross-linkers • In the existence of targets DNAs (tDNA), pDNA hybridises with tDNA to create dual DNA, moving the azide group away from the exterior of MNPs • Cu (I)-catalysed alkyne-azide cycloaddition introduces enablers in to pDNA to activate its ATRP reaction • A huge amount of 9-anthracenylmethyl methacrylate polymers were effectively named on the surface of MNPs, which led to significant fluorescence signal intensification	Human T-lymphotropic virus type II (HTLV-II)	0.22 fM	• The fluorescence signal was proportional to log of tDNA quantity throughout the 1 fm to 1 nm region • Capable of identifying HTLV-II DNA in samples of human serum and distinguishing unmatched bases • High sensitivity, selectivity and simplicity	[143]

(*Continued*)

TABLE 5.3 (*Continued*)
Potential Point of Care DNA Nanoplatforms Based on DNA-Integrated Organic/Inorganic and 2D Nanomaterials

DNA Nanotechnology	Components/Working Mechanism	Target Disease/ Pathogen/ Disease-Related Biomarkers	Detection Limit	Key Features	Ref.
	• Pairing a double coloured graphene quantum dots (blue GQDs and green GQDs) customised DNA probes using carbon nanoparticles (CNPs) to extinguish the fluorescence including both GQDs-DNA probes • Complementary to the Exo III-assisted sequence-independent targeted regeneration and signals amplifying technique	DNA biomarkers For HIV and HBV diagnosis	6.6 pM for HIV and 9.5 pM for HBV	• Signal "off-on" extremely sensitive multiplex diagnostic nanoplatform • High sensitivity • Great selectivity • Concurrent diagnosis of several targets • Can discriminate between precisely matched and unmatched targets in PBS buffer and 1% human serum samples	[144]
	• DNA-bridged gold nanoparticles+quantum dots (QDs) may interact with 2 miRNA molecules at the same time, amplifying the single-molecule input, performing a computation via an AND logic gate, and generating QD photoluminescence (PL) as that of an output signal • Integrated with signal amplifier	miRNA-21 and miRNA-122	46.0 and 39.6 pM, respectively	• Logic sensing of dual miRNA molecules within living cells • High sensitivity • Detects particular cancer cell types through sophisticated detection of miRNA patterns	[145]

(*Continued*)

TABLE 5.3 (*Continued*)
Potential Point of Care DNA Nanoplatforms Based on DNA-Integrated Organic/Inorganic and 2D Nanomaterials

DNA Nanotechnology	Components/Working Mechanism	Target Disease/ Pathogen/ Disease-Related Biomarkers	Detection Limit	Key Features	Ref.
	• A skilfully crafted unimolecular DNA and okay-sized graphene quantum dots are combined • Fluorescence signal in live cells activated by even little amounts of target via multiple enzyme catalysis cycles	Apurinic/apyrimidinic endonuclease 1 (APE1) (for cancer diagnosis)	~29 pM	• Biocompatible functional nanocomposites • Capable of detecting biomarkers in cells of the same kind under various cell circumstances • Applicable to multiple malignant cells • Highly sensitive and specific	[132]
	• Genetic material magnetic nanoparticles dot (QD)-aptamer copolymers • Developed by hybridisation series of reactions and provide enhanced magnetic response, exceptional bonding specificity for target cells across background cells, and super brilliant ensemble QD PL enabling single-cell detection	Circulating tumour cell	-	• Rapid magnetic isolation of CTCs from human blood with high capture efficiency and purity approaching 80% • Free from nonspecific binding • High sensitivity and accuracy	[134]

(*Continued*)

TABLE 5.3 (*Continued*)
Potential Point of Care DNA Nanoplatforms Based on DNA-Integrated Organic/Inorganic and 2D Nanomaterials

DNA Nanotechnology	Components/Working Mechanism	Target Disease/ Pathogen/ Disease-Related Biomarkers	Detection Limit	Key Features	Ref.
	• Combining zirconium metal-organic frameworks (Zr-MOFs) with gold nanoparticles coated with single-stranded DNA (ssDNA-AuNPs) • Zr-MOFs absorb and precipitate AuNPs through single-stranded DNA due to coordination interactions between the Zr6 clusters and the DNA phosphate backbone; stacking and H-bonding • The addition of sperm influences the co-precipitation of Zr-MOFs and ssDNA-AuNPs • Supernatant colour changes	Male infertility diagnosis	-	• Colorimetric sensor array for human semen identification • Can recognise distinct semen instances based on inclusion differences • Rapid and accurate identification • Simple and feasible • Sensitive	[131]

(*Continued*)

TABLE 5.3 (*Continued*)
Potential Point of Care DNA Nanoplatforms Based on DNA-Integrated Organic/Inorganic and 2D Nanomaterials

DNA Nanotechnology	Components/Working Mechanism	Target Disease/ Pathogen/ Disease-Related Biomarkers	Detection Limit	Key Features	Ref.
DNA-integrated organic NPs–based nanoplatforms	• Magnetic beads attached with DNA and nanopores on a liposome membrane generate a duplex with complementary DNA in the presence of target microRNA, which is broken by a duplex-specific nuclease (DSN) • The cleaved DNA, which has a liposome attached to its end, is then freed from the magnetic bead, fuses to the lipid bilayer on chip and generates an electrical signal as a result of the development of a nanopore	microRNAs detection	Above 10 nM	• Detection of target miRNAs from combinations comprising >106 distinct miRNAs sequences • Readily uses blood or urine samples • Purification and labelling not required	[133]

(*Continued*)

TABLE 5.3 (*Continued*)
Potential Point of Care DNA Nanoplatforms Based on DNA-Integrated Organic/Inorganic and 2D Nanomaterials

DNA Nanotechnology	Components/Working Mechanism	Target Disease/ Pathogen/ Disease-Related Biomarkers	Detection Limit	Key Features	Ref.
	• Dandelion-like liposomes-encoded magnetic bead probe-based toehold-mediated DNA circuit • Glucoamylase-encapsulated liposomes (gels)–encoded magnetic bead (gels-MB) probe developed to combine target binding, magnetic separation and signal response • Detecting the target, initiating a toehold-mediated circular strand displacement reaction (TCSDR) with the aid of fuel DNA, building a DNA circuit system and beginning target recycling amplification and liposome deconstruction • Magnetic separation was used to extract disassembled liposomes, and encapsulated glucoamylase was freed to catalyse amylose hydrolysis with numerous turnovers to glucose for PGM reading • Target recycling amplification triggered by toehold-mediated DNA circuit with liposome multiple-label multiplication resulted in the transformation of a tiny amount of target miRNA into a huge glucose signal	miRNA-21	0.7 fM	• Simple and sensitive detection within 1.5 hours • Enzymatic amplification or precise instrumentation not needed • High-confidence quantification • Low cost, ease of use and portability	[146]

(*Continued*)

TABLE 5.3 (*Continued*)
Potential Point of Care DNA Nanoplatforms Based on DNA-Integrated Organic/Inorganic and 2D Nanomaterials

DNA Nanotechnology	Components/Working Mechanism	Target Disease/ Pathogen/ Disease-Related Biomarkers	Detection Limit	Key Features	Ref.
DNA-integrated 2D nanomaterials–based nanoplatforms	• 2D Lu_2O_3–S nanosheets with enough O_2 vacancies were formulated • A crossover-improved electrochemiluminescence cytosensing platform was developed by combining a DNA device cycle-amplification system with signal conversion pretreatment • Transformed target cells into configurable sequencing, using DNA device cycle-amplification over customised electrode interfaces	Acute lymphoblastic leukaemia cancer cell detection	10 cells/mL	• Ag_2S quantum dots used as energy acceptor towards Lu_2O_3–S donor • CCRF-CEM cells (CEM) used as the model CTCs • Displayed good analytical performance	[147]

(*Continued*)

TABLE 5.3 (*Continued*)
Potential Point of Care DNA Nanoplatforms Based on DNA-Integrated Organic/Inorganic and 2D Nanomaterials

DNA Nanotechnology	Components/Working Mechanism	Target Disease/ Pathogen/ Disease-Related Biomarkers	Detection Limit	Key Features	Ref.
	• Rigid 3D DNA "nanosafe-box" (DNB) for containment and deployment of a recognition probe (N3), developed to build an electrochemical biosensor utilising electro-active two-dimensional (2D MOF) nanosheets as signal tags • Blocker DNA holds N3 in the 3D shell of DNB • After hitting the target Hg^{2+}, exonuclease III (Exo III) digestion is started to emancipate the DNA "key" (K); thus, the unrestricted K triggers strand displacement reaction for disclosing prelocked N3 to effectively bind dibenzocyclooctyne (DBCO)-tagged anchor through the use of metal-catalyst-free click chemistry, in which amounts of 2D MOF nanosheets containing Co(II) as electron mediator are given in conjunction with a substantial electrochemical reaction	Mercury ion (Hg2+) detection	33 fM	• Ultrasensitive detection • Enhanced mechanical rigidity and structural stability • Improved accessibility of probes and increased loading amounts of signal tags • Significantly decreased background signal • Outstanding analytical performance • Dynamic linear range of 0.1 pm to 10 nm • Ingenious method for detection of metal ions and biomarkers	[148]

(*Continued*)

TABLE 5.3 (*Continued*)
Potential Point of Care DNA Nanoplatforms Based on DNA-Integrated Organic/Inorganic and 2D Nanomaterials

DNA Nanotechnology	Components/Working Mechanism	Target Disease/ Pathogen/ Disease-Related Biomarkers	Detection Limit	Key Features	Ref.
	• Fluorescent Cu-metal-organic frameworks (MOFs) /aptamer nanoprobe created by integrating 2D Cu-MOF nanosheets with fluorescent dye 6-carboxyfluorescein (FAM) tagged ATP aptamers • ATP disintegrates FAM-aptamer from Cu-MOF nanosheets, resulting in a strong fluorescence signal	Intracellular adenosine triphosphate (ATP) level monitoring	4.24 μM	• Highly sensitive and selective ATP level measurement spanning from 10 to 800 μm • It also detects the undulation of ATP caused by pharmacological stimulation in real time	[149]

(*Continued*)

TABLE 5.3 (*Continued*)
Potential Point of Care DNA Nanoplatforms Based on DNA-Integrated Organic/Inorganic and 2D Nanomaterials

DNA Nanotechnology	Components/Working Mechanism	Target Disease/ Pathogen/ Disease-Related Biomarkers	Detection Limit	Key Features	Ref.
	• Λ exonuclease (λ exo) cleavage reaction and δ-FeOOH nanosheet–based platform • A 5-phosphoryl altered double-stranded DNA probe (5-P-dsDNA) was developed as an ALP substrate, and a 5-dye-labelled single-stranded DNA/-FeOOH system was developed as a detecting device • In absence of ALP, 5-P-dsdna destroyed by exo to produce mononucleotides. The detecting unit's fluorescence is quenched • In the presence of ALP, 5-phosphate functional group of 5-P-dsDNA, which had been removed to create 5-hydroxyl-dsDNA, could no longer be digested by exo. The dye-labelled single-stranded DNA then hybridised with the 5-hydroxyl-dsDNA to produce a triplex DNA (tsDNA), which resulted in enhanced fluorescence due to tsDNA's poor binding to the -FeOOH nanosheet	Alkaline phosphatase (ALP) activity	0.02 mU/mL	• Magnetically controlled 2D nano-DNA fluorescence sensor • Sensitive and selective detection • High signal-to-background ratio through magnetic separation	[150]

a comparison to graphene and graphene oxides, which have minimal or no band gaps, make MoS_2 NSs ideal for sensors capable of detecting DNA, proteins, metal ions, and other biomarkers [135,137,138]. Many recent studies demonstrating the application of such 2D nanomaterials for the successful preparation of POC DNA-nanotechnological platforms are given in Table 5.3·

5.5 CONCLUSION

Over the last few years, several novel POC diagnostic techniques have been introduced in academic research and clinical settings. POC devices optimise diagnosis procedures, improve therapy management, and enable efficient and cost-effective clinical results by offering quick and accurate analysis at the patient's site. Furthermore, a vast amount of research has proved the functioning of DNA as a building block of nanostructures with the establishment of DNA nanotechnology. DNA can self-assemble into a functional nanostructure via the Watson–Crick base pairing, which is being studied extensively for POC diagnostics. Because of the strong programmability of DNA, it is possible to create and assemble a wide range of well-defined 2D and 3D nanostructures. Furthermore, interactions between DNA and biomolecules may be carefully constructed and considerably optimised at the nanoscale, resulting in a large enhancement in biologically responsive sensitivity and selectivity. Different biomarkers and moieties like NAs, proteins, miRNAs, cancer cells, and viruses may be identified using DNA tetrahedron, DNA hydrogel, or signal amplification–based DNA assemblies. Chemical modifications of DNA enable the addition of functional groups to DNA nanostructures, culminating in the development of multifunctional diagnostic nanoplatforms. Moreover, DNA can be used more efficiently in POC diagnostics by integrating it with a range of nanomaterials, such as gold nanomaterials, nanosheets, fluorescent nanoparticles, and magnetic nanoparticles, which reduces their chance of being damaged by intracellular nuclease [151–153].

Although DNA nanotechnology has made significant advances in the domain of diagnostics, there are still some critical difficulties that need to be addressed. For instance, as the size of DNA nanostructures grows, the error rate of self-assembly also increases. As a result, it is critical to explore the kinetic and thermodynamic factors of assembly to build a greatly proficient approach with precise control over the self-assembly approaches. Besides, the biosafety of DNA nanostructures should be thoroughly investigated. DNA is inherently biocompatible and biodegradable. However, when DNA is created as a nanostructure, undesirable immune responses may be generated. As a result, the potential immunostimulatory effects of DNA nanostructures must be thoroughly explored before they are used in healthcare settings. Moreover, modified nucleotides can be developed further to greatly expand the library of DNA sequences and allow access to new features. Finally, intelligent techniques must be devised to commercialise DNA nanotechnology–based POC devices. Overall, we are confident that these issues will be overcome soon and that more functional and intelligent DNA-based nanomaterials for POC diagnostics will be established.

REFERENCES

1. Xiong Y, Zhang J, Yang Z, Mou Q, Ma Y, Xiong Y, et al. Functional DNA regulated CRISPR-Cas12a sensors for point-of-care diagnostics of non-nucleic-acid targets. *J Am Chem Soc.* 2020 Jan 8;142(1):207–13. Available from: https://pubmed.ncbi.nlm.nih.gov/31800219.
2. Tram DTN, Wang H, Sugiarto S, Li T, Ang WH, Lee C, et al. Advances in nanomaterials and their applications in point of care (POC) devices for the diagnosis of infectious diseases. *Biotechnol Adv.* 2016 Dec;34(8):1275–88. Available from: https://pubmed.ncbi.nlm.nih.gov/27686397.
3. Vashist SK. Point-of-care diagnostics: Recent advances and trends. *Biosensors (Basel).* 2017 Dec 18;7(4):62. Available from: https://pubmed.ncbi.nlm.nih.gov/29258285.
4. Sachdeva S, Davis RW, Saha AK. Microfluidic point-of-care testing: Commercial landscape and future directions. *Front Bioeng Biotechnol.* 2021 Jan 15;8:602659. Available from: https://pubmed.ncbi.nlm.nih.gov/33520958.
5. Chandrasekaran AR, Punnoose JA, Zhou L, Dey P, Dey BK, Halvorsen K. DNA nanotechnology approaches for microRNA detection and diagnosis. *Nucleic Acids Res.* 2019 Nov 18;47(20):10489–505. Available from: https://pubmed.ncbi.nlm.nih.gov/31287874.
6. Hu Q, Li H, Wang L, Gu H, Fan C. DNA nanotechnology-enabled drug delivery systems. *Chem Rev.* 2018;119(10):6459–506. Available from: https://doi.org/10.1021/acs.chemrev.7b00663.
7. Norouzi A, Ravan H, Mohammadi A, Hosseinzadeh E, Norouzi M, Fozooni T. Aptamer-integrated DNA nanoassembly: A simple and sensitive DNA framework to detect cancer cells. *Anal Chim Acta.* 2018;1017:26–33. Available from: https://doi.org/10.1016/j.aca.2018.02.037.
8. Shen L, Wang P, Ke Y. DNA nanotechnology-based biosensors and therapeutics. *Adv Healthc Mater.* 2021;10(15):2002205. Available from: https://doi.org/10.1002/adhm.202002205.
9. Zhang J, Wang G, Zhou Y, Chen Y, Ouyang L, Liu B. Mechanisms of autophagy and relevant small-molecule compounds for targeted cancer therapy. *Cellular and Molecular Life Sciences.* 2018;75(10):1803–26. Available from: https://doi.org/10.1007/s00018-018-2759-2.
10. He Y, Ye T, Su M, Zhang C, Ribbe AE, Jiang W, et al. Hierarchical self-assembly of DNA into symmetric supramolecular polyhedra. *Nature.* 2008;452(7184):198–201. Available from: https://doi.org/10.1038/nature06597.
11. Gothelf KV, Brown RS. A modular approach to DNA-programmed self-assembly of macromolecular nanostructures. *Chem A Eur J.* 2005;11(4):1062–9. Available from: https://doi.org/10.1002/chem.200400646.
12. Venkadesh A, Mathiyarasu J, Dave S, Radhakrishnan S. Amine mediated synthesis of nickel oxide nanoparticles and their superior electrochemical sensing performance for glucose detection. *Inorg Chem Commun* 2021;131:108779. https://doi.org/10.1016/j.inoche.2021.108779.
13. Kumar S, Pearse A, Liu Y, Taylor RE. Modular self-assembly of gamma-modified peptide nucleic acids in organic solvent mixtures. *Nat Commun.* 2020 Jun 11;11(1):2960. Available from: https://pubmed.ncbi.nlm.nih.gov/32528008.
14. Liu Y, Yan H. Modular self-assembly of DNA lattices with tunable periodicity. *Small.* 2005;1(3):327–30. Available from: https://doi.org/10.1002/smll.200400104.

15. Zhang F, Jiang S, Li W, Hunt A, Liu Y, Yan H. Self-assembly of complex DNA tessellations by using low-symmetry multi-arm DNA Tiles. *Angew Chem Int Ed*. 2016;55(31):8860–3. Available from: https://doi.org/10.1002/anie.201601944.
16. Bhatia D, Mehtab S, Krishnan R, Indi SS, Basu A, Krishnan Y. Icosahedral DNA nanocapsules by modular assembly. *Angew Chem Int Ed*. 2009;48(23):4134–7. Available from: https://doi.org/10.1002/anie.200806000.
17. Xie N, Liu S, Fang H, Yang Y, Quan K, Li J, et al. Three-dimensional molecular transfer from DNA nanocages to inner gold nanoparticle surfaces. *ACS Nano*. 2019;13(4):4174–82. Available from: https://doi.org/10.1021/acsnano.8b09147.
18. Rothemund PWK. Folding DNA to create nanoscale shapes and patterns. *Nature*. 2006;440(7082):297–302. Available from: https://doi.org/10.1038/nature04586.
19. Qian L, Wang Y, Zhang Z, Zhao J, Pan D, Zhang Y, et al. Analogic China map constructed by DNA. *Chin Sci Bull*. 2006;51(24):2973–6. Available from: https://doi.org/10.1007/s11434-006-2223-9.
20. Pound E, Ashton JR, Becerril HA, Woolley AT. Polymerase chain reaction based scaffold preparation for the production of thin, branched DNA origami nanostructures of arbitrary sizes. *Nano Lett*. 2009;9(12):4302–5. Available from: https://doi.org/10.1021/nl902535q.
21. Zhang F, Jiang S, Wu S, Li Y, Mao C, Liu Y, et al. Complex wireframe DNA origami nanostructures with multi-arm junction vertices. *Nat Nanotechnol*. 2015;10(9):779–84. Available from: https://doi.org/10.1038/nnano.2015.162.
22. Hong F, Jiang S, Wang T, Liu Y, Yan H. 3D framework DNA origami with layered crossovers. *Angew Chem Int Ed*. 2016;55(41):12832–5. Available from: https://doi.org/10.1002/anie.201607050.
23. Andersen ES, Dong M, Nielsen MM, Jahn K, Subramani R, Mamdouh W, et al. Self-assembly of a nanoscale DNA box with a controllable lid. *Nature*. 2009;459(7243):73–6. Available from: https://doi.org/10.1038/nature07971.
24. Kershner RJ, Bozano LD, Micheel CM, Hung AM, Fornof AR, Cha JN, et al. Placement and orientation of individual DNA shapes on lithographically patterned surfaces. *Nat Nanotechnol*. 2009;4(9):557–61. Available from: https://doi.org/10.1038/nnano.2009.220.
25. Maune HT, Han S-P, Barish RD, Bockrath M, Goddard III WA, Rothemund PWK, et al. Self-assembly of carbon nanotubes into two-dimensional geometries using DNA origami templates. *Nat Nanotechnol*. 2009;5(1):61–6. Available from: https://doi.org/10.1038/nnano.2009.311.
26. Steinhauer C, Jungmann R, Sobey T, Simmel F, Tinnefeld P. DNA origami as a nanoscopic ruler for super-resolution microscopy. *Angew Chem Int Ed*. 2009;48(47):8870–3. Available from: https://doi.org/10.1002/anie.200903308.
27. Voigt NV, Tørring T, Rotaru A, Jacobsen MF, Ravnsbæk JB, Subramani R, et al. Single-molecule chemical reactions on DNA origami. *Nat Nanotechnol*. 2010;5(3):200–3. Available from: https://doi.org/10.1038/nnano.2010.5.
28. Douglas SM, Dietz H, Liedl T, Högberg B, Graf F, Shih WM. Self-assembly of DNA into nanoscale three-dimensional shapes. *Nature*. 2009 May 21;459(7245):414–8. Available from: https://pubmed.ncbi.nlm.nih.gov/19458720.
29. Dietz H, Douglas SM, Shih WM. Folding DNA into twisted and curved nanoscale shapes. *Science*. 2009 Aug 7;325(5941):725–30. Available from: https://pubmed.ncbi.nlm.nih.gov/19661424.
30. Han D, Pal S, Nangreave J, Deng Z, Liu Y, Yan H. DNA origami with complex curvatures in three-dimensional space. *Science*. 2011;332(6027):342–6. Available from: https://doi.org/10.1126/science.1202998.

31. Sun W, Boulais E, Hakobyan Y, Wang WL, Guan A, Bathe M, et al. Casting inorganic structures with DNA molds. *Science*. 2014 Nov 7;346(6210):1258361. Available from: https://pubmed.ncbi.nlm.nih.gov/25301973.
32. Ye J, Helmi S, Teske J, Seidel R. Fabrication of metal nanostructures with programmable length and patterns using a modular DNA platform. *Nano Lett.* 2019;19(4):2707–14. Available from: https://doi.org/10.1021/acs.nanolett.9b00740.
33. Bayrak T, Helmi S, Ye J, Kauert D, Kelling J, Schönherr T, et al. DNA-mold templated assembly of conductive gold nanowires. *Nano Lett.* 2018;18(3):2116–23. Available from: https://doi.org/10.1021/acs.nanolett.8b00344.
34. Ye J, Weichelt R, Kemper U, Gupta V, König TAF, Eychmüller A, et al. Casting of gold nanoparticles with high aspect ratios inside DNA molds. *Small.* 2020;16(39):2003662. Available from: https://doi.org/10.1002/smll.202003662.
35. Kuzyk A, Schreiber R, Fan Z, Pardatscher G, Roller EM, Högele A, et al. DNA-based self-assembly of chiral plasmonic nanostructures with tailored optical response. *Nature.* 2012;483(7389):311–4. Available from: https://doi.org/10.1038/nature10889.
36. Liu X, Zhang F, Jing X, Pan M, Liu P, Li W, et al. Complex silica composite nanomaterials templated with DNA origami. *Nature.* 2018;559(7715):593–8. Available from: https://doi.org/10.1038/s41586-018-0332-7.
37. Nguyen L, Döblinger M, Liedl T, Heuer-Jungemann A. DNA-origami-templated silica growth by sol-gel chemistry. *Angew Chem Int Ed.* 2019;58(3):912–6. Available from: https://doi.org/10.1002/anie.201811323.
38. Nguyen MK, Nguyen VH, Natarajan AK, Huang Y, Ryssy J, Shen B, et al. Ultrathin silica coating of DNA origami nanostructures. *Chem Mater.* 2020;32(15):6657–65. Available from: https://doi.org/10.1021/acs.chemmater.0c02111.
39. Meyer TA, Zhang C, Bao G, Ke Y. Programmable assembly of iron oxide nanoparticles using DNA origami. *Nano Lett.* 2020 Apr 8;20(4):2799–805. Available from: https://pubmed.ncbi.nlm.nih.gov/32208663.
40. Zhu D, Pei H, Yao G, Wang L, Su S, Chao J, et al. A surface-confined proton-driven DNA pump using a dynamic 3D DNA scaffold. *Adv Mater.* 2016;28(32):6860–5. Available from: https://doi.org/10.1002/adma.201506407.
41. Li Z, Wang J, Li Y, Liu X, Yuan Q. Self-assembled DNA nanomaterials with highly programmed structures and functions. *Mater Chem Front.* 2018;2(3):423–36. Available from: https://doi.org/10.1039/c7qm00434f.
42. Yu LX, Zhai R, Gong XY, Xie J, Huang ZJ, Liu MY, et al. Progress in DNA tetrahedral nanomaterials and their functionalization research. *Chin J Anal Chem.* 2019;47(11):1742–50. Available from: https://doi.org/10.1016/s1872-2040(19)61198-9.
43. Li Z, Zhao B, Wang D, Wen Y, Liu G, Dong H, et al. DNA nanostructure-based universal microarray platform for high-efficiency multiplex bioanalysis in biofluids. *ACS Appl Mater Interfaces.* 2014;6(20):17944–53. Available from: https://doi.org/10.1021/am5047735.
44. Pei H, Zuo X, Zhu D, Huang Q, Fan C. Functional DNA nanostructures for theranostic applications. *Acc Chem Res.* 2013;47(2):550–9. Available from: https://doi.org/10.1021/ar400195t.
45. Shiu SCC, Fraser LA, Ding Y, Tanner JA. Aptamer display on diverse DNA polyhedron supports. *Molecules.* 2018 Jul 11;23(7):1695. Available from: https://pubmed.ncbi.nlm.nih.gov/29997372.
46. Mo L, Li J, Liu Q, Qiu L, Tan W. Nucleic acid-functionalized transition metal nanosheets for biosensing applications. *Biosens Bioelectron.* 2017 Mar 15;89(Pt 1):201–11. Available from: https://pubmed.ncbi.nlm.nih.gov/27020066.

47. Walsh AS, Yin H, Erben CM, Wood MJA, Turberfield AJ. DNA cage delivery to mammalian cells. *ACS Nano.* 2011;5(7):5427–32. Available from: https://doi.org/10.1021/nn2005574.
48. Zhao Y, Guo LJ, Dai JB, Li Q, Li D, Wang LH. Application progress of DNA nanostructures in drug delivery and smart drug carriers. *Chin J Anal Chem.* 2017;45(7):1078–87. Available from: https://doi.org/10.1016/s1872-2040(17)61027-2.
49. Xie N, Liu S, Yang X, He X, Huang J, Wang K. DNA tetrahedron nanostructures for biological applications: Biosensors and drug delivery. *Analyst.* 2017;142(18):3322–32. Available from: https://doi.org/10.1039/c7an01154g.
50. Ahmed EM. Hydrogel: Preparation, characterization, and applications: A review. *J Adv Res.* 2015 Mar;6(2):105–21. Available from: https://pubmed.ncbi.nlm.nih.gov/25750745.
51. Chai Q, Jiao Y, Yu X. Hydrogels for biomedical applications: Their characteristics and the mechanisms behind them. *Gels.* 2017 Jan 24;3(1):6. Available from: https://pubmed.ncbi.nlm.nih.gov/30920503.
52. Yu X, Jiao Y, Chai Q. Applications of gold nanoparticles in biosensors. *Nano Life.* 2016;06(02):1642001. Available from: https://doi.org/10.1142/s1793984416420010.
53. Pan L, Yu G, Zhai D, Lee HR, Zhao W, Liu N, et al. Hierarchical nanostructured conducting polymer hydrogel with high electrochemical activity. *Proc Natl Acad Sci USA.* 2012 Jun 12;109(24):9287–92. Available from: https://pubmed.ncbi.nlm.nih.gov/22645374.
54. Billiet T, Vandenhaute M, Schelfhout J, Van Vlierberghe S, Dubruel P. A review of trends and limitations in hydrogel-rapid prototyping for tissue engineering. *Biomaterials.* 2012;33(26):6020–41. Available from: https://doi.org/10.1016/j.biomaterials.2012.04.050.
55. Zhu X, Mao X, Wang Z, Feng C, Chen G, Li G. Fabrication of nanozyme@DNA hydrogel and its application in biomedical analysis. *Nano Res.* 2016;10(3):959–70. Available from: https://doi.org/10.1007/s12274-016-1354-9.
56. Marmur J, Doty P. Thermal renaturation of deoxyribonucleic acids. *J Mol Biol.* 1961;3(5):585–94. Available from: https://doi.org/10.1016/s0022-2836(61)80023-5.
57. Choi J, Kim S, Tachikawa T, Fujitsuka M, Majima T. pH-induced intramolecular folding dynamics of i-Motif DNA. *J Am Chem Soc.* 2011;133(40):16146–53. Available from: https://doi.org/10.1021/ja2061984.
58. Kuwahara M, Sugimoto N. Molecular evolution of functional nucleic acids with chemical modifications. *Molecules.* 2010 Aug 9;15(8):5423–44. Available from: https://pubmed.ncbi.nlm.nih.gov/20714306.
59. Li J, Mo L, Lu CH, Fu T, Yang HH, Tan W. Functional nucleic acid-based hydrogels for bioanalytical and biomedical applications. *Chem Soc Rev.* 2016 Mar 7;45(5):1410–31. Available from: https://pubmed.ncbi.nlm.nih.gov/26758955.
60. Khajouei S, Ravan H, Ebrahimi A. DNA hydrogel-empowered biosensing. *Adv Colloid Interface Sci.* 2020 Jan;275:102060. Available from: https://pubmed.ncbi.nlm.nih.gov/31739981.
61. Lu X, Liu J, Wu X, Ding B. Multifunctional DNA origami nanoplatforms for drug delivery. *Chem Asian J.* 2019;14(13):2193–202. Available from: https://doi.org/10.1002/asia.201900574.
62. Kahn JS, Hu Y, Willner I. Stimuli-responsive DNA-based hydrogels: From basic principles to applications. *Acc Chem Res.* 2017;50(4):680–90. Available from: https://doi.org/10.1021/acs.accounts.6b00542.
63. Wang H, Luo D, Wang H, Wang F, Liu X. Construction of smart stimuli-responsive DNA nanostructures for biomedical applications. *Chem A Eur J.* 2020;27(12):3929–43. Available from: https://doi.org/10.1002/chem.202003145.

64. Wang D, Hu Y, Liu P, Luo D. Bioresponsive DNA hydrogels: Beyond the conventional stimuli responsiveness. *Acc Chem Res*. 2017;50(4):733–9. Available from: https://doi.org/10.1021/acs.accounts.6b00581.
65. Pan J, He Y, Liu Z, Chen J. Tetrahedron-based constitutional dynamic network for COVID-19 or other coronaviruses diagnostics and its logic gate applications. *Anal Chem*. 2021;94(2):714–22. Available from: https://doi.org/10.1021/acs.analchem.1c03051.
66. Gao X, Li X, Sun X, Zhang J, Zhao Y, Liu X, et al. DNA tetrahedra-cross-linked hydrogel functionalized paper for onsite analysis of DNA methyltransferase activity using a personal glucose meter. *Anal Chem*. 2020;92(6):4592–9. Available from: https://doi.org/10.1021/acs.analchem.0c00018.
67. Su J, Wu F, Xia H, Wu Y, Liu S. Accurate cancer cell identification and microRNA silencing induced therapy using tailored DNA tetrahedron nanostructures. *Chem Sci*. 2019 Nov 5;11(1):80–6. Available from: https://pubmed.ncbi.nlm.nih.gov/32110359.
68. Wang D, Li S, Zhao Z, Zhang X, Tan W. Engineering a second-order DNA logic-gated nanorobot to sense and release on live cell membranes for multiplexed diagnosis and synergistic therapy. *Angew Chem Int Ed*. 2021;60(29):15816–20. Available from: https://doi.org/10.1002/anie.202103993.
69. Ou D, Sun D, Liang Z, Chen B, Lin X, Chen Z. A novel cytosensor for capture, detection and release of breast cancer cells based on metal organic framework PCN-224 and DNA tetrahedron linked dual-aptamer. *Sens Actuators B Chem*. 2019;285:398–404. Available from: https://doi.org/10.1016/j.snb.2019.01.079.
70. Chen M, Wang Y, Zhao X, Zhang J, Peng Y, Bai J, et al. Target-responsive DNA hydrogel with microfluidic chip smart readout for quantitative point-of-care testing of creatine kinase MB. *Talanta*. 2022;243:123338. Available from: https://doi.org/10.1016/j.talanta.2022.123338.
71. Jiang C, Li Y, Wang H, Chen D, Wen Y. A portable visual capillary sensor based on functional DNA crosslinked hydrogel for point-of-care detection of lead ion. *Sens Actuators B Chem*. 2020;307:127625. Available from: https://doi.org/10.1016/j.snb.2019.127625.
72. Huang D, Ni D, Fang M, Shi Z, Xu Z. Microfluidic ruler-readout and CRISPR Cas12a-responded hydrogel-integrated paper-based analytical devices (μReaCH-PAD) for visible quantitative point-of-care testing of invasive fungi. *Anal Chem*. 2021;93(50):16965–73. Available from: https://doi.org/10.1021/acs.analchem.1c04649.
73. Lin Y, Huang Y, Yang Y, Jiang L, Xing C, Li J, et al. Functional self-assembled DNA nanohydrogels for specific telomerase activity imaging and telomerase-activated antitumor gene therapy. *Anal Chem*. 2020;92(22):15179–86. Available from: https://doi.org/10.1021/acs.analchem.0c03746.
74. Yao S, Xiang L, Wang L, Gong H, Chen F, Cai C. pH-responsive DNA hydrogels with ratiometric fluorescence for accurate detection of miRNA-21. *Anal Chim Acta*. 2022;1207:339795. Available from: https://doi.org/10.1016/j.aca.2022.339795.
75. Mao X, Pan S, Zhou D, He X, Zhang Y. Fabrication of DNAzyme-functionalized hydrogel and its application for visible detection of circulating tumor DNA. *Sens Actuators B Chem*. 2019;285:385–90. Available from: https://doi.org/10.1016/j.snb.2019.01.076.
76. Liu S, Su W, Li Y, Zhang L, Ding X. Manufacturing of an electrochemical biosensing platform based on hybrid DNA hydrogel: Taking lung cancer-specific miR-21 as an example. *Biosens Bioelectron*. 2018;103:1–5. Available from: https://doi.org/10.1016/j.bios.2017.12.021.

77. Zheng L, Qi P, Zhang D. DNA-templated fluorescent silver nanoclusters for sensitive detection of pathogenic bacteria based on MNP-DNAzyme-AChE complex. *Sens Actuators B Chem.* 2018;276:42–7. Available from: https://doi.org/10.1016/j.snb.2018.08.078.
78. Jain KK. Principles of personalized oncology. In: *Textbook of Personalized Medicine*. Cham: Springer International Publishing; 2021. pp. 403–78. https://doi.org/10.1007/978-3-030-62080-6_19.
79. Reisch A, Klymchenko AS. Fluorescent polymer nanoparticles based on dyes: Seeking brighter tools for bioimaging. *Small.* 2016 Apr;12(15):1968–92. Available from: https://pubmed.ncbi.nlm.nih.gov/26901678.
80. Kumar Thiyagarajan S, Raghupathy S, Palanivel D, Raji K, Ramamurthy P. Fluorescent carbon nano dots from lignite: Unveiling the impeccable evidence for quantum confinement. *Phys Chem Chem Phys.* 2016;18(17):12065–73. Available from: https://doi.org/10.1039/c6cp00867d.
81. Wolfbeis OS. An overview of nanoparticles commonly used in fluorescent bioimaging. *Chem Soc Rev.* 2015;44(14):4743–68. Available from: https://doi.org/10.1039/c4cs00392f.
82. McConnell EM, Cozma I, Mou Q, Brennan JD, Lu Y, Li Y. Biosensing with DNAzymes. *Chem Soc Rev.* 2021 Aug 21;50(16):8954–94. Available from: https://pubmed.ncbi.nlm.nih.gov/34227631.
83. Cozma I, McConnell EM, Brennan JD, Li Y. DNAzymes as key components of biosensing systems for the detection of biological targets. *Biosens Bioelectron.* 2021;177:112972. Available from: https://doi.org/10.1016/j.bios.2021.112972.
84. Yue X, Qiao Y, Gu D, Wu Z, Zhao W, Li X, et al. Reliable FRET-ON imaging of telomerase in living cells by a tetrahedral DNA nanoprobe integrated with structure-switchable molecular beacon. *Sens Actuators B Chem.* 2020;312:127943. Available from: https://doi.org/10.1016/j.snb.2020.127943.
85. Liu L, He F, Yu Y, Wang Y. Application of FRET biosensors in mechanobiology and mechanopharmacological screening. *Front Bioeng Biotechnol.* 2020 Nov 9;8:595497. Available from: https://pubmed.ncbi.nlm.nih.gov/33240867.
86. Afzalinia A, Mirzaee M. Ultrasensitive fluorescent miRNA biosensor based on a "Sandwich" oligonucleotide hybridization and fluorescence resonance energy transfer process using an Ln(III)-MOF and Ag nanoparticles for early cancer diagnosis: Application of central composite design. *ACS Appl Mater Interfaces.* 2020;12(14):16076–87. Available from: https://doi.org/10.1021/acsami.0c00891
87. Fu Z, Lu YC, Lai JJ. Recent advances in biosensors for nucleic acid and exosome detection. *Chonnam Med J.* 2019 May;55(2):86–98. Available from: https://pubmed.ncbi.nlm.nih.gov/31161120.
88. Chambers JP, Arulanandam BP, Matta LL, Weis A, Valdes JJ. Biosensor recognition elements. *Curr Issues Mol Biol.* 2008;10:1–12 Available from: https://doi.org/10.21775/cimb.010.001.
89. Tahamtan A, Ardebili A. Real-time RT-PCR in COVID-19 detection: Issues affecting the results. *Expert Rev Mol Diagn.* 2020 May;20(5):453–4. Available from: https://pubmed.ncbi.nlm.nih.gov/32297805.
90. Sánchez Martín D, Oropesa-Nuñez R, de la Torre TZG Formation of visible aggregates between rolling circle amplification products and magnetic nanoparticles as a strategy for point-of-care diagnostics. *ACS Omega.* 2021 Nov 23;6(48):32970–6. Available from: https://pubmed.ncbi.nlm.nih.gov/34901648.
91. Lau HY, Botella JR. Advanced DNA-based point-of-care diagnostic methods for plant diseases detection. *Front Plant Sci.* 2017 Dec 6;8:2016. Available from: https://pubmed.ncbi.nlm.nih.gov/29375588.

92. Li T, Duan R, Duan Z, Huang F, Xia F. Fluorescence signal amplification strategies based on DNA nanotechnology for miRNA detection. *Chem Res Chin Univ.* 2019;36(2):194–202. Available from: https://doi.org/10.1007/s40242-019-0031-4.
93. Dirks RM, Pierce NA. Triggered amplification by hybridization chain reaction. *Proc Natl Acad Sci USA.* 2004 Oct 26;101(43):15275–8. Available from: https://pubmed.ncbi.nlm.nih.gov/15492210.
94. Li B, Ellington AD, Chen X. Rational, modular adaptation of enzyme-free DNA circuits to multiple detection methods. *Nucleic Acids Res.* 2011 Sep 1;39(16):e110–e110. Available from: https://pubmed.ncbi.nlm.nih.gov/21693555.
95. Luo Z, Li Y, Zhang P, He L, Feng Y, Feng Y, et al. Catalytic hairpin assembly as cascade nucleic acid circuits for fluorescent biosensor: Design, evolution and application. *TrAC Trends Anal Chem.* 2022;151:116582. Available from: https://doi.org/10.1016/j.trac.2022.116582.
96. Weng S, Lin D, Lai S, Tao H, Chen T, Peng M, et al. Highly sensitive and reliable detection of microRNA for clinically disease surveillance using SERS biosensor integrated with catalytic hairpin assembly amplification technology. *Biosens Bioelectron.* 2022;208:114236. Available from: https://doi.org/10.1016/j.bios.2022.114236.
97. Liu J, Zhang Y, Xie H, Zhao L, Zheng L, Ye H. Applications of catalytic hairpin assembly reaction in biosensing. *Small.* 2019;15(42):1902989. Available from: https://doi.org/10.1002/smll.201902989.
98. Zheng AX, Li J, Wang JR, Song XR, Chen GN, Yang HH. Enzyme-free signal amplification in the DNAzyme sensor via target-catalyzed hairpin assembly. *Chem Commun.* 2012;48(25):3112. Available from: https://doi.org/10.1039/c2cc30305a.
99. Li F, Zhang H, Wang Z, Li X, Li XF, Le XC. Dynamic DNA assemblies mediated by binding-induced DNA strand displacement. *J Am Chem Soc.* 2013 Feb 20;135(7):2443–6. Available from: https://pubmed.ncbi.nlm.nih.gov/23360527.
100. Wei J, Gong X, Wang Q, Pan M, Liu X, Liu J, et al. Construction of an autonomously concatenated hybridization chain reaction for signal amplification and intracellular imaging. *Chem Sci.* 2017 Oct 23;9(1):52–61. Available from: https://pubmed.ncbi.nlm.nih.gov/29629073.
101. Li B, Chen X, Ellington AD. Adapting enzyme-free DNA circuits to the detection of loop-mediated isothermal amplification reactions. *Anal Chem.* 2012 Oct 2;84(19):8371–7. Available from: https://pubmed.ncbi.nlm.nih.gov/22947054.
102. Jiang YS, Li B, Milligan JN, Bhadra S, Ellington AD. Real-time detection of isothermal amplification reactions with thermostable catalytic hairpin assembly. *J Am Chem Soc.* 2013 May 22;135(20):7430–3. Available from: https://pubmed.ncbi.nlm.nih.gov/23647466.
103. Kimura Y, de Hoon MJL, Aoki S, Ishizu Y, Kawai Y, Kogo Y, et al. Optimization of turn-back primers in isothermal amplification. *Nucleic Acids Res.* 2011 May;39(9):e59. Available from: https://pubmed.ncbi.nlm.nih.gov/21310714.
104. Bi S, Yue S, Zhang S. Hybridization chain reaction: A versatile molecular tool for biosensing, bioimaging, and biomedicine. *Chem Soc Rev.* 2017;46(14):4281–98. Available from: https://doi.org/10.1039/c7cs00055c.
105. Wang W, Cai X, Li Q, Zheng L, Yu X, Zhang H, et al. Application of a microfluidic paper-based bioimmunosensor with laser-induced fluorescence detection in the determination of alpha-fetoprotein from serum of hepatopaths. *Talanta.* 2021;221:121660. Available from: https://doi.org/10.1016/j.talanta.2020.121660.
106. Chai H, Cheng W, Jin D, Miao P. Recent progress in DNA hybridization chain reaction strategies for amplified biosensing. *ACS Appl Mater Interfaces.* 2021;13(33):38931–46. Available from: https://doi.org/10.1021/acsami.1c09000.

107. Wang L, Zeng L, Wang Y, Chen T, Chen W, Chen G, et al. Electrochemical aptasensor based on multidirectional hybridization chain reaction for detection of tumorous exosomes. *Sens Actuators B Chem.* 2021;332:129471. Available from: https://doi.org/10.1016/j.snb.2021.129471.
108. Ji Y, Zhang L, Zhu L, Lei J, Wu J, Ju H. Binding-induced DNA walker for signal amplification in highly selective electrochemical detection of protein. *Biosens Bioelectron.* 2017;96:201–5. Available from: https://doi.org/10.1016/j.bios.2017.05.008.
109. Liu S, Wang Y, Ming J, Lin Y, Cheng C, Li F. Enzyme-free and ultrasensitive electrochemical detection of nucleic acids by target catalyzed hairpin assembly followed with hybridization chain reaction. *Biosens Bioelectron.* 2013;49:472–7. Available from: https://doi.org/10.1016/j.bios.2013.05.037.
110. Qu X, Zhu D, Yao G, Su S, Chao J, Liu H, et al. An exonuclease III-powered, on-particle stochastic DNA walker. *Angew Chem Int Ed.* 2017;56(7):1855–8. Available from: https://doi.org/10.1002/anie.201611777.
111. Yehl K, Mugler A, Vivek S, Liu Y, Zhang Y, Fan M, et al. High-speed DNA-based rolling motors powered by RNase H. *Nat Nanotechnol.* 2016 Feb;11(2):184–90. Available from: https://pubmed.ncbi.nlm.nih.gov/26619152.
112. Pan J, Li F, Cha TG, Chen H, Choi JH. Recent progress on DNA based walkers. *Curr Opin Biotechnol.* 2015;34:56–64. Available from: https://doi.org/10.1016/j.copbio.2014.11.017.
113. Awaja F, Wakelin EA, Sage J, Altaee A. Description of DNA molecular motion for nanotechnology applications. *Prog Mater Sci.* 2015;74:308–31. Available from: https://doi.org/10.1016/j.pmatsci.2015.03.001.
114. Jung C, Allen PB, Ellington AD. A stochastic DNA walker that traverses a microparticle surface. *Nat Nanotechnol.* 2016 Feb;11(2):157–63. Available from: https://pubmed.ncbi.nlm.nih.gov/26524397.
115. Xu H, Xia A, Wang D, Zhang Y, Deng S, Lu W, et al. An ultraportable and versatile point-of-care DNA testing platform. *Sci Adv.* 2020 Apr 22;6(17):eaaz7445. Available from: https://pubmed.ncbi.nlm.nih.gov/32426466.
116. Park BH, Oh SJ, Jung JH, Choi G, Seo JH, Kim DH, et al. An integrated rotary microfluidic system with DNA extraction, loop-mediated isothermal amplification, and lateral flow strip based detection for point-of-care pathogen diagnostics. *Biosens Bioelectron.* 2017;91:334–40. Available from: https://doi.org/10.1016/j.bios.2016.11.063.
117. Yin C, Wu Y, Li X, Niu J, Lei J, Ding X, et al. Highly selective, naked-eye, and trace discrimination between perfect-match and mismatch sequences using a plasmonic nanoplatform. *Anal Chem.* 2018;90(12):7371–6. Available from: https://doi.org/10.1021/acs.analchem.8b00756.
118. Wang L, Liu ZJ, Cao HX, Liang GX. Ultrasensitive colorimetric miRNA detection based on magnetic 3D DNA walker and unmodified AuNPs. *Sens Actuators B Chem.* 2021;337:129813. Available from: https://doi.org/10.1016/j.snb.2021.129813.
119. Deng X, Liu X, Wu S, Zang S, Lin X, Zhao Y, et al. Ratiometric fluorescence imaging of intracellular MicroRNA with NIR-assisted signal amplification by a Ru-SiO_2@Polydopamine nanoplatform. *ACS Appl Mater Interfaces.* 2021;13(38):45214–23. Available from: https://doi.org/10.1021/acsami.1c11324.
120. Li P, Yu X, Han W, Kong Y, Bao W, Zhang J, et al. Ultrasensitive and reversible nanoplatform of urinary exosomes for prostate cancer diagnosis. *ACS Sens.* 2019;4(5):1433–41. Available from: https://doi.org/10.1021/acssensors.9b00621.

121. Sivakumar R, Dinh VP, Lee NY. Ultraviolet-induced *in situ* gold nanoparticles for point-of-care testing of infectious diseases in loop-mediated isothermal amplification. *Lab Chip.* 2021;21(4):700–9. Available from: https://doi.org/10.1039/d1lc00019e.
122. Liu L, Rong Q, Ke G, Zhang M, Li J, Li Y, et al. Efficient and reliable MicroRNA imaging in living cells via a FRET-based localized hairpin-DNA cascade amplifier. *Anal Chem.* 2019;91(5):3675–80. Available from: https://doi.org/10.1021/acs.analchem.8b05778.
123. Zhao H, Wang M, Xiong X, Liu Y, Chen X. Simultaneous fluorescent detection of multiplexed miRNA of liver cancer based on DNA tetrahedron nanotags. *Talanta.* 2020;210:120677. Available from: https://doi.org/10.1016/j.talanta.2019.120677.
124. Cheong J, Yu H, Lee CY, Lee JU, Choi HJ, Lee JH, et al. Fast detection of SARS-CoV-2 RNA via the integration of plasmonic thermocycling and fluorescence detection in a portable device. *Nat Biomed Eng.* 2020 Dec;4(12):1159–67. Available from: https://pubmed.ncbi.nlm.nih.gov/33273713.
125. Lu Y, Liu J. Functional DNA nanotechnology: emerging applications of DNAzymes and aptamers. *Curr Opin Biotechnol.* 2006;17(6):580–8. Available from: https://doi.org/10.1016/j.copbio.2006.10.004.
126. Xing H, Hwang K, Li J, Torabi SF, Lu Y. DNA aptamer technology for personalized medicine. *Curr Opin Chem Eng.* 2014 May 1;4:79–87. Available from: https://pubmed.ncbi.nlm.nih.gov/24791224.
127. Breaker RR. DNA aptamers and DNA enzymes. *Curr Opin Chem Biol.* 1997;1(1):26–31. Available from: https://doi.org/10.1016/s1367-5931(97)80105-6.
128. Li L, Xing H, Zhang J, Lu Y. Functional DNA molecules enable selective and stimuli-responsive nanoparticles for biomedical applications. *Acc Chem Res.* 2019 Sep 17;52(9):2415–26. Available from: https://pubmed.ncbi.nlm.nih.gov/31411853.
129. Yrad FM, Castañares JM, Alocilja EC. Visual detection of Dengue-1 RNA using gold nanoparticle-based lateral flow biosensor. *Diagnostics (Basel).* 2019 Jul 11;9(3):74. Available from: https://pubmed.ncbi.nlm.nih.gov/31336721.
130. Campos EVR, de Oliveira JL, Abrantes DC, Rogério CB, Bueno C, Miranda VR, et al. Recent developments in nanotechnology for detection and control of aedes aegypti-borne diseases. *Front Bioeng Biotechnol.* 2020 Feb 20;8:102.
131. Sun Z, Wu S, Ma J, Shi H, Wang L, Sheng A, et al. Colorimetric sensor array for human semen identification designed by coupling zirconium metal-organic frameworks with dna-modified gold nanoparticles. *ACS Appl Mater Interfaces.* 2019;11(40):36316–23. Available from: https://doi.org/10.1021/acsami.9b10729.
132. Zhang H, Ba S, Yang Z, Wang T, Lee JY, Li T, et al. Graphene quantum dot-based nanocomposites for diagnosing cancer biomarker APE1 in living cells. *ACS Appl Mater & Interfaces.* 2020;12(12):13634–43. Available from: https://doi.org/10.1021/acsami.9b21385.
133. Fujii S, Kamiya K, Osaki T, Misawa N, Hayakawa M, Takeuchi S. Purification-free MicroRNA detection by using magnetically immobilized nanopores on liposome membrane. *Anal Chem.* 2018;90(17):10217–22. Available from: https://doi.org/10.1021/acs.analchem.8b01443.
134. Li Z, Wang G, Shen Y, Guo N, Ma N. DNA-templated magnetic nanoparticle-quantum dot polymers for ultrasensitive capture and detection of circulating tumor cells. *Adv Funct Mater.* 2018;28(14):1707152. Available from: https://doi.org/10.1002/adfm.201707152.

135. Nandwana V, Huang W, Li Y, Dravid VP. One-pot green synthesis of Fe_3O_4/MoS_2 0D/2D nanocomposites and their application in noninvasive point-of-care glucose diagnostics. *ACS Appl Nano Mater.* 2018;1(4):1949–58. Available from: https://doi.org/10.1021/acsanm.8b00429.
136. Jin H, Zhu T, Huang X, Sun M, Li H, Zhu X, et al. ROS-responsive nanoparticles based on amphiphilic hyperbranched polyphosphoester for drug delivery: Light-triggered size-reducing and enhanced tumor penetration. *Biomaterials.* 2019 Aug 1;211:68–80.
137. Singhal C, Khanuja M, Chaudhary N, Pundir CS, Narang J. Detection of chikungunya virus DNA using two-dimensional MoS(2) nanosheets based disposable biosensor. *Sci Rep.* 2018 May 16;8(1):7734. Available from: https://pubmed.ncbi.nlm.nih.gov/29769549.
138. Geldert A, Kenry, Lim CT. Paper-based MoS(2) nanosheet-mediated FRET aptasensor for rapid malaria diagnosis. *Sci Rep.* 2017 Dec 13;7(1):17510. Available from: https://pubmed.ncbi.nlm.nih.gov/29235484.
139. Miao P, Tang Y. Gold nanoparticles-based multipedal DNA walker for ratiometric detection of circulating tumor cell. *Anal Chem.* 2019;91(23):15187–92. Available from: https://doi.org/10.1021/acs.analchem.9b04000.
140. Steinmetz M, Lima D, Viana AG, Fujiwara ST, Pessôa CA, Etto RM, et al. A sensitive label-free impedimetric DNA biosensor based on silsesquioxane-functionalized gold nanoparticles for Zika Virus detection. *Biosens Bioelectron.* 2019;141:111351. Available from: https://doi.org/10.1016/j.bios.2019.111351.
141. Kshirsagar P, Seshacharyulu P, Muniyan S, Rachagani S, Smith LM, Thompson C, et al. DNA-gold nanoprobe-based integrated biosensing technology for non-invasive liquid biopsy of serum miRNA: A new frontier in prostate cancer diagnosis. *Nanomedicine.* 2022 Jul;43:102566. Available from: https://pubmed.ncbi.nlm.nih.gov/35569810.
142. Kiplagat A, Martin DR, Onani MO, Meyer M. Aptamer-conjugated magnetic nanoparticles for the efficient capture of cancer biomarker proteins. *J Magn Magn Mater.* 2020;497:166063. Available from: https://doi.org/10.1016/j.jmmm.2019.166063.
143. Zheng X, Zhao L, Wen D, Wang X, Yang H, Feng W, et al. Ultrasensitive fluorescent detection of HTLV-II DNA based on magnetic nanoparticles and atom transfer radical polymerization signal amplification. *Talanta.* 2020;207:120290. Available from: https://doi.org/10.1016/j.talanta.2019.120290.
144. Wang S, Kang G, Cui F, Zhang Y. Dual-color graphene quantum dots and carbon nanoparticles biosensing platform combined with Exonuclease III-assisted signal amplification for simultaneous detection of multiple DNA targets. *Anal Chim Acta.* 2021;1154:338346. Available from: https://doi.org/10.1016/j.aca.2021.338346.
145. Yue R, Li Z, Wang G, Li J, Ma N. Logic sensing of MicroRNA in living cells using DNA-programmed nanoparticle network with high signal gain. *ACS Sens.* 2018;4(1):250–6. Available from: https://doi.org/10.1021/acssensors.8b01422.
146. Kong Y, Liu X, Liu C, Xue Q, Li X, Wang H. A dandelion-like liposomes-encoded magnetic bead probe-based toehold-mediated DNA circuit for the amplification detection of MiRNA. *Analyst.* 2019;144(15):4694–701. Available from: https://doi.org/10.1039/c9an00887j.
147. Gao H, Zhang J, Wei X, Zhu Q, Wei T. Enhanced electrochemiluminescence cytosensing based on abundant oxygen vacancies contained 2D nanosheets emitter coupled with DNA device cycle-amplification. *Talanta.* 2021;228:122230. Available from: https://doi.org/10.1016/j.talanta.2021.122230.

148. Qing M, Chen S, Xie S, Tang Y, Zhang J, Yuan R. Encapsulation and release of recognition probes based on a rigid three-dimensional DNA "Nanosafe-box" for construction of a electrochemical biosensor. *Anal Chem*. 2019;92(2):1811–7. Available from: https://doi.org/10.1021/acs.analchem.9b03627.
149. Shi X, Xu H, Wu Y, Zhao Y, Meng HM, Li Z, et al. Two-dimension (2D) Cu-MOFs/aptamer nanoprobe for in situ ATP imaging in living cells. *J Anal Test*. 2021;5(2):165–73. Available from: https://doi.org/10.1007/s41664-021-00172-1.
150. Li X, Fu Y, Ding X, Li Z, Zhu G, Fan J. Magnetically controlled 2D nano-DNA fluorescent biosensor for selective and sensitive detection of alkaline phosphatase activity. *Sens Actuators B Chem*. 2021;327:128914. Available from: https://doi.org/10.1016/j.snb.2020.128914.
151 Santhamoorthy M, Thirupathi K, Krishnan S, Guganathan L, Dave S, Phan TTV, Kim SC. Preparation of Magnetic Iron Oxide Incorporated Mesoporous Silica Hybrid Composites for pH and Temperature-Sensitive Drug Delivery. *Magnetochemistry* 2023;9(3):81.
152. Dave S, Dave S, Mathur A, Das J. Biological synthesis of magnetic nanoparticles. In *Nanobiotechnology* (pp. 225–234). Elsevier, 2021.
153. Dave S, Das Jayshankar. *Advanced Nanomaterials for Point of Care Diagnosis and Therapy*. Elsevier, 2022. https://doi.org/10.1016/C2020-0-02584-3.

6 Strategic Synthesis of Diagnostic Novel Materials against Infectious Diseases

Past, Present, and Future

Maheswata Moharana, Fahmida Khan, and Subrat Kumar Pattanayak

6.1 INTRODUCTION

The term "infectious diseases" refers to contagious illness spread by various pathogens such as fungi, virus, and bacteria. Infectious diseases are the vital problems worldwide causing millions of fatalities every year, most of which occur in underdeveloped countries [1]. Through direct or indirect contact, these diseases can transmit from one person to another, causing a wide range of illness. Bacterial infections continue to be the leading causes of death globally despite the availability of antibiotics. This is due to the emergence of bacterial resistance that affects the public health [2]. About one-third of infectious deaths are caused by different dangerous microorganisms such as *Escherichia coli*, *Salmonella*, and *Listeria* [3]. Decreased antibiotic absorption, biofilm development, and inactivation of antibiotic degradation enzymes are some of the few examples of bacterial resistance mechanism [4]. Numerous antimicrobial substances, including cationic polymers [5], antimicrobial peptides [6], silver nanoparticles (AgNPs) [7], and metal-containing NPs [8], have recently been developed to treat drug-resistant bacterial infections.

The significant increase in the frequency and variety of fungal infections is caused due to the changes in medical and surgical care, particularly the use of invasive catheters along with the use of more potent immunosuppressive antibiotic agents. The adoption of organ support techniques such as parental hyper alimentation, mechanical ventilation, hemodialysis, and venovenous hemofiltration is included as additional support for fungal infection [9]. Some of the severe and most common infections in the world are caused by parasitic organisms, usually referred to as tropical/subtropical in nature. The protozoans (such as *Plasmodium* and *Leishmania*), helminths, and *Schistosoma* are among the causative agents

DOI: 10.1201/9781003316435-6

of diseases that belong to the parasitic group [10]. Infectious diseases are also largely caused by viral pathogens. In recent decades, the novel influenza A flu, the novel Ebola hemorrhagic fever, and the Zika virus diseases are few of the severe viral infectious diseases that had significant adverse effects on both human health and economy [11]. The severe acute respiratory coronavirus disease-2019 pandemic has recently created an emergency situation worldwide [12].

Inappropriate use of antibiotics, the emergence of new infectious agents, the spread of multidrug-resistant pathogens, and easy and quick spread due to population growth and globalization are the main obstacles to the management of infectious diseases [13]. For the therapeutic management of infectious diseases to be successful, early identification and commencement of targeted antimicrobial treatment are worth necessary. The conventional procedure for diagnosing common infectious diseases includes collection and transport of biological samples like urine, blood, tissue swabs, etc. from the point of care (POC) to the laboratory for sample processing by trained individuals. The laboratory contacts the clinicians when the reports are ready, then clinicians discuss the details with the patients, and finally alterations in treatment plans were made as necessary. This intrinsic inefficiency makes providing patients timely evidence-based therapy is more difficult and has led to the inappropriate use of medications [14].

At present, different laboratory tests such as culture, microscopy, nucleic acid amplification, and immunoassays are frequently used clinically for the diagnosis of significant diseases caused by different infectious agents like viruses, bacteria, fungi, and parasites [15].

Even though these methods have been used very frequently, many of the *in vitro* diagnostics have well-known drawbacks such as microscopy is insensitive and culture takes a long time to develop. Multiplex detection is labor-intensive and difficult to deploy for immunoassays like enzyme-linked immunosorbent assay (ELISA) [16]. Although molecular specificity is a benefit of nucleic acid amplification assays like polymerase chain reaction (PCR), sample preparation is difficult and false-positive results may possible [17].

6.2 CONVENTIONAL DETECTION STRATEGY

6.2.1 Microscope and Culture-Based Method

Most pathogens, such as bacteria, fungi, protozoa, and worms, have traditionally been detected microscopically, usually after growth in pure culture. Usually, samples from the infected person are taken and observed under the microscope to detect the presence of pathogens. Likewise, the presence of bacteria and fungi was confirmed by different biochemical tests based on their growth patterns [18]. Despite being highly specific, these methods have a number of drawbacks. First, the only samples with high content of pathogens can be analyzed using microscopy-based techniques. Second, the typical incubation time for growth pattern methods is at least 24 hours after the pathogen has grown in a specific medium. Third, not all pathogens can easily be grown in culture. These restrictions are highly important in the identification of viruses because viruses due to their smaller size (~100 nm) cannot be analyzed with a conventional optical microscope.

6.2.2 Nucleic Acid–Based Method

The PCR methods are widely used for nucleic acid detection. These methods utilize primers and the enzyme DNA polymerase to amplify, isolate, and quantify a small DNA sequence on the genetic structure of the targeted bacteria from the overall DNA sequence. The reverse transcription PCR [19] and real-time quantitative PCR [20] are two examples of the sophisticated nucleic acid amplification techniques that were created based on the PCR concept. These methods are sensitive and highly specific, and require very small volume of samples for detection. The detection methods are also very rapid that even within 5–24 hours, one can get the analysis results. These techniques are very well known to identify pathogens in the samples, including faces from different living organisms and processed food samples. The method has excellent specificity and sensitivity for measuring viruses in both symptomatic and asymptomatic patients. Recently, SARS-CoV-2 coronavirus, the primary cause of the COVID-19 pandemic, has been identified using the RT-PCR and qT-PCR methods globally [21,22].

6.2.3 Antibody- and Antigen-Based Methods

Various infections are detected using immunological techniques such as ELISA. The fundamental tenet of antibody–antigen interactions is that each antibody has the tendency to bind with a unique antigen. The degree to which the antibody binds to the antigen determines how sensitive and precise this approach is. This method is widely used as a conventional technique that enables individuals to detect and measure cells, viruses, and molecular antigens [23]. The three different forms of ELISA like direct, indirect, and sandwich methods have been widely employed with the accessibility of ELISA kits for the identification of infectious pathogens in different food products [24,25]. Because of long hour incubation and blocking times, the conventional ELISA takes longer time to complete. This method is not an appropriate one for POC diagnosis because of its high sample and reagent consumption rates and dependency on costly laboratory settings [26].

6.3 POINT OF CARE DIAGNOSIS FOR INFECTIOUS DISEASES

For the sake of enhancing human health and sustaining a high standard of living, it is crucial to detect specific species in samples like water, saliva, blood, and food at low concentrations. Applications of medicine, forensic science, food safety, and drug development all place a high priority on the accurate diagnosis of infectious diseases caused by different pathogens. On the other side, reducing mortality rate due to infectious diseases has become a major global problem. For accurate and consistent pathogen detection and for constant monitoring, a high-precision and sensitive analytical approach is needed. POC tools for pathogen detection have been mostly used in clinical management and in many fields including pathology, food safety, and drug discovery [27]. POC systems, often by miniaturization and simplification, have been designed to address the limitations associated with the traditional diagnosis methods of infectious diseases.

The POC system is regarded as a comprehensive diagnostic platform, including sample collection, analysis, data generation, and diagnosis in a single unit. Additionally, these systems ought to be rapid to deliver results, portable (or at least transportable), and simple to use by both the end user and a field-deployed care professional [28]. Different foundations supported the development of POC diagnostic technology for the developing world [29]. Utilizing smart phones, nanotechnology, and microfluidic technologies, various novel POC methods have been developed and made available for commercial use such as glucose meters and pregnancy test kits [30].

The POC detection of nucleic acid is gaining interest as it uses DNA and RNA as primary targets for disease diagnosis. Genotyping, genetic prognostics, expression profiling, and infectious disease detection are some of the examples of the applications of nucleic acid detection. Nucleic acids, for instance, are utilized in the diagnosis of infectious disease and cancer as well as in the surveillance of epidemics and the emergence of novel diseases (e.g., H7N9). By simulating retroviral RNA replication, the partial isothermal method of nucleic acid sequence–based amplification results in the formation of ssRNA. This method maintained its popularity due to the fact that it naturally interacts with RNA instead of DNA, which makes it perfect for spotting single-stranded viral RNA or endogenous RNA. This is an effective amplification method that can be used to amplify RNA.

Although DNAs and proteins are both utilized as biomarkers to identify certain diseases, use of DNA frequently fails in terms of providing a predicted and consistent diagnosis. This is due to further regulation of translation that affects the interaction between the levels of expression of mRNAs and the related proteins. Furthermore, one gene may produce several proteins, each with a distinct biological significance, and the proteins produced by the gene may go through a variety of post-translational modifications, some of which may be essential in different disease processes. On the other hand, proteins are considered to be useful sources for diagnosis. This is because proteins are the ultimate forms of gene and hence linked with biological processes [31].

Phenotypic techniques, such as staining and culture, were traditionally used for bacterial detection. However, a significant drawback is that it can take a longer time (~48 hour) to deliver the results, and sometimes the results are insufficient to guide the prescription of an antibiotic at correct time.

The demand for quick diagnosis necessitates the development of novel diagnostic tools that may be used in both primary care and community settings and are based on the recognition and quantification of certain analytes by biorecognition components [32]. An electrochemiluminescence-based POC targets the 5-methythio-D-xylofuranose-lipoarabinomannan epitope of *Mycobacterium tuberculosis*. Lateral flow immunoassay (LFIA) or immune chromatography is straightforward, speedy, and transferable. Although LFIA has been used commercially for many years, recent improvements in its sensitivity, reproducibility, and ability to detect numerous analytes make it appropriate for the identification of hospital-acquired infections [33]. Another diagnostic tool that has been widely utilized to find viruses and bacteria is surface plasmon resonance. The vibrating electrons on metallic surfaces can be triggered by light beams with a specified wavelength when certain conditions are satisfied. In most cases, a prism employing total internal reflection (TIR) is used to excite electrons and produce surface plasmon resonance (SPR). In SPR biosensors, biorecognition components (such as antibodies and aptamers) are attached to thin metal films that are typically made of gold, silver, or aluminum, and the light wave excites plasmons on their surface [34]. For the early diagnosis of various chronic diseases, cancers, and metabolic abnormalities, monitoring of biomarkers is crucial. Any element, structure, or mechanism that may be detected in the body or its products that denotes the chance of diseases is referred to as a biomarker. In tumor tissues, serum, or body fluids, it may be genes, proteins, lipids, or metabolites. Since biomarkers are challenging to identify, the procedures are often labor- and time-intensive. Analytical platforms ranging from complex instruments such as immunoassays and PCR to simple paper-based analytical devices (PADs) can be used to identify biomarkers.

The basis of immunoassays, which include radio-immunoassays, enzyme-linked immunosorbent assays, and chemiluminescence immunoassays, is the interaction of an antibody with a particular antigen in a solution. In order to detect antibodies or antigens, they are chemically attached to conjugated labels (such as enzymes, radioactive isotopes, or chemical probes). Their interactions result in quantifiable signals that can be picked up by particular detectors (such as radiation, color change, fluorescence, or light emission) [35]. Immunoassays produce precise qualitative and quantitative results because they are very sensitive and specific. In developed countries, immunoassays and PCR are typically established in modern laboratories. Both methods need a certain instrument and several procedures to process the sample. Due to lack of skilled operators, resources, and financial assistance, they are not frequently used in remote locations. Therefore, new POC devices for biomarker detection should be designed in order to provide immediate measurements that are accurate enough and help doctors interact with patients in a proper way. To solve these issues, several analytical procedures are combined onto a single microchip in lab-on-chip (LOC) devices, which include PADs. These procedures involve a number of common laboratory procedures, such as handling samples, combining samples and reagents, reacting, separating, and detecting [36]. Figure 6.1 provides a visual representation of numerous POC technology applications.

6.4 BIOSENSOR-BASED NOVEL MATERIALS

The concept of biosensor was first introduced by Clark and Lyons in 1962 with the development of oxidase enzyme electrode for glucose detection. Since bacterial and viral infections have become key threats for human health, pathogen detection has become one of the most relevant goals of biosensor devices [37]. Biosensing

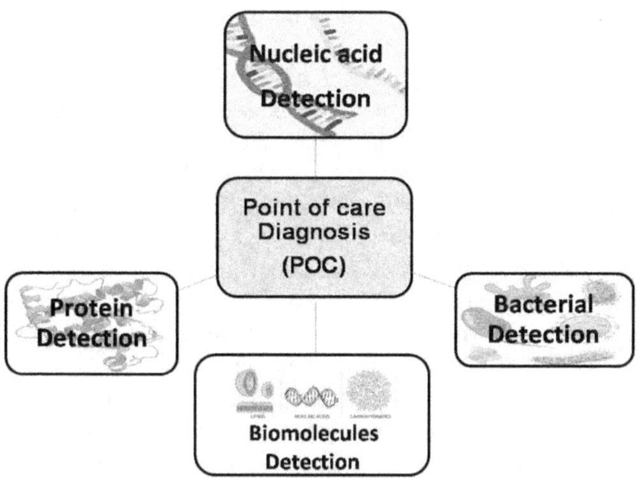

FIGURE 6.1 Different applications of point of care (POC) technology.

technology has become more popular over the decades as a potential diagnostic instrument due to its various advantages [38]. The rapid development of biosensor technology has been facilitated by the focus on the development of susceptible, quick, and inexpensive identification methods that may be implemented at or close to the POC. These are analytical tools that identify target specimens and translate molecular recognition processes into quantifiable signals. The biosensor technique constitutes a receptor that captures target molecules and a transducer method that generates electrical signals in response to target identification. As a quick diagnostic tool for infectious disorders, biosensors are superior to conventional assays because they offer a less expensive platform for detection and have easier operational procedures that may be carried out at the POC [39]. Biosensors are bio-electromechanical systems and can be classified into different categories. Recently, electrochemical biosensing devices have developed for disease diagnosis with a variety of advantages including cheap cost, high sensitivity, high selectivity, and quick response. The electrochemical biosensors are composed of an electrochemical transducer and a biological sensing system. These devices are mainly concerned with detecting current or upcoming changes associated to interactions occurring at the sample–matrix interface of the sensor.

The targeted analyte is preferentially reacted with the recognition factors like enzymes, tissues, antibodies, and biomolecules, which helps generate electrical signals that are sent to the signal processing units via the transducer. Before the collection of data, the signals are amplified and the noise is removed [40]. Voltammetric biosensors, a type of electrochemical sensors, convert the data from a biological system into an electronic signal. These electroanalytical sensing techniques produce current between the working electrode and a counter-electrode. The process of biorecognition between the recognition layer and the analytes in voltammetric biosensors results in the current response either through redox processes or by labeling. It has been utilized to identify a variety of toxins and infections. Simple to complicate sensing platforms, such as particular nanomaterials and nanostructures, have been used [41]. For decades, electrochemical impedance spectroscopy methods have been used by electrochemists as effective tools in biosensing application due to the label-free detection. The technology uses the charge transfer resistance of the interfacial capacitance to identify the biochemical changes that take place at the electrode–electrode interface. These changes follow the change of various physical and chemical properties of the electrode–electrolyte interface. It is a non-destructive technology because it uses small amplitude perturbations, in contrast to other electrochemical techniques like cyclic voltammetry, which use large amplitude perturbations [42]. The quartz crystal microbalance (QCM) is a type of biosensor instrument that comprises a transducer that functions according to the mass detection principle. Because of their capacity to identify almost any sort of biomolecule using a label-free technique, this type of biosensors have attracted considerable interest in the field of pathogen detection. The development of these new diagnostic tools is particularly appealing due to the quick detection process and great sensitivity. These systems are a dynamic platform for identifying the various kinds of disease biomarkers because mass is an intrinsic attribute of all substances and may be used to detect virtually any type of molecule [43]. It works on the basis of the piezoelectric effect, wherein applying an external electric field to quartz causes the crystal to experience mechanical stresses [44]. The optical detection technique of backscattering interferometry (BI) is also applied in the field of biosensing. The devices contain a light source having single wavelength aimed onto a microfluidic channel and a detector to measure the intensity of the light reflected. It enables real-time assessment of binding constants ranging from micro to pico mole. It can detect molecule interactions in free solution or on surfaces immobilized with exceptional precision in microfluidic device [45]. Recently, the potential of glycans (polymers based on carbohydrates) was used to find biomarkers for infectious diseases. Attomolar-level sensitivity was demonstrated for a glycan-immobilized field effect transistor biosensor in the detection and differentiation of human (H1) and avian (H5) influenza viruses. QCM, optical wave guides, and SPR were used for glycan-based influenza virus detection. Development of multifunctional paper devices is essentially helpful in detecting prevalent and endemic diseases in areas with limited resources. Sample treatment, RNA extraction, automatic flow control, and reverse transcription LAMP can all be done by the equipment. The three main components of this lab-on-paper were serum treatment, fluidic flow of the target RNA, and RNA amplification [46]. Electrochemical transduction or amplifying elements have been incorporated into paper microfluidic devices. For instance, an NP enhanced cellulose paper microchip with screen-printed graphene–silver electrodes, which was intended for the detection of the Zika virus [47]. Because of their high specificity, aptamer-based biosensors have become a viable option for viral detection. The aptamer is chosen based on how well it binds to the target molecule. As a result, aptamer-based sensors are frequently very

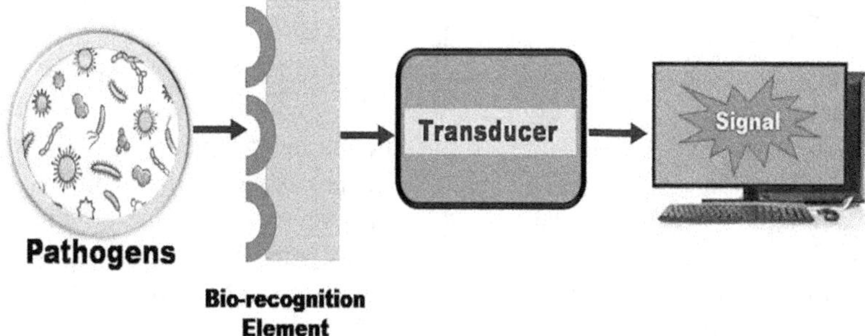

FIGURE 6.2 A schematic representation of biosensors for the detection of pathogens.

precise and selective. A selective biosensor was created using aptamers and gold NPs with catalytic activity (Figure 6.2) [48].

6.5 NANOTECHNOLOGY-BASED DIAGNOSTIC STRATEGY

The development of drug-resistant pathogens and the emergence of co-infections limit the effectiveness of current treatments for infections, and developing nations in particular face a major challenge in the fight against infectious disease. The potential effects of nanotechnology on global health have long been recognized, leading to the development of a variety of techniques for identifying and monitoring diseases, delivering drug, and preventing diseases. The aim of nanotechnology is to improve the treatment regimens by reducing the tablet load and targeted drug delivery to the disease reservoirs or at the pathogenic sites [49]. By modifying the shape, size, composition, and surface modification of nanomaterials, it is possible to specifically regulate their properties for pathogen detection. The structural parameters of NP, such as their size, composition, self-assembly, and binding properties, can be used to modify specific properties, such as their electronic, spectroscopic, conductive, and light scattering [50]. The development of distinctive nanomaterials, including monolithic and hybrid structures like photon-up conversion NPs, has been supported by advancements in nanoscience and nanotechnology (for example, lanthanide-doped nanocrystals) [51,52]. They can also be used as substrate materials, labels in bioassays, amplification tools, and bulk/surface modifiers in biosensors [53]. Because of their plasmonic (in the case of optical sensors) or electrocatalytic (for electrochemical sensors) properties, metals (such as gold, platinum, and silver), magnetic NPs, quantum dots (QDs), and carbon-based nanomaterials are the most commonly used nanomaterials [54]. NPs with size smaller than 100 nm can be categorized as inorganic, liposomes, polymeric, immunostimulant complexes, virus-like particles, depending on their chemical composition. They have been demonstrated to promote immunological responses, including cell recruitment, activation of antigen (Ag)-presenting cells (APCs), production of cytokine, and release of chemokine [55]. Metallic nanoparticles (MeNPs) have rigid structures, have a simple synthesis process, and are generally not biodegradable. The immunological properties of MeNPs have already been investigated earlier days [56]. Gold nanoparticles (AuNPs) are widely mentioned as suitable for a variety of biosensing usages. Their distinctive electric, photonic, and catalytic features along with the molecular interaction selectivity of various biomolecules represent the design principles of a variety of virus detection systems [57]. The AuNPs have special chemical as well as physical characteristics that make them suitable for a variety of biological applications. These undergo an SPR, or electron oscillation with lights, to produce a color change or localized heating. Previously, the researchers in Ref. [58] utilized AuNPs to develop vaccines in their study of the efficacy of a prototype vaccination against tick-borne encephalitis. The vaccine was produced by conjugating AuNPs with a soluble antigen that had an average diameter of 15 nm. Silver is considered as a Lewis acid and has a natural tendency to react with a Lewis base, such as biomolecules containing phosphorus and sulfur, which are important building blocks for proteins, DNA, and cell membranes. AgNPs can build up on cell walls and membranes, generating immediately noticeable morphological alterations such as cytoplasmic shrinkage, membrane separation, multiple electron density, and ultimately disrupted membrane. Due to its broad-spectrum antimicrobial properties and potent antimicrobial efficacy against a variety of pathogens, including bacteria, viruses, and fungi, AgNP is the most studied antibacterial nanoagent [59].

AgNPs are one of the most significant and fascinating nanomaterials among the many MeNPs employed in biomedical application. Additionally, AgNPs are crucial to nanotechnology and nanoscience, particularly in nanomedicine. The biological activity AgNPs is influenced by a number of variables, including surface chemistry, size distribution, coating, shape or agglomeration, capping, dissolving rate, particle reactivity in solution, ion release efficiency, and cell type. Cytotoxicity is also greatly influenced by the type of reducing agents used to synthesize AgNPs. Recently, it has been shown that AgNPs have the potential to be powerful antiviral agents that can combat numerous fatal viruses, including COVID-19. AgNPs have the ability to produce free radicals and reactive oxygen species (ROS), which cause cells to die through apoptosis, preventing viral infection [60]. Due to the numerous advantages, including biocompatibility, bioavailability, cytotoxicity, biodegradability, and precise distribution at the desired site of action, polymeric NPs have the potential for a wide range of therapeutic applications. Colloid solids, known as polymeric NPs, range in size from 10 to 1,000 nm and can be produced using polyacrylate, polycaprolactone, natural polymers like chitosan and alginate, and even proteins like albumin [61]. Recent advances in polymeric nanomedicine have enabled the delivery of therapeutic drugs and the promotion of tissue development of lung in inflammatory organs. Among the numerous nano- and biosensing approaches, molecularly imprinted polymers provide promise application and physicochemical resilience for detecting viral infections. Molecularly imprinted polymer (MIPs) are created by new molecularly imprinted functional polymers with molecular target selectivity that has already been established. For the detection of the SARS-CoV-2 virus,

MIP-based sensors can be used because of their distinctive selectivity and sensitivity [62]. Innovation in materials is essential to the development of new technologies. Particularly, 2D materials have recently gained a great deal of interest in biomedical science and technology. Graphene and related 2D materials have excellent antiviral and antibacterial properties, high surface area, and photothermal and photocatalytical properties for sensing and detection. They can also be integrated with cutting-edge manufacturing techniques like additive manufacturing due to the ability of their surfaces to be functionalized with different functional groups. These qualities make it possible for them to be used directly or indirectly in different biomedical systems. A number of components based on graphene and its derivatives have been developed recently to combat COVID-19, according to recent studies. In particular, within a short span of time, face masks, three-dimensionally printed medical components, diagnosis tools, sterilizers, gloves, grapheme/grapheme composite–based antiviral coatings, etc. have been produced [63]. A grapheme oxide chitosan nanocomposite is used to create a DNA-based electrochemical biosensor for typhoid diagnosis. For better biosensor performance, graphene oxide and its nanocomposites have been used. According to studies, grapheme oxide nanosheets dispersed in a polymer matrix like chitosan improve electrochemical performance, biocompatibility, ease of immobilization, and microenvironment for the development of enzymatic biosensors [64]. An area in a semiconductor crystal known as a quantum dot (QD) has electrons, holes, or both in three dimensions. All the three matters have the dimensions in nanometer scale. Light scattering is the main feature of these QDs. Due to their smaller size, QDs are regarded as the unique class of semiconductors. Globally, biosensors are utilized to identify viral infections linked to the molecular identification of biomarkers. As a result, QDs biomarker–based virus detection is low cost and has a lot of potential. QDs seem to be a potential choice as biological probes to identify the ultrasensitive biomarkers of viral infections [65]. Carbon quantum dots (CQDs), a new class of nanomaterials, have drawn more interest in the past decades because of their unique properties. CQDs are small particles, often smaller than 10 nm, with important properties such as photostability, biocompatibility, high water solubility, photoluminescence, no toxicity, and high sustainability. Some investigations have recently revealed that specific CQD types have strong and powerful antiviral activity against human norovirus, herpesvirus, and corona virus. A broad-spectrum agent to inhibit viral infectivity against deadly flaviviruses and non-enveloped viruses (porcine parvovirus and adenovirus-associated virus) has recently been reported to be generated from benzoxazine monomer CQDs [66]. The semiconductor QD have special optical and electric characteristics, such as size-tunable light emission, a limited emission spectrum, great brightness, and photostability. QDs are successfully utilized with recent scientific developments that have reduced their toxicity. The *in vivo* identification of tumors and cancer cells was made possible by encapsulating QDs in polymeric NPs and attaching target ligands to them. They have shown successful applications in the monitoring and diagnosis of myocardial infarction [67]. Recent developments in smart phone technology, isothermal amplification, and QD barcode engineering were

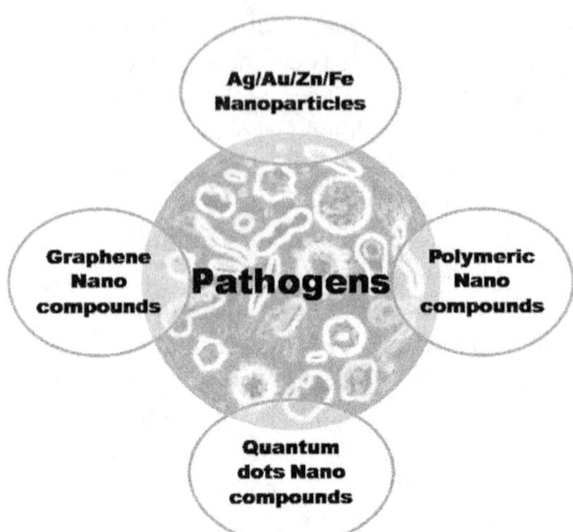

FIGURE 6.3 Application of nanoparticles in the diagnosis of infectious diseases.

combined to create a simple, inexpensive chip-based wireless multiplex diagnostic device. The combination of QD bar-coding technology and a smart phone reader enables real-time knowledge shift of emerging or urgent disease threats with healthcare and defense sector, as well as the capacity for global infectious disease surveillance [68]. NPs, including polymeric nanocompounds, used for diagnosis of infectious disease causing pathogens are shown in Figure 6.3.

6.6 CONCLUSIONS AND FUTURE PERSPECTIVE

Infectious diseases continue to be a significant global health issue. In order to detect infectious diseases, many strategies have used the special features of non-material. A perfect diagnostic platform may be quicklyand effectively re targeted to numerous diseases with minor operational changes. Different conventional detection strategies such as microscopy, culture-based methods, nucleic acid–based methods, antibody- and antigen-based methods, and biosensor-based novel materials were employed for identification of infectious diseases. Phenotypic techniques, such as staining and culture, were traditionally used for the detection of bacterial infections. Colorimetric biosensors have received much attention for the diagnosis of infectious diseases due to their low cost and quick diagnostic procedures. Electrochemical biosensing methods such as voltammetric biosensor, amperometric biosensor, and impedance biosensor are used for the diagnosis of infectious diseases. Polymeric materials, especially dendrimers, have also an extensive biomedical application. Protein-coupled magnetic beads were used in semiconductor-based biological sensors to identify target molecules in biomedical sector [69–73]. In the past couple of years, different NP-based compounds and biosensors played vital roles in the diagnosis of infectious diseases. Silver, gold, zinc, and iron NPs; graphene nanocompounds; QD nanocompounds; and polymeric nanocompounds were also applied in the diagnosis of infectious diseases. In general, the use of these effective techniques points to the adoption of nanotechnology-based diagnosis methods for the identification of infectious diseases.

REFERENCES

1. Markwalter CF, Kantor AG, Moore CP, Richardson KA, Wright DW. Inorganic complexes and metal-based nanomaterials for infectious disease diagnostics. *Chemical Reviews.* 2018 Dec 4;119(2):1456–518.
2. Spellberg B, Guidos R, Gilbert D, Bradley J, Boucher HW, Scheld WM, Bartlett JG, Edwards Jr. J, Infectious Diseases Society of America. The epidemic of antibiotic-resistant infections: A call to action for the medical community from the Infectious Diseases Society of America. *Clinical Infectious Diseases.* 2008 Jan 15;46(2):155–64.
3. Bai X, Nakatsu CH, Bhunia AK. Bacterial biofilms and their implications in pathogenesis and food safety. *Foods.* 2021 Sep 8;10(9):2117.
4. Sionov RV, Steinberg D. Targeting the holy triangle of quorum sensing, biofilm formation, and antibiotic resistance in pathogenic bacteria. *Microorganisms.* 2022 Jun 16;10(6):1239.
5. Pan Y, Xia Q, Xiao H. Cationic polymers with tailored structures for rendering polysaccharide-based materials antimicrobial: An overview. *Polymers.* 2019 Aug 1;11(8):1283.
6. Toke O. Antimicrobial peptides: New candidates in the fight against bacterial infections. *Peptide Science: Original Research on Biomolecules.* 2005;80(6):717–35.
7. Skóra B, Krajewska U, Nowak A, Dziedzic A, Barylyak A, Kus-Liśkiewicz M. Noncytotoxic silver nanoparticles as a new antimicrobial strategy. *Scientific Reports.* 2021 Jun 29;11(1):1–3.
8. Yeroslavsky G, Lavi R, Alishaev A, Rahimipour S. Sonochemically-produced metal-containing polydopamine nanoparticles and their antibacterial and antibiofilm activity. *Langmuir.* 2016 May 24;32(20):5201–12.
9. Van Thiel DH, George M, Moore CM. Fungal infections: Their diagnosis and treatment in transplant recipients. *International Journal of Hepatology.* 2012 Jan 1;2012:106923.
10. Ricciardi A, Ndao M. Diagnosis of parasitic infections: What's going on? *Journal of Biomolecular Screening.* 2015 Jan;20(1):6–21.
11. Trovato M, Sartorius R, D'Apice L, Manco R, De Berardinis P. Viral emerging diseases: Challenges in developing vaccination strategies. *Frontiers in Immunology.* 2020 Sep 3;11:2130.
12. Acter T, Uddin N, Das J, Akhter A, Choudhury TR, Kim S. Evolution of severe acute respiratory syndrome coronavirus 2 (SARS-CoV-2) as coronavirus disease 2019 (COVID-19) pandemic: A global health emergency. *Science of the Total Environment.* 2020 Aug 15;730:138996.
13. Karam G, Chastre J, Wilcox MH, Vincent JL. Antibiotic strategies in the era of multidrug resistance. *Critical Care.* 2016 Dec;20(1):1–9.
14. Nayak S, Blumenfeld NR, Laksanasopin T, Sia SK. Point-of-care diagnostics: Recent developments in a connected age. *Analytical Chemistry.* 2017 Jan 3;89(1):102–23.
15. Siddiqi K, Lambert ML, Walley J. Clinical diagnosis of smear-negative pulmonary tuberculosis in low-income countries: The current evidence. *The Lancet Infectious Diseases.* 2003 May 1;3(5):288–96.

16. Chin CD, Laksanasopin T, Cheung YK, Steinmiller D, Linder V, Parsa H, Wang J, Moore H, Rouse R, Umviligihozo G, Karita E. Microfluidics-based diagnostics of infectious diseases in the developing world. *Nature Medicine*. 2011 Aug;17(8):1015–9.
17. Craw P, Balachandran W. Isothermal nucleic acid amplification technologies for point-of-care diagnostics: A critical review. *Lab on a Chip*. 2012;12(14):2469–86.
18. Stetzenbach LD, Buttner MP, Cruz P. Detection and enumeration of airborne biocontaminants. *Current Opinion in Biotechnology*. 2004 Jun 1;15(3):170–4.
19. Bachman J. Reverse-transcription PCR (rt -PCR). In *Methods in Enzymology*, 2013 Jan 1 (Vol. 530, pp. 67–74). Academic Press, Cambridge, MA.
20. Pabinger S, Rödiger S, Kriegner A, Vierlinger K, Weinhäusel A. A survey of tools for the analysis of quantitative PCR (qPCR) data. *Biomolecular Detection and Quantification*. 2014 Sep 1;1(1):23–33.
21. Brandolini M, Taddei F, Marino MM, Grumiro L, Scalcione A, Turba ME, Gentilini F, Fantini M, Zannoli S, Dirani G, Sambri V. Correlating qRT-PCR, dPCR and viral titration for the identification and quantification of SARS-CoV-2: A new approach for infection management. *Viruses*. 2021 May 28;13(6):1022.
22. Vasudevan HN, Xu P, Servellita V, Miller S, Liu L, Gopez A, Chiu CY, Abate AR. Digital droplet PCR accurately quantifies SARS-CoV-2 viral load from crude lysate without nucleic acid purification. *Scientific Reports*. 2021 Jan 12;11(1):780.
23. Sanjay ST, Li M, Zhou W, Li X, Li X. A reusable PMMA/paper hybrid plug-and-play microfluidic device for an ultrasensitive immunoassay with a wide dynamic range. *Microsystems & Nanoengineering*. 2020 Jun 15;6(1):28.
24. Aydin S. A short history, principles, and types of ELISA, and our laboratory experience with peptide/protein analyses using ELISA. *Peptides*. 2015 Oct 1;72:4–15.
25. Kumar BK, Raghunath P, Devegowda D, Deekshit VK, Venugopal MN, Karunasagar I, Karunasagar I. Development of monoclonal antibody based sandwich ELISA for the rapid detection of pathogenic Vibrio parahaemolyticus in seafood. *International Journal of Food Microbiology*. 2011 Jan 31;145(1):244–9.
26. Ma L, Abugalyon Y, Li X. Multicolorimetric ELISA biosensors on a paper/polymer hybrid analytical device for visual point-of-care detection of infection diseases. *Analytical and Bioanalytical Chemistry*. 2021 Jul;413(18):4655–63.
27. Roy S, Arshad F, Eissa S, Safavieh M, Alattas SG, Ahmed MU, Zourob M. Recent developments towards portable point-of-care diagnostic devices for pathogen detection. *Sensors & Diagnostics*. 2022;1(1):87–105.
28. Suea-Ngam A, Bezinge L, Mateescu B, Howes PD, deMello AJ, Richards DA. Enzyme-assisted nucleic acid detection for infectious disease diagnostics: Moving toward the point-of-care. *ACS Sensors*. 2020 Aug 25;5(9):2701–23.
29. Ahmed MU, Saaem I, Wu PC, Brown AS. Personalized diagnostics and biosensors: A review of the biology and technology needed for personalized medicine. *Critical Reviews in Biotechnology*. 2014 Jun 1;34(2):180–96.
30. Shu T, Hunter H, Zhou Z, Sun Y, Cheng X, Ma J, Su L, Zhang X, Serpe MJ. Portable point-of-care diagnostic devices: An updated review. *Analytical Methods*. 2021;13(45):5418–35.
31. Choi S, Goryll M, Sin LY, Wong PK, Chae J. Microfluidic-based biosensors toward point-of-care detection of nucleic acids and proteins. *Microfluidics and Nanofluidics*. 2011 Feb;10:231–47.
32. Furst AL, Francis MB. Impedance-based detection of bacteria. *Chemical Reviews*. 2018 Dec 17;119(1):700–26.

33. Reali S, Najib EY, Balázs KE, Tan AC, Váradi L, Hibbs DE, Groundwater PW. Novel diagnostics for point-of-care bacterial detection and identification. *RSC Advances*. 2019;9(37):21486–97.
34. Nath P, Kabir A, Khoubafarin Doust S, Kreais ZJ, Ray A. Detection of bacterial and viral pathogens using photonic point-of-care devices. *Diagnostics*. 2020 Oct 19;10(10):841.
35. Patel KR, Gan SD. Enzyme immunoassay and enzyme-linked immunosorbent assay. *J Invest Dermatol*. 2013 Sep 1;133(9):e12.
36. Suntornsuk W, Suntornsuk L. Recent applications of paper-based point-of-care devices for biomarker detection. *Electrophoresis*. 2020 Mar;41(5–6):287–305.
37. Castillo-Henríquez L, Brenes-Acuña M, Castro-Rojas A, Cordero-Salmerón R, Lopretti-Correa M, Vega-Baudrit JR. Biosensors for the detection of bacterial and viral clinical pathogens. *Sensors*. 2020 Dec 4;20(23):6926.
38. Rodovalho V, Alves L, Castro A, Madurro J, Brito-Madurro A, Santos A. Biosensors applied to diagnosis of infectious diseases: An update. *Austin Journal of Biosensors & Bioelectronics*. 2015;1(3):10–5.
39. Sin ML, Mach KE, Wong PK, Liao JC. Advances and challenges in biosensor-based diagnosis of infectious diseases. *Expert Review of Molecular Diagnostics*. 2014 Mar 1;14(2):225–44.
40. Lazcka O, Del Campo FJ, Munoz FX. Pathogen detection: A perspective of traditional methods and biosensors. *Biosensors and Bioelectronics*. 2007 Feb 15;22(7):1205–17.
41. Thomas A, Kumar KG. Communication-Electrooxidation of dopamine at CoNP-pAHNSA modified electrode: A sensitive approach to its determination. *Journal of the Electrochemical Society*. 2018 Jul 31;165(10):B466.
42. Liustrovaite V, Drobysh M, Rucinskiene A, Baradoke A, Ramanaviciene A, Plikusiene I, Samukaite-Bubniene U, Viter R, Chen CF, Ramanavicius A. Towards an electrochemical immunosensor for the detection of antibodies against SARS-CoV-2 spike protein. *Journal of the Electrochemical Society*. 2022 Mar 1;169(3):037523.
43. Afzal A, Mujahid A, Schirhagl R, Bajwa SZ, Latif U, Feroz S. Gravimetric viral diagnostics: QCM based biosensors for early detection of viruses. *Chemosensors*. 2017 Feb 13;5(1):7.
44. Lim HJ, Saha T, Tey BT, Tan WS, Ooi CW. Quartz crystal microbalance-based biosensors as rapid diagnostic devices for infectious diseases. *Biosensors and Bioelectronics*. 2020 Nov 15;168:112513.
45. Kussrow A, Baksh MM, Bornhop DJ, Finn MG. Universal sensing by transduction of antibody binding with backscattering interferometry. *ChemBioChem*. 2011 Feb 11;12(3):367–70.
46. Seok Y, Batule BS, Kim MG. Lab-on-paper for all-in-one molecular diagnostics (LAMDA) of zika, dengue, and chikungunya virus from human serum. *Biosensors and Bioelectronics*. 2020 Oct 1;165:112400.
47. Draz MS, Shafiee H. Applications of gold nanoparticles in virus detection. *Theranostics*. 2018;8(7):1985.
48. Weerathunge P, Ramanathan R, Torok VA, Hodgson K, Xu Y, Goodacre R, Behera BK, Bansal V. Ultrasensitive colorimetric detection of murine norovirus using NanoZyme aptasensor. *Analytical Chemistry*. 2019 Jan 14;91(5):3270–6.
49. Mitchell SL, Carlson EE. Tiny things with enormous impact: Nanotechnology in the fight against infectious disease. *ACS Infectious Diseases*. 2018 Aug 2;4(10):1432–5.
50. Sau TK, Rogach AL, Jäckel F, Klar TA, Feldmann J. Properties and applications of colloidal nonspherical noble metal nanoparticles. *Advanced Materials*. 2010 Apr 22;22(16):1805–25.

51. Wu Y, Ang MJY, Sun M, Huang B, Liu X. Expanding the toolbox for lanthanide-doped upconversion nanocrystals. *Journal of Physics D: Applied Physics*. 2019;52(38):383002.
52. Hlavacek A, Mickert MJ, Soukka T, Lahtinen S, Tallgren T, Pizúrová N, Król A, Gorris HH. Large-scale purification of photon-upconversion nanoparticles by gel electrophoresis for analogue and digital bioassays. *Analytical Chemistry*. 2018 Dec 10;91(2):1241–6.
53. Malekzad H, Sahandi Zangabad P, Mirshekari H, Karimi M, Hamblin MR. Noble metal nanoparticles in biosensors: Recent studies and applications. *Nanotechnology Reviews*. 2017 Jun 27;6(3):301–29.
54. Heydari-Bafrooei E, Ensafi AA. Typically used carbon-based nanomaterials in the fabrication of biosensors. In *Electrochemical Biosensors* 2019 Jan 1 (pp. 77–98). Elsevier. doi: 10.1016/B978-0-12-816491-4.00004-8.
55. Liang A, Riaz H, Dong F, Luo X, Yu X, Han Y, Chong Z, Han L, Guo A, Yang L. Evaluation of efficacy, biodistribution and safety of antibiotic-free plasmid encoding somatostatin genes delivered by attenuated Salmonella enterica serovar Choleraesuis. *Vaccine*. 2014 Mar 10;32(12):1368–74.
56. Hofmann-Amtenbrink M, Grainger DW, Hofmann H. Nanoparticles in medicine: Current challenges facing inorganic nanoparticle toxicity assessments and standardizations. *Nanomedicine: Nanotechnology, Biology and Medicine*. 2015 Oct 1;11(7):1689–94.
57. Draz MS, Venkataramani M, Lakshminarayanan H, Saygili E, Moazeni M, Vasan A, Li Y, Sun X, Hua S, Xu GY, Shafiee H. Nanoparticle-enhanced electrical detection of Zika virus on paper microchips. *Nanoscale*. 2018;10(25):11841–9.
58. Demenev VA, Shchinova MA, Ivanov LI, Vorob'eva RN, Zdanovskaia NI, Nebaĭkina NV. Perfection of methodical approaches to designing vaccines against tick-borne encephalitis. *Voprosy Virusologii*. 1996 May 1;41(3):107–10.
59. Tang S, Zheng J. Antibacterial activity of silver nanoparticles: Structural effects. *Advanced Healthcare Materials*. 2018 Jul;7(13):1701503.
60. Allawadhi P, Singh V, Khurana A, Khurana I, Allwadhi S, Kumar P, Banothu AK, Thalugula S, Barani PJ, Naik RR, Bharani KK. Silver nanoparticle based multifunctional approach for combating COVID-19. *Sensors International*. 2021 Jan 1;2:100101.
61. Aguilera-Correa JJ, Esteban J, Vallet-Regí M. Inorganic and polymeric nanoparticles for human viral and bacterial infections prevention and treatment. *Nanomaterials*. 2021 Jan 8;11(1):137.
62. Rana MM. Polymer-based nano-therapies to combat COVID-19 related respiratory injury: Progress, prospects, and challenges. *Journal of Biomaterials Science, Polymer Edition*. 2021 Jun 13;32(9):1219–49.
63. Seo G, Lee G, Kim MJ, Baek SH, Choi M, Ku KB, Lee CS, Jun S, Park D, Kim HG, Kim SJ. Rapid detection of COVID-19 causative virus (SARS-CoV-2) in human nasopharyngeal swab specimens using field-effect transistor-based biosensor. *ACS Nano*. 2020 Apr 15;14(4):5135–42.
64. Singh A, Sinsinbar G, Choudhary M, Kumar V, Pasricha R, Verma HN, Singh SP, Arora K. Graphene oxide-chitosan nanocomposite based electrochemical DNA biosensor for detection of typhoid. *Sensors and Actuators B: Chemical*. 2013 Aug 1;185:675–84.
65. Mousavi SM, Hashemi SA, Yari Kalashgrani M, Omidifar N, Lai CW, Vijayakameswara Rao N, Gholami A, Chiang WH. The pivotal role of quantum dots-based biomarkers integrated with ultra-sensitive probes for multiplex detection of human viral infections. *Pharmaceuticals*. 2022 Jul 17;15(7):880.

66. Xue Y, Liu C, Andrews G, Wang J, Ge Y. Recent advances in carbon quantum dots for virus detection, as well as inhibition and treatment of viral infection. *Nano Convergence.* 2022 Apr 2;9(1):15.
67. Mukherjee A, Shim Y, Myong Song J. Quantum dot as probe for disease diagnosis and monitoring. *Biotechnology Journal.* 2016 Jan;11(1):31–42.
68. Ming K, Kim J, Biondi MJ, Syed A, Chen K, Lam A, Ostrowski M, Rebbapragada A, Feld JJ, Chan WC. Integrated quantum dot barcode smartphone optical device for wireless multiplexed diagnosis of infected patients. *ACS Nano.* 2015 Mar 24;9(3):3060–74.
69. Santhamoorthy M, Thirupathi K, Krishnan S, Guganathan L, Dave S, Phan TTV and Kim SC. Preparation of Magnetic Iron Oxide Incorporated Mesoporous Silica Hybrid Composites for pH and Temperature-Sensitive Drug Delivery. *Magnetochemistry* 2023;9(3):81.
70. Dave S, Dave S, Mathur A, Das J. Biological synthesis of magnetic nanoparticles. In *Nanobiotechnology* (pp. 225–234). Elsevier, 2021.
71. Dave S, Das Jayshankar. *Advanced Nanomaterials for Point of Care Diagnosis and Therapy.* Elsevier, 2022. https://doi.org/10.1016/C2020-0-02584-3.
72. Dhanalakshmi M, Sruthi D, Jinuraj KR, Das K, Dave S, Andal NM, Das J. Mannose: a potential saccharide candidate in disease management. *Medicinal Chemistry Research*, 2023;32(3):391–408.
73. Jagtap P, Nath H, Kumari PB, Dave S, Mohanty P, Das J, Dave S. Mycogenic fabrication of nanoparticles and their applications in modern agricultural practices & food industries. In *Fungi Bio-Prospects in Sustainable Agriculture, Environment and Nano-Technology* (pp. 475–488) 2021.

7 Carbon Nanobots as Biosensors for Infectious Diseases

Medha Pandya, Urja Desai, and Shreya Modi

7.1 INTRODUCTION

Despite the advancement in medical sciences, some diseases like cancer [1,2], diabetes, some infectious diseases, autoimmune diseases [3], and chronic pain have not been treated efficiently due to lack of proper diagnosis and treatment techniques [4]. One of the most dangerous causes of illnesses in humans today is emerging pathogenic bacteria and viruses. Infectious illnesses (like coronavirus disease 2019) are a significant threat to worldwide public health. Early detection of infectious disease can help patients' conditions be effectively controlled and treated. Because of this, the invention of novel diagnostic technology that is high-throughput, ultra-sensitive, and cost-effective has become a popular research area. The creation of detection systems utilizing complicated materials is a difficult but essential area of investigation for illness diagnosis due to the discovery of novel materials and the viability of processing and modification. Any global health system that promotes health care entails the diagnosis, treatment, and prevention of any human disease [5]. Through point of care (POC) technology, which helps with better on-site diagnostics, it has been continuously improved. POC testing implies that every test can be performed at or close to the location of patient care [6]. Nanotechnology has been proved as an efficient technology and widely exploited in recent times for the different medical and diagnosis applications. Different areas of diagnosis, medicine, and treatment have also focused on the use of nano-derived products [7]. With the determination of the biocompatibility of nanomaterials within the immune system it is widely fulfilled according to their surface chemistry. Recently, nanotechnology is widely applied to enhance targeted immune responses to the prevention and treatment of a number of infectious and non-infectious diseases [8]. The notion of nanomaterials has been adopted by science as a result of the connection between medical diagnostics, therapies, and monitoring with nanorobots [9]. Researchers in molecular biology, chemistry, medicine, math, engineering, and computer science all work in the field of nanotechnology, which is vastly multidisciplinary and involves many analytical hurdles. Carbon nanomaterials (CNs) are promising for multiple biological applications due to their structural variety, large surface area-to-volume

 DOI: 10.1201/9781003316435-7

ratios, ease of functionalization, peculiar optical characteristics, and biocompatibility. The variety of nanocarbon structures is remarkable. Graphene, fullerenes, carbon nanotubes (CNTs), graphene quantum dots (GQDs), carbon dots (CDs), carbon fibers (CFs), nanodiamonds, carbon nano-onions, and amorphous carbon nanostructures are allotropes of only one element, carbon [10]. Recent developments in the field of biosensing by CNs are introduced and discussed, highlighting the significance of their special properties in the diagnosis and treatment of infectious diseases as well as the difficulties and possibilities for potential clinical applications. The use of CNs in the biosensing of many diseases is still in its early stages, but biosensor technologies based on CNs represent a new generation.

7.2 BIOSENSORS

Biosensors are analytical instruments that detect biological components. There are mainly two types of biosensors: electrochemical and optical. Chemical sensors that belong to the subclass of electrochemical biosensors combine the high specificity of biological recognition processes with the sensitivity of electrochemical transducers, as shown by their low detection limits [11]. These devices have a biological recognition component that reacts with the target analyte only when it is present, resulting in the production of an electrical signal that is correlated with the quantity of the analyte under investigation. The signal is created and then sent as an electrical charge to the signal processor through the transducer. Useful information is made available in a legible form after a sequence of stages, including amplification and separation. Electrochemical biosensors are gaining popularity and are being developed extensively; some of them have already reached the commercial stage and are often utilized in agricultural and environmental applications [12]. Optical biosensors have excellent performance in identifying biological systems and support critical developments in clinical diagnostics, treatments, food process management, and environmental monitoring. High sensitivity, durability, and reliability of optical biosensors allow them to be incorporated into a single chip without trouble during pretreatment with little risk of changing the nature of the biological entity [13]. The transducing device transforms the recognition from the target molecules into a distinct visual signal. Optical signals are particularly sensitive, steady, and disturbance-resistant in comparison to other physical signals. Consequently, these biosensors benefit from the conventional sensors with labels.

In general, biosensors are composed of three components: a receptor (disease-specific) that detects the analyte, a transducer that turns the bio-recognition event into a quantifiable signal, and a readout. A biosensor commonly contains natural active compounds that are integrated into equipment that empowers the transformation of biochemical signals into quantifiable signals. Specifically, there are (i) bioreceptor (e.g., antibody, aptamer, nucleic acid) enabling the selectivity and specificity of the equipment, (ii) a transducer (e.g., cathode, fluorophore) promoting the physical or chemical changes subsequent to detecting analytes, and (iii) a signal-processing unit (signal output) [14]. Since the biomarker may some

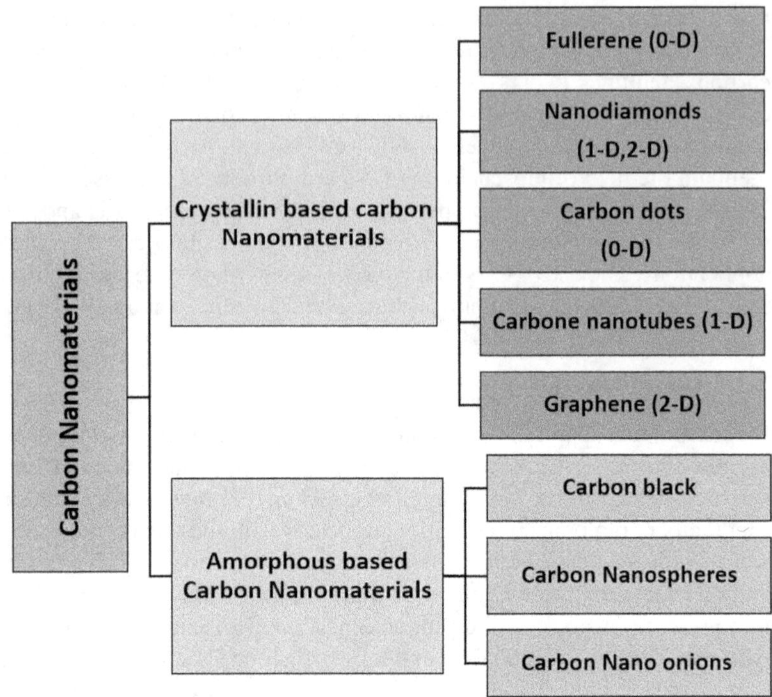

FIGURE 7.1 List of carbon-based materials applied for biosensor application.

of the time be found at extremely low fixations, the reasonableness, reproducibility, and strength of transducers are basically significant. Because of the special properties depicted above, various carbon-based nanomaterials (Figure 7.1) are ideal candidates for developing transducing components. Here, relying upon the signals produced by the transducers, nanomaterials can be efficiently applied for detection of a number of diseases [15].

7.3 CARBON NANOBOTS FOR BIOSENSING

Nanobots/nanorobot is a tiny device that is designed to carry out a specific function or sometimes can be used to perform tasks with precision at nanoscale dimensions of 1–100 nm [16–18]. Nanobots are widely used as sensors as well as for maintaining and protecting the human body against pathogenic microbes. Nanobots have ideal characteristics like they have exterior passive diamond coating especially to get rid of attack by the host immune system [19]. Generally, sensors provide two functions to the surface for the detection of the presence of target molecules and indirectly know the amount of damage that exists from the change in the functional properties of nanobots. Nanobots possess a high and rapid analysis. Currently, nano-cantilevers are being used as sensors to be applied in nanobots. The main significance of using cantilevers in nanobots is that it gives real-time detection, directly and quickly. Apart from these, they are capable of measuring cell mass, biomolecules, nucleic acids and others, as well as detecting specific molecules, and even manipulate and place nano-objects in predefined arrangements [20]. Nanobots implanted with chemical biosensors can be utilized to perform detection of tumor cells in beginning phases of development inside the patient's body. Coordinated nanosensors can be used for such a task in order to find the power of E-cadherin signals [21]. Patients having diabetes must take blood tests quite often to control glucose levels in their blood. Such strategies are awkward and extremely inconvenient. To avoid such sort of issues, the level of sugar in the body can be noticed by means of constant glucose monitoring by using medical nanorobots. Drinking water is the major concern all around the world. It has been reported that even a very low degree of fecal contamination in drinking water is adequate to cause a public health risk, and it remains challenging to rapidly detect bacteria such as *Escherichia coli.* As the current strategies require long incubation periods, are costly, and have impractical equipment, they cannot fulfill regulatory standards. To solve such issues, bacteriophages, tuned by billions of years of evolution to bind viable bacteria and designed to promptly create custom proteins, are exceptionally fit to bacterial identification. Researchers have developed a biosensor stage based on magnetized phages encoding brilliant correspondent compounds. The developed framework uses bio-symmetrically functionalized phages to empower site-specific conjugation to magnetic nanoparticles. The subsequent phage-based nanobots, when joined with standard, portable field equipment, take into account detection of <10 cfu/100 mL of viable *E. coli* within 7 hours, which is quicker than any methods distributed to date [22].

7.3.1 Graphene

Graphene, a carbon allotrope, has sparked a new "gold rush" since its discovery by the Nobel Prize winners Novoselov and Geim in 2010 [23] Graphene, a single-layer form of graphite, is a one-atom-thick sheet of carbon atoms located in a hexagonal lattice and bound by sp2. A monatomic layer of graphite is meant by the term "graphene." It is the fundamental building block of other allotropes like graphite, charcoal, carbon nanotubes, and fullerenes.

Nanomaterials in the graphene family have shown promising results in several areas of science. There has been a growing potential use of graphene and its derivatives [graphene oxide (GO) and reduced graphene oxide (rGO)] in several biomedical areas, such as drug delivery systems, biosensors, and imaging systems, especially due to their excellent optical, electronic, thermal, and mechanical properties [24,25]. GO is an intermediate product during the synthesis of rGO and prepared by oxidative exfoliation of graphite. At present, the dominant type of graphene used in adsorption applications is prepared via the GO route not only because of its potential for large-scale production, but also because it produces a functional form of graphene that is attractive for adsorption applications.

Graphene and its derivatives are particularly well suited to be used for designing nanobiosensors [26]. They can also be used to selectively bind to the SARS-CoV-2 virus through chemical functionalization with specific functional groups, and this can be harnessed to detect, capture, and even neutralize the viral pathogen. The use of plasmonic biosensors for the detection of viral pathogens (Dengue virus, Zika, Ebola, HIV, Hepatitis B, Avian influenza, Norovirus, etc.) has been the subject of several extensive and comprehensive reviews [27,28]. Recently, graphene biosensors were used to create POC testing tools for the detection of coronavirus disease-19 (COVID-19), a pandemic that is still running strong and affecting the entire world. SARS-CoV-2, the virus responsible for COVID-19, must be quickly and sensitively detected in order to control its spread within populations [29,30].

7.3.2 Carbon Nanotubes

Sumio Iijima, in his groundbreaking study published in *Nature* in 1991 titled "Helical Microtubules of Graphitic Carbon," reported the discovery of multi-walled carbon nanotubes and is credited with discovering carbon nanotubes (CNTs) [31]. Since Iijima's report on multi-walled carbon nanotubes (MWNTs), reports on single-walled carbon nanotubes (SWNTs) also followed [32,33]. CNTs have become one of the most intensively studied nanostructured materials [34], with thousands of papers published annually, promising new applications that have attracted academic and industrial interest.

CNTs are ideal for use in a multitude of fields, including engineering, electronics, optoelectronics, photonics, space, defense, medicine, molecular and biological systems, and many more due to their nanoscale sizes and extraordinary mechanical, electronic, transport, electrical, and optical properties, and they have been acknowledged as the material of the 21st century.

CNTs are hollow carbon structures with one or more walls, with a diameter measured in nanometers and a length that is more significant than the diameter. They are the stiffest and strongest fibers known due to their well-ordered arrangement of carbon atoms connected by sp2 bonds. Their distinct combination of electrical, magnetic, optical, mechanical, and chemical capabilities gives them an edge over other nanomaterials and holds great potential for a variety of applications, including biosensing [35,36]. CNs are carbon materials with a dispersive relative scale of at least one dimension less than 100 nm, including mainly CDs (0D), fullerenes (0D), carbon nanotubes (1D), carbon felts (1D), graphene (2D), and nanodiamonds (3D). Carbon nanotubes are classified into two types: single-walled carbon nanotubes (SWCNTs) and multi-walled carbon nanotubes (MWCNTs). Despite their striking similarities, SWCNTs and MWCNTs have drastically different physical properties due to their structural variations. These distinctions between single-walled and multi-walled carbon nanotubes result in significantly diverse characteristics and subsequent implications on materials. The different physical properties of SWCNTs vs MWCNTs are described in Table 7.1.

TABLE 7.1
Different Physical Properties of SWCNTs vs MWCNTs

Parameter	SWCNTs	MWCNTs
Key parameters		
Typical diameter	1–2 nm[a]	7–100 nm
Typical length	Up to 1 mm[b]	Up to 1 mm
Aspect ratio	Up to 10,000	50–4000
Mechanical properties		
Elastic modulus	1000–3000 GPa	300–1000 GPa
Tensile strength	50–100 GPa	10–50 GPa
Electronic structure properties		
Thermal conductivity at 300K	3000–6000 W/(m·K)	2000–3000 W/(m·K)
Minimum working dosage as an anti-static additive	0.01%	0.5%

[a] Larger diameters are possible but could lead to an increased number of defects.

[b] Longer lengths are possible but only at laboratory scale.

The COVID-19 pandemic, caused by a coronavirus, exemplifies the continued importance of these human-pathogenic viruses as a leading cause of illness and death around the world in 2020. Primary diagnostics are essential for making effective and timely treatment decisions for diseases. Diagnostic tests that are sensitive, specific, and quick are crucial in laying the groundwork for effective treatments and also in reducing the spread of infectious diseases [37] (Figure 7.2).

Though carbon nanotubes (CNTs) have been present for less than 30 years, and they continue to garner significant interest from researchers. Current global CNT production capacity exceeds several thousand tons per year. CNTs have attracted a lot of attention in numerous sensing applications due to their outstanding mechanical, electric, and optoelectronic capabilities and high aspect ratio [38].

To aid in the early detection, monitoring, and containment of disease outbreaks, nanosensors based on carbon nanotubes and graphene technology can play a significant role in the expansion of existing diagnostic capabilities around the world. Because of their unique physical, chemical, mechanical, and optoelectronic properties, as well as their vast surface area, these low-dimensional nanomaterials, such as carbon nanotubes and graphene, are highly useful for biological applications. The remarkable scalability, functional tunability, photostability, and optoelectronic features of carbon nanostructures make them a promising platform for biosensor creation.

Nanobiosensors use the principle of signal amplification based on the transduction of weak signals to detect the presence of biomolecules or microorganisms such as bacteria and viruses [39]. Various types of biosensors have been investigated based on their detection mechanism. These include resonant biosensors (coupled acoustic waves), optical biosensors (light), thermal biosensors (heat), ion-sensitive biosensors (change in surface potential), electrochemical biosensors

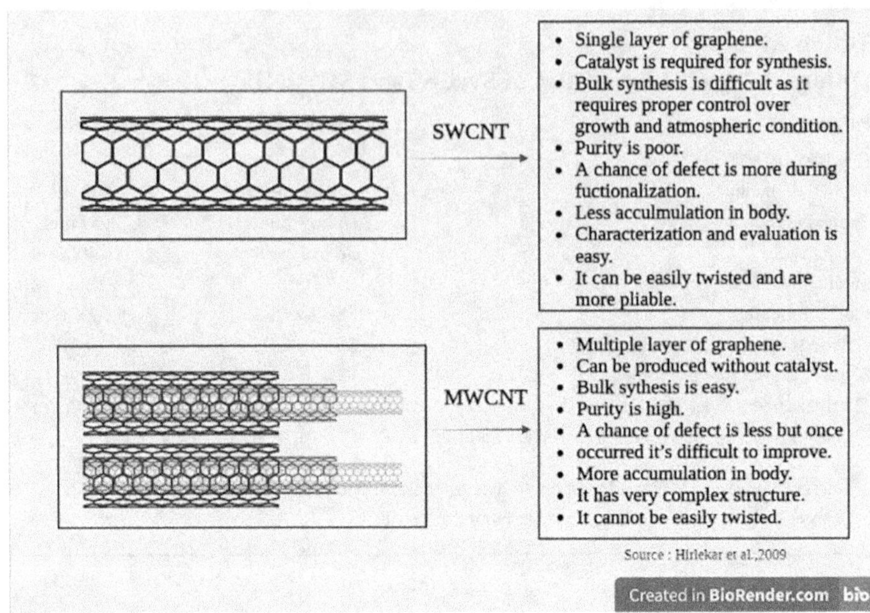

FIGURE 7.2 Characteristics of multi-walled carbon nanotubes (MWNTs) and single-walled carbon nanotubes (SWNTs).

(change in electrical characteristics of the medium), and amperometric or potentiometric biosensors (electron activity or redox potential) [40]. Plasmonic biosensors have been extensively reviewed for their use in the detection of viral (Dengue, Zika, Ebola, HIV, Hepatitis B, Avian influenza, Norovirus, etc.) infections, and it has added knowledge with recent publications of plasmonic biosensors [27,28]. High sensitivity, low cost, little sample pretreatment, rapid turnaround time from sample collection to assay result, and simple equipment are just some of the benefits that sensors based on plasmonic phenomena including surface plasmon resonance, localized surface plasmon resonance, surface-enhanced Raman scattering, surface-enhanced fluorescence, and IR absorption spectroscopy can provide [41]. These CNs are showing promise as candidates for a variety of scalable technologies, particularly in the field of biosensors for rapid diagnostics, due to the advancements in synthesis, sorting, purification, characterization, and functionalization techniques [42,43].

These low-dimensional nanomaterials, like carbon nanotubes and graphene, have unique physical, chemical, mechanical, and optoelectronic properties, a large surface area, and dimensions that are comparable to those of important biomolecules like DNA, proteins, and viruses. These properties make them especially advantageous for biomedical applications.

For the detection of viral infections including Zika, Ebola, MERS, and HIV, graphene and its derivatives (such GO or rGO) have been investigated in a variety of approaches [44,45] reported using a graphene-based field-effect transistor

(FET) covered with an antibody against the spike protein of the virus as one of the first electrochemical sensors used to detect SARS-CoV-2.

In 2020, it was stated that a graphene sensor platform coated with Au nanoparticles, resulting in surface-enhanced Raman scattering, might be used to create a quick (5 minutes), low-cost electrochemical sensor. A nanoparticle-based electrochemical sensor on graphene that targets the N-gene of SARS-CoV-2. The sensor had a 100% sensitivity, specificity, and accuracy in differentiating between COVID-19 positive and negative samples (as verified with an FDA EUA-approved RT-PCR diagnostic kit) [12].

In recent years, CRISPR-Cas/gRNA complexes have been employed for sensitive detection of nucleic acids, including those generated from human infections [46–52]. Using a CRISPR-Cas12a method (DNA endonuclease-targeted CRISPR trans reporter; DETECTOR), one team was able to properly detect 25/25 and 23/25 clinical specimens carrying human papillomavirus 16 (HPV16) and HPV18, respectively [47].

Recently, great progress has been made toward the application of methods like CRISPR-associated nuclease (Cas) proteins, in the form of a CRISPR-enhanced, graphene-based FET manufactured as a "CRISPR-Chip" to allow for rapid and selective detection of a target sequence contained inside genomic DNA [53]. In order to control the spread of the coronavirus pandemic and protect large populations, rapid, portable, and inexpensive diagnostics of COVID-19 are urgently required, particularly in resource-limited situations. Indian scientists have developed an innovative biosensor, eCovSens, an electrochemical device that can detect the SARS-CoV-2 virus's spike protein domain I with extreme sensitivity [54]. CalTech engineers developed RapidPlex, a multiplexed wireless telemedicine technology based on graphene [55]. Biomarkers such as SARS-CoV-2 nucleocapsid protein, antibodies against the spike protein (S1-IgM and S1-IgG), and C-reactive protein can be detected quantitatively in human blood and saliva using a mass-produced, laser-engraved graphene platform with four working electrodes [30]. This enables for the diagnostic testing of viral infection (NP) and immune response (IgG and Ig (CRP).

7.3.3 Carbon Dots

Among the different CNs, CDs with their size typically fewer than 10 nm represent an arising class of profoundly fluorescent 0D nanomaterials [56]. CDs belong to a family of quantum dots that are semiconductor nanoparticles commonly coated by a capping ligand as a passivating agent to maintain its colloidal stability [57]. On account of their smaller size and exceptional design, CDs show extraordinary fluorescence properties and can accordingly transmit light with high photoluminescent quantum yield (QY) after suitable illumination [58]. It has been shown that the fluorescence of CDs is profoundly steady and impervious to photobleaching and photo-blinking, which is beneficial, particularly when contrasted with normally utilized natural colors or polymer spots [59]. Generally, optical biosensors function by converting intangible data regarding target analysts into detectable optical signals. As ultraviolet rays are harmful to living organisms and

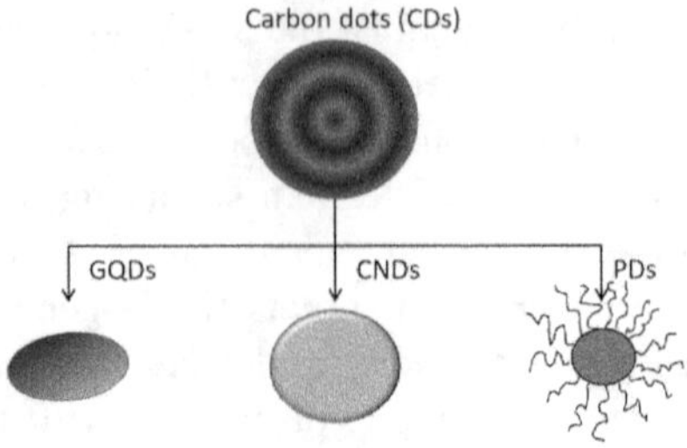

FIGURE 7.3 Three types of fluorescent CDs: graphene quantum dots (GQDs), carbon nanodots (CNDs), and polymer dots (PDs).

visible light is easily absorbed by living tissues, the nanoprobe should be working in the near-infrared (NIR) region. Compared to other nanomaterials, CDs can be tuned from the visible region to NIR range via careful selection of carbon precursor, manipulation of their synthesis process, and heteroatom doping. Due to such reasons, CDs are immensely suitable for optical biosensor development. CDs remain stable in the body and are not utilized without any problem by cells. Subsequent to detecting, CDs can be released from the body. Apart from these, their chemical inertness, hydrophobicity, and excellent biocompatibility make them more favorable for applications in biological and biomedical fields [60,61]. As compared to other nanomaterials, CDs represent numerous novel advantages in biosensing (Figure 7.3).

Raveendran and Kizhakayil [62] derived carbon dots from Mint leaf extract (M-CDs) and applied then for fluorimetric sensing of biologically relevant folic acid via quenching response originating from the inner filter effect, with a limit of detection of 280 nM. It has been reported that CDs are highly selective toward folic acid in a collection of 16 biomolecules. As per MTT assay, the M-CDs were found to be non-cytotoxic against primary H8 cells. Boronic acid–modified CDs are applied for various biomedical applications including biosensing, HIV therapy, cancer therapy, bioimaging, and as antiviral.

7.3.4 Graphene Quantum Dots (GQDs)

Nanomaterials successfully improve the sensor execution concerning their reproducibility, selectivity, and responsiveness. Specifically, GQDs, which are preferably graphene sections of nanometer size, comprise discrete highlights, like acting as attractive fluorophores and excellent electro catalysts inferable from their photostability, water-dissolvability, biocompatibility, non-harmfulness and favorable candidate that make them great possibility for many novel biomedical applications [63].

7.3.4.1 Novel Characteristics of Graphene Quantum Dots

GQDs are zero-dimensional, carbon-based, anisotropic nanomaterials having a texture homologous to graphene. The morphological elements of GQDs emulate the two CDs as well as graphene. They are extremely utilized as smart probes for environmental, optoelectronics, electrochemical, and organic activities. Their edge aspect is greater than their vertex, delivering single or complex boards of graphene with compound moieties on their horizontal surface, which convey countless destinations for synthetic functionalization [64]. GQDs can be effortlessly formed with a few nanomaterials through π–π cooperation, with a reason to create crossover nanomaterials [65]. Moreover, GQDs can likewise be united with a number of antibiotics, proteins, and small nucleic acids because of their layered similarities to such particles. GQDs are reported for successful upgradation of the outer layer of biosensors for retaining a noticeable number of receptors [63,66]. Different approaches are applied to synthesize GQDs which are listed in Figure 7.4.

Yersinia causes serious yersiniosis, a bacterial infection having the symptoms of fever, abdominal pain, cramps, diarrhea, joint pain, and other symptoms similar to appendicitis in older children and adults. To diagnose, GQOs-based immunosensor has been developed and used for the detection of the bacterium in milk and human serum. The GOD immunosuppression empowered the measurement of *Y. enterocolitica* in a wide fixation range with a high responsiveness (LODmilk = 5 cfu/mL and LODserum = 30 cfu/mL) and specificity. The developed method can be used for any pathogenic bacteria detection for food and clinical samples

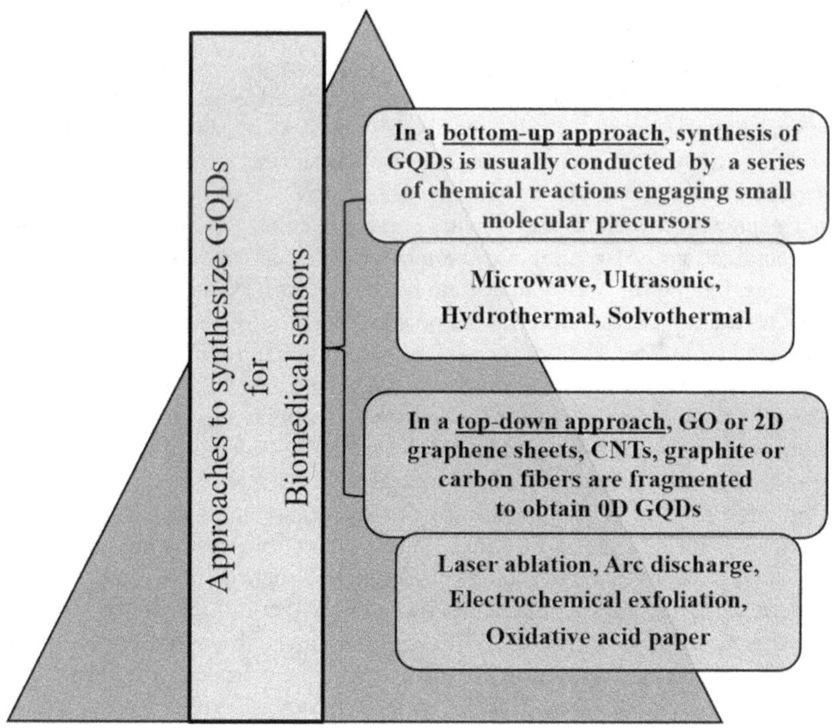

FIGURE 7.4 Approaches used to synthesize GQD.

without any pre-sample treatment. It has been stated that GQDs-based immunosensors are a more efficient, rapid, specific, and sensitive method compared to current methods used for pathogen detection like ELISA, PCR, and SPR-based tests [67]. In another study, researchers had developed field-effect transistors (FET)–based immunoassay techniques for the identification of inactivated Ebola viral (EBOV) infection. During the study, the surface of the FET was modified with rGO. The antibody against EBOV was immobilized on the surface of charged FET, and the reaction to EBOV was estimated as a component of the shift of Dirac voltage. The strategy can distinguish the EBOV over the focus range from 2.4×10^{-12} to $1–1.2\times10^{-7}$ g/mL and with a constraint of location as low as 2.4 pg/mL which represent satisfactory results [95]. The number of materials has been combined to enhance the efficiency of graphene-based biosensors which are represented in Table 7.2.

7.3.5 Fullerenes

Fullerenes are normal zero-dimensional carbon materials prepared by heating graphite under specific temperatures. In the current era, buckminsterfullerenes (C60) [105] and (C70) are the most broadly involved fullerene materials in research. The following stable homologue is C70 followed by higher fullerenes C74, C76, C78, C80, C82, C84, etc. [106]. Fullerenes have comparative properties to other CNs giving them an efficient role in disease diagnosis [107]. The outer layer of fullerenes can be functionalized by recognition atoms, for example, antibodies to focus on specific biomarkers specifically. Apart from these, one more particular property of fullerenes is the one of a kind 18π-electron aromatic structure, which empowers them to absorb photons across the solar spectrum in order to have a suitable direct band gap (2.0–2.6 eV) and a strong electron giver and acceptor limit with respect to photocurrent reaction balance through various functionalizations. Also, they are the most widely recognized spherical hollow molecules, having the ability to chelate heavy metals to their spherical interiors, in this way, altogether decreasing the poisonousness of different agents made by heavy metals and working on the safety of bioimaging techniques. The water solvency and *in vivo* biocompatibility of fullerenes are vital issues that should be tinted to, and various examinations have been performed to foster fullerene materials altered with hydrophilic groups (including fullerenol) to upgrade their application in the diagnosis of various diseases [108,109].

Fullerene-C60 is generally utilized for the development of electrochemical biosensors [110]. For the most part, electrochemical biosensors are logical gadgets which are comprised of a bioreceptor, an electrochemical dynamic point of interaction, a transducer component which convert natural responses to an electrical signal, and a signal processor [111]. Different electrode materials like gold, carbon paste, CFs, glassy fibers, and screen-printed electrodes have been utilized widely to immobilize DNA. But, because of advanced properties of CNs like fullerenes, they have attracted much attraction as the material for DNA sensors. In 2007, Shiraishi et al. [112] developed a new fullerene-based, DNA-modified

TABLE 7.2
Graphene-Based Biosensors for the Detection of Nucleic Acids and Genes

Type of Immunosensor	Target Molecule	Detection Methods	Detection Limit	References
Armchair graphene nanoribbon-Au electrode-FET	DNA hybridization	Electrical	-	[68]
Zirconia-reduced graphene oxide-thionine (ZrO2-rGO-Thi)	Nucleic acids	Electrochemical detection	24 fM	[69]
Crumpled graphene FET	miRNA let-7b	Electrical	600 zM	[70]
Deformed monolayer graphene channel	Nucleic acids	Electrochemical detection	600 zM and 20 aM	[70]
Polyaniline/graphene biosensor	HIV-1 gene	Electrochemical detection	1×10^{-16} M	[71]
Graphene field-effect transistor biosensor	RNA HIV-1 gene	Electrochemical detection	0,1 fM	[72]
AuNPs-GO nanocomposite	HIV-1 gene	Fluorescence detection	15 fM	[73]
Thionine-functionalized rGO (Thi-rGO) and rGO-graphene double-layer electrode	ssDNA	Electrochemical detection	$4.28 \times 10^{-19 M}$ and 1.58×10^{-13}	[74]
Glassy carbon electrode modified with rGO (GCE/RGO)	Amelogenin gene (AMEL)	Electrochemical detection	3.2×10^{-21} M	[75]
GO-DNA sensor	DNA of *Staphylococcus aureus*	Fluorescence detection	0.00625 nM	[76]
GO ethidium bromide	DNA and exonuclease activity	Electrochemical detection	32 nM	[77]
GO	ssDNA	Fluorescence detection	200 nM	[78]
Pencil graphite electrode modified with GO (GO/PGE)	Hepatitis B virus gene (HIV) gene	Electrochemical detection	2.02 μM	[79]
GO	T antigen gene of SV40 DNA	Fluorescence detection	14.3 nM	[80]
GQDs for the detection of viruses				
GQDs	Adenovirus	Optoelectronic	8.75 PFU/mL	[81]
MWCNT-NH2-IL-rGO	Human papillomavirus (HPV)	Electrochemical	1.3 nM	[82]
AuNP-MoS2-rGO	Porcine epidemic diarrhea virus	Electrochemical	-	[83]

(Continued)

TABLE 7.2 (*Continued*)

Graphene-Based Biosensors for the Detection of Nucleic Acids and Genes

Type of Immunosensor	Target Molecule	Detection Methods	Detection Limit	References
AuNPs-Graphene	*E.coli* O157	Electrochemical	10^2 CFU/mL	[84]
AuNPs-Graphene	*E.coli* K12	Electrochemical	12 CFU/mL	[85]
rGO, rGO/CuNPs	Hepatitis C virus (HCV)	Optical, electrochemical	10 fM, 0.4 nM	[86]
Magnetic rGO-CuNCs	HCV	Electrochemical	405.0 pM	[87]
APTMS-ZnO/c-GO	*E. coli* O157	Electrochemical	0.1 fM	[88]
GO	*Bacillus anthracis*	Fluorescence	0.625 μM	[89]
Graphene-AuNPs	*Staphylococcus aureus*	Surface acoustic wave	12.4 pg/mL	[90]
rGO, rGO/PAMAM	Dengue virus	Optical	0.08 pM	[91–92]
G/CVD, GO/PANi	HIV	Electrochemical	0.1 ng/mL, 100 aM	[93]
rGO	Ebola virus	Electrochemical	2.4 pg/mL and 1 μg/mL	[94–95]
rGO	*E. coli*	Electrical	10^3 CFU/mL	[96]
Graphene	Zika virus	Electrical	0.45 nM	[97]
rGO/AuNPs, quantum dots	Hepatitis B virus	Electrochemical	3.8 ng/mL, 1 nM	[98–99]
GO-AgNPs Nanocomposite	*Salmonella typhimurium*	Cyclic voltammetry (CV)	10 cfu/mL	[100]
GQDs on AuNPs with polyamidoamine dendrimer embedded on MWCNTs	Celiac disease	Electrochemical	0.1 gf/6 μL	[101]
Graphene oxide-MB-chitosan	Influenza A virus	Electrochemical	9.4 and 8.4 pM	[102]
Graphene-polypyrrole	Cholera toxin	Surface plasmon resonance	4 pg/mL	[103]
GO	Rotavirus	Photoluminescence	10^5 PFU/mL	[104]

electrode for the electrochemical detection of 16S rDNA extracted from *E. coli* (JCM1649). During the study, the electrodes were fabricated by screen printing a fullerene-impregnated carbon ink onto a poly(methyl methacrylate) substrate and mobilizing a probe DNA on the surface subsequent to enacting the electrode with air plasma. The outcomes represented that by immobilizing the probe onto the fullerene-impregnated, screen-printed electrodes, the PCR product of the 16s DNA separated from *E. coli* was straightforwardly identified without any pretreatment.

7.4 SUMMARY

The emergence and spread of infectious diseases continue to be a pervasive risk to public health worldwide, especially in a number of countries, and rural and backward areas of cities. The basic reason behind the genesis of severe diseases can be the scarcity of efficient and reliable diagnostic techniques and consequent therapeutic approaches, resulting from the inappropriate availability of consolidated and fortified healthcare procedure and equipment for analysis. The recent advances in various ranges of CNs, especially nanocarbon-based biosensors, graphene, fullerene, carbon nanotubes, and other bioimaging approaches for the detection of infectious diseases and tumors, were described in this chapter. The unique electrochemical, optical, surface tenability, and surface area-to-volume ratio of CNs make them extraordinarily suitable for various applications in the field of medical science. The outbreaks of epidemic and pandemic diseases (like SARS-CoV-2) and the necessity of early diagnosis methods stimulated the application of CNs in diagnosis and biomedicine.

REFERENCES

1. Mozaffari H, Izadi B, Sadeghi M, Rezaei F, Sharifi R, Jalilian F. Prevalence of oral and pharyngeal cancers in Kermanshah province, Iran: A ten-year period. *International Journal of Cancer Research*. 2016;12(3–4):169–75.
2. Moyer E, Hardon A. A disease unlike any other? Why HIV remains exceptional in the age of treatment. *Medical Anthropology*. 2014 Jul 4;33(4):263–9.
3. Mozaffari HR, Zavattaro E, Saeedi M, Lopez-Jornet P, Sadeghi M, Safaei M, Imani MM, Nourbakhsh R, Moradpoor H, Golshah A, Sharifi R. Serum and salivary interleukin-4 levels in patients with oral lichen planus: A systematic review and meta-analysis. *Oral Surgery, Oral Medicine, Oral Pathology and Oral Radiology*. 2019 Aug 1;128(2):123–31.
4. Rezaei R, Safaei M, Mozaffari HR, Moradpoor H, Karami S, Golshah A, Salimi B, Karami H. The role of nanomaterials in the treatment of diseases and their effects on the immune system. *Open Access Macedonian Journal of Medical Sciences*. 2019 Jun 6;7(11):1884.
5. Acharya D, Satapathy S, Dixit PK, Mishra G, Mohanty P, Das J, Dave S. Biological nanomaterials for toxicity of bacteria. In K. Pal, T. Zaheer (eds.) *Nanomaterials in the Battle Against Pathogens and Disease Vectors*, 2022 (pp. 187–204). CRC Press, Boca Raton, FL.

6. Panwar R, Churi H, Dave S. Point-of-care electrochemical biosensors using CRISPR/Cas for RNA analysis. In *Biosensors for Emerging and Re-Emerging Infectious Diseases*, 2022 Jan 1 (pp. 317–333). Academic Press. doi:10.1016/B978-0-323-88464-8.00003-8.
7. Rezaei R, Safaei M, Mozaffari HR, Moradpoor H, Karami S, Golshah A, Salimi B, Karami H. The role of nanomaterials in the treatment of diseases and their effects on the immune system. *Open access Macedonian Journal of Medical Sciences*. 2019 Jun 6;7(11):1884.
8. Chai LX, Fan XX, Zuo YH, Zhang B, Nie GH, Xie N, Xie ZJ, Zhang H. Low-dimensional nanomaterials enabled autoimmune disease treatments: Recent advances, strategies, and future challenges. *Coordination Chemistry Reviews*. 2021 Apr 1;432:213697.
9. Ghosh S, Nag M, Lahiri D, Mukherjee D, Garai S, Ray RR. Advanced nanomaterials for point-of-care diagnosis and therapy. In *Advanced Nanomaterials for Point of Care Diagnosis and Therapy*. 2022 Jan 1:423–50. doi: 10.1016/B978-0-323-85725-3.00010-6.
10. Holban AM, Grumezescu AM, editors. *Materials for Biomedical Engineering: Nanomaterials-based Drug Delivery*, 2019. Elsevier. doi: 10.1016/C2017-0-04563-9.
11. Das J, Dave S, Radhakrishnan S, Mohanty P. *Biosensors for Emerging and Re-emerging Infectious Diseases*, 2022. Elsevier, San Diego, CA.
12. Alafeef M, Dighe K, Moitra P, Pan D. Rapid, ultrasensitive, and quantitative detection of SARS-CoV-2 using antisense oligonucleotides directed electrochemical biosensor chip. *ACS Nano*. 2020 Oct 20;14(12):17028–45.
13. Ahmed SR, Mogus J, Chand R, Nagy E, Neethirajan S. Optoelectronic fowl adenovirus detection based on local electric field enhancement on graphene quantum dots and gold nanobundle hybrid. *Biosensors and Bioelectronics*. 2018 Apr 30;103:45–53.
14. Shah S, Maharshi A, Pandya M, Dhanalakshmi M, Das K. Nucleic acid based biosensor as a cutting edge tool for point of care diagnosis. In *Biosensors for Emerging and Re-Emerging Infectious Diseases* 2022 Jan 1 (pp. 265–301). Academic Press. doi: 10.1016/B978-0-323-88464-8.00014-2.
15. Yu Z, Cai G, Liu X, Tang D. Pressure-based biosensor integrated with a flexible pressure sensor and an electrochromic device for visual detection. *Analytical Chemistry*. 2021 Jan 25;93(5):2916–25.
16. Safaei M, Karimi N, Alavi M, Taran M. Application of nanomaterial in nutrition and food sciences. *Journal of Advances in Applied Science Research*. 2017;1(12):1–6.
17. Pandya M, Jani S, Dave V, Rawal R. Nanoinformatics: An emerging trend in cancer therapeutics. *Nanobiotechnology*. 2020 Mar 19:135–62.
18. Dave V, Pandya M, Rawal R, Bhatnagar SP, Mehta R. Smart and intelligent vehicles for drug delivery: Theranostic nanorobots. In *Advanced Nanomaterials for Point of Care Diagnosis and Therapy*, 2022 Jan 1 (pp. 541–564). Elsevier. doi: 10.1016/B978-0-323-85725-3.00004-0.
19. Sivasankar M, Durairaj R. Brief review on nano robots in bio medical applications. *Advances in Robotics and Automation*. 2012 Feb 27;1(101):2.
20. Johnson BN, Mutharasan R. Biosensing using dynamic-mode cantilever sensors: A review. *Biosensors and Bioelectronics*. 2012 Feb 15;32(1):1–8.
21. Kumar SS, Nasim BP, Abraham E. Nanorobots a future device for diagnosis and treatment. *Journal of Pharmacy and Pharmacology*. 2018 Feb 1;5:44–9.
22. Zurier HS, Duong MM, Goddard JM, Nugen SR. Engineering biorthogonal phage-based nanobots for ultrasensitive, in situ bacteria detection. *ACS Applied Bio Materials*. 2020 Jun 23;3(9):5824–31.

23. Geim AK, Novoselov KS. The rise of graphene. *Nature Materials.* 2007 Mar;6(3):183–91.
24. Magne TM, de Oliveira Vieira T, Alencar LMR, Junior FFM, Gemini-Piperni S, Carneiro SV, Fechine LM, Freire RM, Golokhvast K, Metrangolo P, Fechine P. Graphene and its derivatives: Understanding the main chemical and medicinal chemistry roles for biomedical applications. *Journal of Nanostructure in Chemistry.* 2021;12:1–35.
25. Reina G, González-Domínguez JM, Criado A, Vázquez E, Bianco A, Prato M. Promises, facts and challenges for graphene in biomedical applications. *Chemical Society Reviews.* 2017;46(15):4400–16.
26. Novoselov KS, Colombo L, Gellert PR, Schwab MG, Kim K. A roadmap for graphene. *Nature.* 2012 Oct;490(7419):192–200.
27. Hassan MM, Sium FS, Islam F, Choudhury SM. A review on plasmonic and metamaterial based biosensing platforms for virus detection. *Sensing and Bio-Sensing Research.* 2021 Aug 1;33:100429.
28. Shrivastav AM, Cvelbar U, Abdulhalim I. A comprehensive review on plasmonic-based biosensors used in viral diagnostics. *Communications Biology.* 2021 Jan 15;4(1):1–2.
29. Alafeef M, Dighe K, Moitra P, Pan D. Rapid, ultrasensitive, and quantitative detection of SARS-CoV-2 using antisense oligonucleotides directed electrochemical biosensor chip. *ACS Nano.* 2020;14(12):17028–17045.
30. Torrente-Rodríguez RM, Lukas H, Tu J, Min J, Yang Y, Xu C, Rossiter HB, Gao W. SARS-CoV-2 RapidPlex: A graphene-based multiplexed telemedicine platform for rapid and low-cost COVID-19 diagnosis and monitoring. *Matter.* 2020 Dec 2;3(6):1981–98.
31. Iijima S. Helical microtubules of graphitic carbon. *Nature.* 1991 Nov;354(6348):56–8.
32. Iijima S, Ichihashi T. Single-shell carbon nanotubes of 1-nm diameter. *Nature.* 1993 Jun;363(6430):603–5.
33. Journet C, Maser WK, Bernier P, Loiseau A, de La Chapelle ML, Lefrant DS, Deniard P, Lee R, Fischer JE. Large-scale production of single-walled carbon nanotubes by the electric-arc technique. *Nature.* 1997 Aug;388(6644):756–8.
34. Balasubramanian K, Burghard M, Kern K, Scolari M, Mews A. Photocurrent imaging of charge transport barriers in carbon nanotube devices. *Nano Letters.* 2005 Mar 9;5(3):507–10.
35. Holzinger M, Le Goff A, Cosnier S. Carbon nanotube/enzyme biofuel cells. *Electrochimica Acta.* 2012 Nov 1;82:179–90.
36. Biju V. Chemical modifications and bioconjugate reactions of nanomaterials for sensing, imaging, drug delivery and therapy. *Chemical Society Reviews.* 2014;43(3):744–64.
37. Chen H, Cheng Z, Zhou X, Wang R, Yu F. Emergence of surface-enhanced raman scattering probes in near-infrared windows for biosensing and bioimaging. *Analytical Chemistry.* 2021;94(1):143–164.
38. Camilli L, Passacantando M. Advances on sensors based on carbon nanotubes. *Chemosensors.* 2018 Dec 6;6(4):62.
39. Sharma PK, Dorlikar S, Rawat P, Malik V, Vats N, Sharma M, Rhyee JS, Kaushik AK. Nanotechnology and its application: A review. *Nanotechnology in Cancer Management.* 2021 Jan 1:1–33. doi: 10.1016/B978-0-12-818154-6.00010-X.
40. Bardhan NM, Jansen P, Belcher AM. Graphene, carbon nanotube and plasmonic nanosensors for detection of viral pathogens: opportunities for rapid testing in pandemics like COVID-19. *Frontiers in Nanotechnology.* 2021;3:733126.

41. Anker JN, Hall WP, Lyandres O, Shah NC, Zhao J, Duyne RV. Biosensing with plasmonic nanosensors. *Nature Materials*. 2008;7:442.
42. Hong G, Diao S, Antaris AL, Dai H. Carbon nanomaterials for biological imaging and nanomedicinal therapy. *Chemical Reviews*. 2015 Oct 14;115(19):10816–906.
43. Bardhan NM, Kumar PV, Li Z, Ploegh HL, Grossman JC, Belcher AM, Chen GY. Enhanced cell capture on functionalized graphene oxide nanosheets through oxygen clustering. *ACS Nano*. 2017 Feb 28;11(2):1548–58.
44. Jiang Z, Feng B, Xu J, Qing T, Zhang P, Qing Z. Graphene biosensors for bacterial and viral pathogens. *Biosensors and Bioelectronics*. 2020 Oct 15;166:112471.
45. Seo G, Lee G, Kim MJ, Baek SH, Choi M, Ku KB, Lee CS, Jun S, Park D, Kim HG, Kim SJ. Rapid detection of COVID-19 causative virus (SARS-CoV-2) in human nasopharyngeal swab specimens using field-effect transistor-based biosensor. *ACS Nano*. 2020 Apr 15;14(4):5135–42.
46. Bruch R, Baaske J, Chatelle C, Meirich M, Madlener S, Weber W, Dincer C, Urban GA. CRISPR/Cas13a-powered electrochemical microfluidic biosensor for nucleic acid amplification-free miRNA diagnostics. *Advanced Materials*. 2019 Dec;31(51):1905311.
47. Chen JS, Ma E, Harrington LB, Da Costa M, Tian X, Palefsky JM, Doudna JA. CRISPR-Cas12a target binding unleashes indiscriminate single-stranded DNase activity. *Science*. 2018 Apr 27;360(6387):436–9.
48. Gootenberg JS, Abudayyeh OO, Lee JW, Essletzbichler P, Dy AJ, Joung J, Verdine V, Donghia N, Daringer NM, Freije CA, Myhrvold C. Nucleic acid detection with CRISPR-Cas13a/C2c2. *Science*. 2017 Apr 28;356(6336):438–42.
49. Hajian R, Balderston S, Tran T, DeBoer T, Etienne J, Sandhu M, Wauford NA, Chung JY, Nokes J, Athaiya M, Paredes J. Detection of unamplified target genes via CRISPR-Cas9 immobilized on a graphene field-effect transistor. *Nature Biomedical Engineering*. 2019 Jun;3(6):427–37.
50. Lucia A, Guzmán E. Emulsions containing essential oils, their components or volatile semiochemicals as promising tools for insect pest and pathogen management. *Advances in Colloid and Interface Science*. 2021 Jan 1;287:102330.
51. Pardee K, Green AA, Takahashi MK, Braff D, Lambert G, Lee JW, Ferrante T, Ma D, Donghia N, Fan M, Daringer NM. Rapid, low-cost detection of Zika virus using programmable biomolecular components. *Cell*. 2016 May 19;165(5):1255–66.
52. Li H, Gao H, Meng H, Wang Q, Li S, Chen H, Li Y, Wang H. Detection of pulmonary infectious pathogens from lung biopsy tissues by metagenomic next-generation sequencing. *Frontiers in Cellular and Infection Microbiology*. 2018 Jun 25;8:205.
53. Hajian R, Balderston S, Tran T, DeBoer T, Etienne J, Sandhu M, Wauford NA, Chung JY, Nokes J, Athaiya M, Paredes J. Detection of unamplified target genes via CRISPR-Cas9 immobilized on a graphene field-effect transistor. *Nature Biomedical Engineering*. 2019 Jun;3(6):427–37.
54. Mahari S, Roberts A, Shahdeo D, Gandhi S. eCovSens-ultrasensitive novel in-house built printed circuit board based electrochemical device for rapid detection of nCovid-19 antigen, a spike protein domain 1 of SARS-CoV-2. BioRxiv. 2020 Jan 1. doi: 10.1101/2020.04.24.059204.
55. Zhang Z, Tang Z, Farokhzad N, Chen T, Tao W. Sensitive, rapid, low-cost, and multiplexed COVID-19 monitoring by the wireless telemedicine platform. *Matter*. 2020 Dec 2;3(6):1818–20.
56. Xia C, Zhu S, Feng T, Yang M, Yang B. Evolution and synthesis of carbon dots: From carbon dots to carbonized polymer dots. *Advanced Science*. 2019 Dec;6(23):1901316.

57. Aung YY, Kristanti AN, Lee HV, Fahmi MZ. Boronic-acid-modified nanomaterials for biomedical applications. *ACS Omega*. 2021 Jul 6;6(28):17750–65.
58. Issa MA, Abidin ZZ, Sobri S, Rashid SA, Mahdi MA, Ibrahim NA. Fluorescent recognition of Fe^{3+} in acidic environment by enhanced-quantum yield N-doped carbon dots: Optimization of variables using central composite design. *Scientific Reports*. 2020 Jul 16;10(1):1–8.
59. Wang K, Gao Z, Gao G, Wo Y, Wang Y, Shen G, Cui D. Systematic safety evaluation on photoluminescent carbon dots. *Nanoscale Research Letters*. 2013 Dec;8(1):1–9.
60. Lim CS, Hola K, Ambrosi A, Zboril R, Pumera M. Graphene and carbon quantum dots electrochemistry. *Electrochemistry Communications*. 2015 Mar 1;52:75–9.
61. Langer M, Paloncýová M, Medveď M, Pykal M, Nachtigallová D, Shi B, Aquino AJ, Lischka H, Otyepka M. Progress and challenges in understanding of photoluminescence properties of carbon dots based on theoretical computations. *Applied Materials Today*. 2021 Mar 1;22:100924.
62. Raveendran V, Kizhakayil RN. Fluorescent carbon dots as biosensor, green reductant, and biomarker. *ACS Omega*. 2021 Aug 27;6(36):23475–84.
63. Mansuriya BD, Altintas Z. Applications of graphene quantum dots in biomedical sensors. *Sensors*. 2020 Feb 16;20(4):1072.
64. Faridbod F, Sanati AL. Graphene quantum dots in electrochemical sensors/biosensors. *Current Analytical Chemistry*. 2019 Apr 1;15(2):103–23.
65. Tachi S, Morita H, Takahashi M, Okabayashi Y, Hosokai T, Sugai T, Kuwahara S. Quantum yield enhancement in graphene quantum dots via esterification with benzyl alcohol. *Scientific Reports*. 2019 Oct 1;9(1):1–7.
66. Roushani M, Valipour A, Bahrami M. The potentiality of graphene quantum dots functionalized by nitrogen and thiol-doped (GQDs-NS) to stabilize the antibodies in designing of human chorionic gonadotropin immunosensor. *Nanochemistry Research*. 2019;4:20–6.
67. Savas S, Altintas Z. Graphene quantum dots as nanozymes for electrochemical sensing of Yersinia enterocolitica in milk and human serum. *Materials*. 2019 Jul 8;12(13):2189.
68. Bagherzadeh-Nobari S, Kalantarinejad R. Real-time label-free detection of DNA hybridization using a functionalized graphene field effect transistor: A theoretical study. *Journal of Nanoparticle Research*. 2021 Aug;23(8):1–6.
69. Chen Z, Liu X, Liu D, Li F, Wang L, Liu S. Ultrasensitive electrochemical DNA biosensor fabrication by coupling an integral multifunctional zirconia-reduced graphene oxide-thionine nanocomposite and exonuclease I-assisted cleavage. *Frontiers in Chemistry*. 2020 Jul 9;8:521.
70. Hwang MT, Heiranian M, Kim Y, You S, Leem J, Taqieddin A, Faramarzi V, Jing Y, Park I, van der Zande AM, Nam S. Ultrasensitive detection of nucleic acids using deformed graphene channel field effect biosensors. *Nature Communications*. 2020 Mar 24;11(1):1.
71. Gong Q, Han H, Yang H, Zhang M, Sun X, Liang Y, Liu Z, Zhang W, Qiao J. Sensitive electrochemical DNA sensor for the detection of HIV based on a polyaniline/graphene nanocomposite. *Journal of Materiomics*. 2019 Jun 1;5(2):313–9.
72. Tian M, Xu S, Zhang J, Wang X, Li Z, Liu H, Song R, Yu Z, Wang J. RNA detection based on graphene field-effect transistor biosensor. *Advances in Condensed Matter Physics*. 2018 Jun 3;2018:1–6.
73. Qaddare SH, Salimi A. Amplified fluorescent sensing of DNA using luminescent carbon dots and AuNPs/GO as a sensing platform: A novel coupling of FRET and DNA hybridization for homogeneous HIV-1 gene detection at femtomolar level. *Biosensors and Bioelectronics*. 2017;89:773–80.

74. Ye Y, Xie J, Ye Y, Cao X, Zheng H, Xu X, Zhang Q. A label-free electrochemical DNA biosensor based on thionine functionalized reduced graphene oxide. *Carbon*. 2018 Apr 1;129:730–7.
75. Benvidi A, Rajabzadeh N, Mazloum-Ardakani M, Heidari MM, Mulchandani A. Simple and label-free electrochemical impedance Amelogenin gene hybridization biosensing based on reduced graphene oxide. *Biosensors and Bioelectronics*. 2014 Aug 15;58:145–52.
76. Jia F, Duan N, Wu S, Ma X, Xia Y, Wang Z, Wei X. Impedimetric aptasensor for Staphylococcus aureus based on nanocomposite prepared from reduced graphene oxide and gold nanoparticles. *Microchimica Acta*. 2014 Jul;181:967–74.
77. Jiang Y, Tian J, Chen S, Zhao Y, Wang Y, Zhao S. A graphene oxide-based sensing platform for the label-free assay of DNA sequence and exonuclease activity via long range resonance energy transfer. *Journal of Fluorescence*. 2013 Jul;23(4):697–703.
78. Liu H, Wang Y, Shen A, Zhou X, Hu J. Highly selective and sensitive method for cysteine detection based on fluorescence resonance energy transfer between FAM-tagged ssDNA and graphene oxide. *Talanta*. 2012 May 15;93:330–5.
79. Muti M, Sharma S, Erdem A, Papakonstantinou P. Electrochemical monitoring of nucleic acid hybridization by single-use graphene oxide-based sensor. *Electroanalysis*. 2011 Jan;23(1):272–9.
80. He S, Song B, Li D, Zhu C, Qi W, Wen Y, Wang L, Song S, Fang H, Fan C. A graphene nanoprobe for rapid, sensitive, and multicolor fluorescent DNA analysis. *Advanced Functional Materials*. 2010 Feb 8;20(3):453–9.
81. Ahmed SR, Mogus J, Chand R, Nagy E, Neethirajan S. Optoelectronic fowl adenovirus detection based on local electric field enhancement on graphene quantum dots and gold nanobundle hybrid. *Biosensors and Bioelectronics*. 2018 Apr 30;103:45–53.
82. Farzin L, Sadjadi S, Shamsipur M, Sheibani S. Electrochemical genosensor based on carbon nanotube/amine-ionic liquid functionalized reduced graphene oxide nanoplatform for detection of human papillomavirus (HPV16)-related head and neck cancer. *Journal of Pharmaceutical and Biomedical Analysis*. 2020 Feb 5;179:112989.
83. Li J, Li Y, Zhai X, Cao Y, Zhao J, Tang Y, Han K. Sensitive electrochemical detection of hepatitis C virus subtype based on nucleotides assisted magnetic reduced graphene oxide-copper nano-composite. *Electrochemistry Communications*. 2020 Jan 1;110:106601.
84. You Z, Qiu Q, Chen H, Feng Y, Wang X, Wang Y, Ying Y. Laser-induced noble metal nanoparticle-graphene composites enabled flexible biosensor for pathogen detection. *Biosensors and Bioelectronics*. 2020 Feb 15;150:111896.
85. Zhao W, Xing Y, Lin Y, Gao Y, Wu M, Xu J. Monolayer graphene chemiresistive biosensor for rapid bacteria detection in a microchannel. *Sensors and Actuators Reports*. 2020 Nov 1;2(1):100004.
86. Fan J, Yuan L, Liu Q, Tong C, Wang W, Xiao F, Liu B, Liu X. An ultrasensitive and simple assay for the Hepatitis C virus using a reduced graphene oxide-assisted hybridization chain reaction. *Analyst*. 2019;144(13):3972–9.
87. Li JY, You Z, Wang Q, Zhou ZJ, Qiu Y, Luo R, Ge XY. The epidemic of 2019-novel-coronavirus (2019-nCoV) pneumonia and insights for emerging infectious diseases in the future. *Microbes and Infection*. 2020 Mar 1;22(2):80–5.
88. Jaiswal N, Pandey CM, Solanki S, Tiwari I, Malhotra BD. An impedimetric biosensor based on electrophoretically assembled ZnO nanorods and carboxylated graphene nanoflakes on an indium tin oxide electrode for detection of the DNA of Escherichia coli O157: H7. *Microchimica Acta*. 2020 Jan;187(1):1–8.

89. Ziółkowski R, Oszwałdowski S, Kopyra KK, Zacharczuk K, Zasada AA, Malinowska E. Toward fluorimetric-paired-emitter-detector-diode test for Bacillus anthracis DNA based on graphene oxide. *Microchemical Journal.* 2020 May 1;154:104592.
90. Ji J, Pang Y, Li D, Wang X, Xu Y, Mu X. Single-layered graphene/Au-nanoparticles-based love wave biosensor for highly sensitive and specific detection of Staphylococcus aureus gene sequences. *ACS Applied Materials & Interfaces.* 2020 Jan 24;12(11):12417–25.
91. Omar NAS, Fen YW, Abdullah J, Mustapha Kamil Y, Daniyal WMEMM, Sadrolhosseini AR, Mahdi MA. Sensitive detection of dengue virus type 2 E-proteins signals using self-assembled monolayers/reduced graphene oxide-PAMAM dendrimer thin film-SPR optical sensor. *Scientific Reports.* 2020;10(1):1–15.
92. Kanagavalli P, Veerapandian M. Opto-electrochemical functionality of Ru (II)-reinforced graphene oxide nanosheets for immunosensing of dengue virus non-structural 1 protein. *Biosensors and Bioelectronics.* 2020 Feb 15;150:111878.
93. Islam S, Shukla S, Bajpai VK, Han YK, Huh YS, Kumar A, Ghosh A, Gandhi S. A smart nanosensor for the detection of human immunodeficiency virus and associated cardiovascular and arthritis diseases using functionalized graphene-based transistors. *Biosensors and Bioelectronics.* 2019;126:792–799.
94. Maity A, Sui X, Jin B, Pu H, Bottum KJ, Huang X, Chang J, Zhou G, Lu G, Chen J. Resonance-frequency modulation for rapid, point-of-care Ebola-Glycoprotein diagnosis with a graphene-based field-effect biotransistor. *Analytical Chemistry.* 2018 Nov 6;90(24):14230–8.
95. Jin X, Zhang H, Li YT, Xiao MM, Zhang ZL, Pang DW, Wong G, Zhang ZY, Zhang GJ. A field effect transistor modified with reduced graphene oxide for immunodetection of Ebola virus. *Microchimica Acta.* 2019 Apr;186(4):1–9.
96. Thakur B, Zhou G, Chang J, Pu H, Jin B, Sui X, Yuan X, Yang CH, Magruder M, Chen J. Rapid detection of single E. coli bacteria using a graphene-based field-effect transistor device. *Biosensors and Bioelectronics.* 2018 Jul 1;110:16–22.
97. Afsahi S, Lerner MB, Goldstein JM, Lee J, Tang X, Bagarozzi Jr. DA, Pan D, Locascio L, Walker A, Barron F, Goldsmith BR. Novel graphene-based biosensor for early detection of Zika virus infection. *Biosensors and Bioelectronics.* 2018 Feb 15;100:85–8.
98. Abd Muain MF, Cheo KH, Omar MN, Hamzah AS, Lim HN, Salleh AB, Tan WS, Tajudin AA. Gold nanoparticle-decorated reduced-graphene oxide targeting anti hepatitis B virus core antigen. *Bioelectrochemistry.* 2018 Aug 1;122:199–205.
99. Xiang Q, Huang J, Huang H, Mao W, Ye Z. A label-free electrochemical platform for the highly sensitive detection of hepatitis B virus DNA using graphene quantum dots. *RSC Advances.* 2018;8(4):1820–5.
100. Sign C, Sumana G. Antibody conjugated graphene nanocomposites for pathogen detection. *Journal of Physics: Conference Series.* 2016 Apr 1;704(1):012014.
101. Gupta S, Kaushal A, Kumar A, Kumar D. Ultrasensitive transglutaminase based nanosensor for early detection of celiac disease in human. *International Journal of Biological Macromolecules.* 2017 Dec 1;105:905–11.
102. Veerapandian M, Hunter R, Neethirajan S. Dual immunosensor based on methylene blue-electroadsorbed graphene oxide for rapid detection of the influenza A virus antigen. *Talanta.* 2016 Aug 1;155:250–7.
103. Singh M, Holzinger M, Tabrizian M, Winters S, Berner NC, Cosnier S, Duesberg GS. Noncovalently functionalized monolayer graphene for sensitivity enhancement of surface plasmon resonance immunosensors. *Journal of the American Chemical Society.* 2015 Mar 4;137(8):2800–3.

104. Jung JH, Cheon DS, Liu F, Lee KB, Seo TS. A graphene oxide based immunobiosensor for pathogen detection. *Angewandte Chemie*. 2010 Aug 2;122(33):5844–7.
105. Gergeroglu H, Yildirim S, Ebeoglugil MF. Nano-carbons in biosensor applications: An overview of carbon nanotubes (CNTs) and fullerenes (C60). *SN Applied Sciences*. 2020 Apr;2(4):1–22.
106. Pilehvar S, De Wael K. Recent advances in electrochemical biosensors based on fullerene-C60 nano-structured platforms. *Biosensors*. 2015 Nov 23;5(4):712–35.
107. Alagarsamy KN, Mathan S, Yan W, Rafieerad A, Sekaran S, Manego H, Dhingra S. Carbon nanomaterials for cardiovascular theranostics: Promises and challenges. *Bioactive Materials*. 2021 Aug 1;6(8):2261–80.
108. Gao Z, Nakanishi Y, Noda S, Omachi H, Shinohara H, Kimura H, Nagasaki Y. Development of Gd3N@ C80 encapsulated redox nanoparticles for high-performance magnetic resonance imaging. *Journal of Biomaterials Science,* Polymer Edition. 2017 Aug 13;28(10–12):1036–50.
109. He Y, Hu C, Li Z, Wu C, Zeng Y, Peng C. Multifunctional carbon nanomaterials for diagnostic applications in infectious diseases and tumors. *Materials Today Bio*. 2022 Mar 5:100231.
110. Kurbanoglu S, Cevher SC, Toppare L, Cirpan A, Soylemez S. Electrochemical biosensor based on three components random conjugated polymer with fullerene (C60). *Bioelectrochemistry*. 2022 Oct 1;147:108219.
111. Pilehvar S, De Wael K. Recent advances in electrochemical biosensors based on fullerene-C60 nano-structured platforms. *Biosensors*. 2015 Nov 23;5(4):712–35.
112. Shiraishi H, Itoh T, Hayashi H, Takagi K, Sakane M, Mori T, Wang J. Electrochemical detection of *E. coli* 16S rDNA sequence using air-plasma-activated fullerene-impregnated screen printed electrodes. *Bioelectrochemistry*. 2007 May 1;70(2):481–7. Akhavan O, Ghaderi E, Rahighi R. Toward single-DNA electrochemical biosensing by graphene nanowalls. *ACS Nano*. 2012 Apr 24;6(4):2904–16.

8 Artificial Intelligence – The Imperative Tool in Healthcare Innovations Employing Nanotechnology

Dhanalakshmi, M., Kajari Das, Muhammed Iqbal, Mohanan, V. P., and Sushma Dave

8.1 INTRODUCTION

Artificial intelligence (AI) is the intelligence manifested by machines in understanding, producing, and deriving information, and machine learning (ML) is a subset of AI. Apart from predicting drug–protein interactions and 3D structure of biological targets, data mining in drug discovery and de novo drug design are also gaining momentum with cutting-edge ML algorithms [1]. In polypharmacology, AI is applied to design bio-specific and multi-target drug molecules. In drug repurposing, therapeutic target identification and new usage for existing drugs are two avenues blooming through the assistance of AI/ML technology [2]. Predicting the reaction yield, developing retro-synthesis pathways, finding possible reaction mechanisms, and designing synthetic routes for reactions are a few areas to be explored by chemical synthesis groups using this technology [3]. Improvements in techniques of nanomedicine fabrication, coupled with a surge in understanding cancer biology, stimulated the rational design of targeted therapy procedures employing endogenous and external stimuli for better drug delivery mechanisms [4].

In order to solve tedious problems in basic science, with the advancement of computers, new tools and techniques are evolved based on computational methods which have both quantum mechanics and classical mechanics as their backbone [5]. ML algorithms can have a transformative impact, amplifying the potential insights accumulated from computational chemistry [6]. Traditional computational chemistry methods required expert end users who should decide on the work plan with high-end theoretical support along with a good computational facility. Nowadays, any "instrument" that is able to think logically using curated data can produce the most reasonable pattern/important trend/feature that

DOI: 10.1201/9781003316435-8

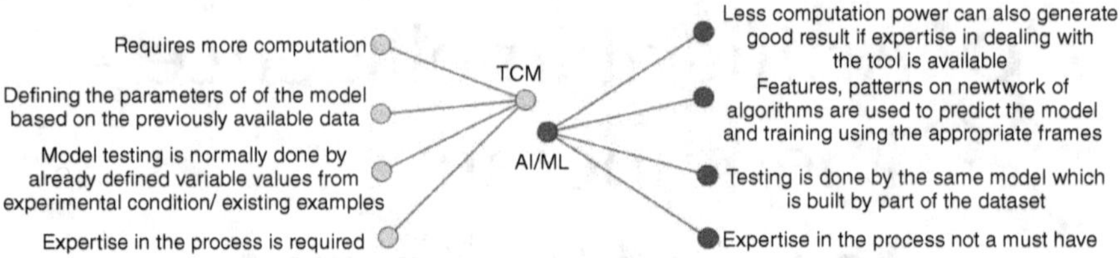

FIGURE 8.1 A comparison between AI/ML and traditional computational methods (TCMs).

is hidden in the data without much of the subject expertise [7]. The important changes brought about by AI/ML techniques are depicted in Figure 8.1.

8.1.1 Artificial Intelligence/Machine Learning

ML first identifies valid, potentially useful, easily understandable information and then generates the dependencies hidden in data using computing facilities that have an inbuilt capacity to learn and unlearn. ML tools use computational algorithms "to learn" from the data they are exposed without depending on equations that are predetermined as a model, and these algorithms improve their performance adaptively, as the amount of samples accessible for learning increases [8]. In data mining, it finds hidden patterns, whereas in statistical analysis, it helps understand the process of generating the data in order to test hypotheses. In drug discovery, the potential of AI-based algorithms plays an imperative role in predictive modeling of data to mimic the existing phenomena or to find new characteristics/activities of the available data [9]. In short, the properties of "y" are predicted by using a sample variable "x" considering the training set of "T", where training is the process by which the system learns.

8.1.2 Classification of Machine Learning

The ML methods can be classified as "supervised" if the training set T consists of samples with labels and "unsupervised" if it comprises data without labels [8]. If the training set has both labeled and unlabeled data, then it can fall in the category of "semi-supervised" learning methodology. A training dataset is usually comprised of examples with target values (e.g., bioassays with known activities). A validation dataset is used to estimate the error and improve the model performance parameters along with a test set. The purpose is to assess the performance of data sets which belong to the initial dataset and are not part of the training set to provide an unbiased error estimation [10].

8.1.3 Supervised Machine Learning

The aim of supervised machine learning (SML) is to build a model, in the presence of uncertainty, that makes predictions based on evidence. It takes a known set of input and response data to generate a data output, and trains a model to make

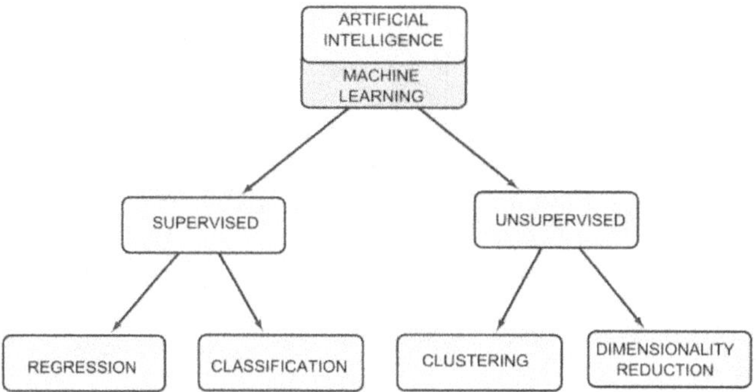

FIGURE 8.2 Classification of machine learning techniques.

predictions on new data. SML uses classification based on categorical labels and regression techniques to develop predictive models on numerical labels, whereas clustering and dimensionality reduction techniques come under unsupervised machine learning (UML) methodology as shown in Figure 8.2 [10].

8.1.3.1 Regression

Here the predicted response is continuous. The mapping and statistical correlation is made primarily without assuming the functional form of distributed data [8]. It is an attempt to generate a function to model the data with minimal errors (Figure 8.3).

The main objective of regression analysis is to define the regression equation explicitly to establish a meaningful/valid relation between the study variable and the explanatory variable [8]. It could be used to understand the role of any explanatory variables and to forecast the study variable or the response variable for the given set of data.

The model is validated by the performance which can be measured from the confusion matrix (Figure 8.4) in terms of precision, recall accuracy, etc. The area under the ROC curve (AUC) is another widely used measure that gives the dependence between the recall and false positive rate [10]. If the value of AUC is larger, it corresponds to a better performance of the predicting model. Biosensing uses three other measures, namely, the relative error of prediction (REP), the correlation coefficient (R2), and the root-mean-square difference (RMSD), in order to

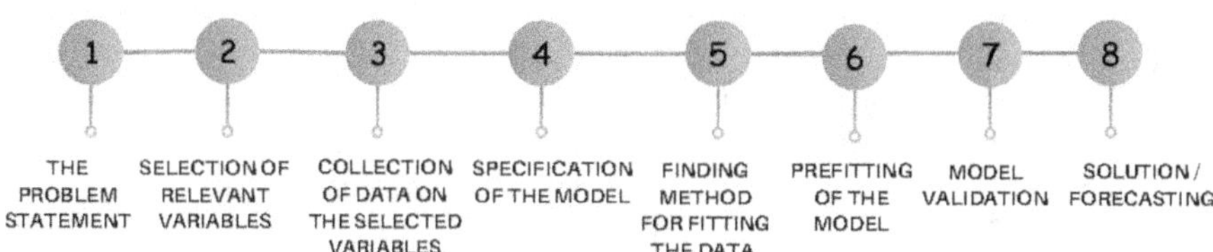

FIGURE 8.3 The steps in any regression analysis.

	Predicted Positive	Predicted Negative	Measurement
Actual Positive	True Positive (TP)	False Negative (FN)	Recall $= \frac{TP}{TP+FN}$ True Positive Rate (TPR)
Actual Negative	False Positive (FP)	True Negative (TN)	Specificity $= \frac{TN}{FP+TN}$ True Negative Rate (TNR)
Measurement	Precision $= \frac{TP}{TP+FP}$	False Negative Rate (FNR) $= \frac{FN}{FN+TP}$	False Positive Rate (FPR) $= \frac{FP}{FP+TN}$
$F1\ score = 2 * \frac{Precision * Recall}{Precision + Recall}$		$Accuracy = \frac{\#\ of\ correct\ predictions}{\#\ of\ total\ predictions} = \frac{TP+TN}{TP+FP+TN+FN}$	

FIGURE 8.4 The terms and measurements of confusion matrix.

evaluate the performance of the model and the metric calculations provided by Cui et al. [11].

$$\text{Accuracy} = \frac{\#\text{ of correct predictions}}{\#\text{ of total predictions}} = \frac{\text{TP}+\text{TN}}{\text{TP}+\text{FP}+\text{TN}+\text{FN}}$$

8.1.3.2 Classification

Classification is a process of generalizing the known structure to apply to any new data. In this technique, discrete responses are predicted. The predicted model categorizes the given data, e.g., whether the tumor is benign or cancerous and Covid-19 is positive or negative.

Pre-processing of data is a crucial step in classification to improve accuracy, as well as scalability and efficiency. Data cleaning is the process used to reduce noise. For example, if there is a missing value in the given data, it is replaced by "the most commonly used value of that particular attribute" or "the most probable value proposed by statistics". Relevance analysis can help remove redundant values and irrelevant attributes, and correlation analysis identifies if any two attributes are statistically related [8].

Data reduction techniques, such as principal component analysis (PCA), clustering normalization and generalization, can be adopted to transform to improve scalability and efficiency. In case distance measurements or neural networks are involved, a normalization is used in the "learning" step. Normalization involves making all values of a selected attribute within a specified range, say, for example, –1 to +1. For continuous-valued attributes concept hierarchy may be utilized to generalize the data. Usually, numeric values for attributes can be generalized such as affinity (or income in the case of financial studies), low, medium, and high.

The criteria of a good classifier algorithm are accuracy, speed, robustness, scalability, and interpretability. Accuracy refers to the ability of the classifier to predict the values of new attributes in order to classify previously unseen data correctly. The rate of prediction of a given ML algorithm is proportional to the number of computational resources it consumes. If the classifier is robust, it can accurately predict noisy data such as missing values. The classifier's ability to efficiently predict large amounts of data is achieved through scalability. Interpretability is the level of understanding that is provided by the classifier to get an insight into the data and is difficult to evaluate as it is subjective.

Classification can be done in many ways. Fundamental and widely used ones are decision tree (DT), induction, Bayesian statistics, and support vector machines (SVMs). Classification techniques which are majorly used with their working principal along with pros and cons have been discussed in detail by Soofi and Awan [12].

8.1.3.2.1 Decision Tree

The DT classifier construction does not require any domain knowledge or parameter settings, and therefore, it is suitable for exploratory knowledge discovery. DTs can process high-dimensional data. The knowledge obtained in the tree form is intuitive and easy to assimilate. The classification steps and the learning process in the DT induction are simple and fast. It is widely used in medicinal research, manufacturing and production, financial analysis, astronomy and molecular biology. DT techniques, which resemble our own logical reasoning, are widely used to build classification models. Kotsiantis in his review discussed in detail its relevance in the current research scenario and issues of DT [13].

8.1.3.2.2 Support Vector Machine

SVM is a widely used and highly sensitive classification algorithm that creates a separation line dividing the data into two classes in the best possible way. The detailed understanding of this theory is well documented by Vapnik in the book *The Nature of Statistical Learning Theory* [16].

The original input space should be mapped into some higher dimensional feature space where the training set is possible to separate. The similarity function flexibility and sparseness of solution while dealing with large datasets are advantages and well suited for feature selection. Hypertext categorization, image classification, bio/cheminformatics classifications, and handwritten character recognition are well handled by SVM. The SVM could produce a lower error during prediction even with methods employing artificial neural networks when the features to be analyzed are large. Evgeny Byvatov explained the role of SVMs and their broad areas of applications in the field of bioinformatics [17].

8.1.4 Unsupervised Machine Learning

Clustering and dimensionality reduction are the two important unsupervised data analyzing ML techniques widely used in drug development science, and a fundamental understanding of them can help identify their potential areas of usage. In the clustering method, the relevant subgroups are identified in a given dataset without a defined hypothesis.

8.1.4.1 Clustering

Clustering is the task of grouping data based on similarity/differences, a process in which a set of patterns are partitioned. In clustering, larger datasets are grouped into smaller groups based on some similarity. It can organize data, partition a dataset and can even compress large datasets into processable clusters. There are many methodologies used to get the data clustered. The two broad categories are hierarchical and partitional.

Hierarchical clustering can be done in two ways: bottom-up (agglomerative) and top-down (divisive) methods. The former combines feature vectors of different dimensions hierarchically. If it begins with N clusters, the first step is to discover the most comparable pair of clusters and merge them into one cluster. This process is repeated up to N-1 times forming binary trees. In this process, one can decide the number of clusters as well as terminate at any time at a desired step. A pattern will be formed from similar features in the "d"-dimensional space of feature vectors. The measure of similarities between each pattern can be determined through certain distances, which decides the shape of the cluster measured. The common distances used for this purpose are Euclidian distance, Manhattan distance and cosine similarity. If the distance is very high, the similarity will be less and vice versa.

Graph-based clustering, iterative clustering (K-means clustering), artificial neural network-based clustering, etc. are different ways to convert unsupervised data into processable information to generate knowledge. An overview of important steps and techniques that must be taken care of while conducting any cluster analysis studies, particularly on biomedical data, is given by Richard Rottge [18]. Discussing each one will be beyond the scope of this chapter, but Kohonen's self-organizing maps are widely in use as they reduce dimensions [nonlinear/multidimensional to 1D/2D] and help understand the relationship of structure to biological activity easily [19]. In many pharmaceutical researches, it can be employed since the artificial neural network identifies the nonlinear connections of arbitrary dimensions into simple one or two dimensions [20–22].

The important neural networks that are in use today, based on network structures and learning types, are classified as shown in Figure 8.5. Artificial neural networks (ANNs) are found to have an imperative role in medical science as their mapping and optimization are comparatively effortless and demonstrative in real-time issues. A detailed review of ANNs in medical sciences is a good reference in this regard [23].

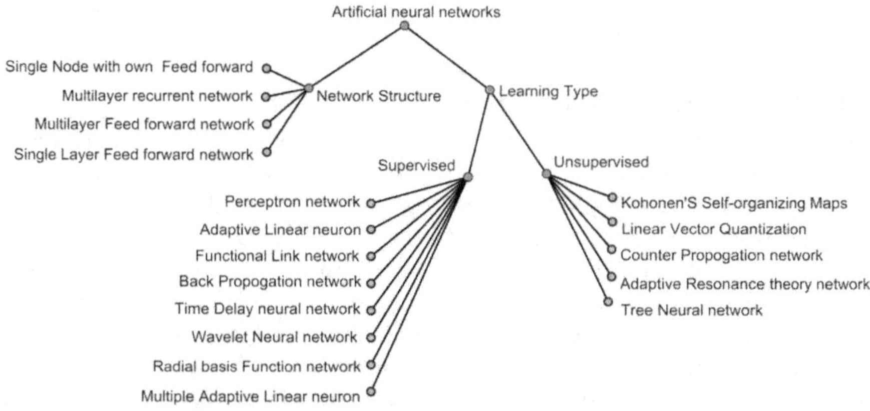

FIGURE 8.5 Classification of artificial neural networks.

8.1.4.1.1 Deep Learning

Deep learning, a branch of ML which uses "deep ANN", is gaining increasing popularity among researchers in recent years. The key parameter is the size of the hidden layer which significantly affects the performance of the ANN model. Engineers and scientists can now have the access to many deep learning tools that are open source like Theano, TensorFlow, CNTK and Pytorch.

One type of widely used deep learning algorithm is convolutional neural network (CNN) which is usually good at analyzing images of MRI (magnetic resonance images), CT (computed tomography) and X-ray. The CNN model has three layers, namely, the convolutional layer which filters slipping across preprocessed signals, the pooling layer also known as a down-sampling layer which does a dimensionality reduction and thus limits the phenomenon of overfitting and reduces the computational intensity, and a fully connected layer. Activation functions are incorporated in order to establish non-linearity into the output data such as Tanh and Sigmoid. Initially, CNN was developed for 2D image recognition. There are many advancements that improved the performance of spatial relation data such as electroencephalograms (EEGs), spectra and audio signals. The accuracy and repeatability reveal that CNN-based spectral analysis needs a larger sample size for better performance.

Recurrent neural networks (RNN), another deep learning method, has connections forming a directed cycle which permits it to show dynamic and temporal nature, enabling it to process sequential data. RNN's network topology is specially created to represent historical data in each recurrent round, making it well suited for the analysis of time series or sequential data. RNN is frequently used for sequence mapping problems like sequence creation, speech recognition, handwriting recognition, reinforcement learning and other sequence mapping problems because it has the ability to propagate past information over time through recurrent connections. It has been used by biomedical researchers to identify connections between genes and proteins. The RNNs known as long short-term memory (LSTM) networks are a specific kind that can handle long-term dependency [11,23].

8.1.4.2 Dimensionality Reduction

The dimensionality (in other words, the number of features that feature space occupies) is high most of the time in the provided sample. Challenges due to this are not just in data interpretation or visualization but equally toughness of its analysis. In fact, in most cases, it can be avoided. PCA was theoretically known before the term machine learning, but it is well utilized for dimensionality reduction [10]. Uniform manifold approximation and projection or t-distributed stochastic neighbor embedding and autoencoder are recent additions in this area. Lan Huong Nguyen and Susan Holmes discussed in their review about effective dimensionality reduction tips in biomedical data processing [24].

8.1.4.2.1 Principal Component Analysis (PCA)

Any prediction becomes valid, if a huge amount of data is effortlessly interpreted through smaller variables retaining maximum accuracy. PCA is a dimensionality reduction procedure that operates by reducing the number of variables that may be redundant or not very significant [24–26]. The variable redundancy enables a linear combination among themselves to form comparatively smaller but more accountable artificial variables, the principle components having maximum variances shown by the natural variables [27]. In other words, it analyses all possible variances in the original variables and transforms them into components with reduced variance, least redundancy and independence.

8.2 ARTIFICIAL INTELLIGENCE TOOLS IN DRUG DISCOVERY

AI and ML are revolutionizing drug discovery and drug development processes in healthcare addressing the bottleneck of chemical space with innumerable compounds (more than 10^{60}) to be analyzed [28]. The large datasets are developed by pharma companies involving innumerable compounds. Predictions of complex biological properties using traditional quantitative structure–activity relationship (QSAR) methodologies often fail in efficacy and cause adverse effects. Moreover, they can only deal with smaller datasets effectively and incorporate a lesser number of molecular descriptors. Thus, the model's performance can also be poor compared to ANNs and deep learning algorithms. An intelligent selection of AI/ML methods can make the structure- and ligand-based virtual screening techniques more effective. It can enhance the selection of lead molecules and their optimization from the data provided by the chemical space, by analyzing the physical, chemical and toxicological aspects of the available candidates [29].

In ligand-based virtual screening, an active molecule or a group of potential candidates can be designed against certain target proteins from the available biological activity data by analyzing the structural/physicochemical properties which may be responsible for the activity. Selection and appropriate analog designing, pharmacophore modeling, QSAR, etc. can be utilized to their fullest with ML

TABLE 8.1
AI Tools for *In Silico* Drug Discovery

Name of the Tool	Application	Reference
AlphaFold	Can predict proteins' 3D structures	https://deepmind.com/blog/alphafold
Chemputer	Procedure for chemical synthesis can be predicted in standardized format	https://zenodo.org/record/1481731
DeepChem	To discover an appropriate candidate drug	https://github.com/deepchem/deepchem
DeepNeuralNetQSAR	Molecular activity of materials	https://github.com/Merck/DeepNeuralNet-QSAR
DeepTox	To forecast toxicity drugs	www.bioinf.jku.at/research/DeepTox
DeltaVina	Scoring–ligand binding affinity	https://github.com/chengwang88/deltavina
Hit Dexter	To predict possible molecules having action on biochemical assays	http://hitdexter2.zbh.uni-hamburg.de
Neural graph fingerprint	Novel molecule's properties can be predicted	https://github.com/HIPS/neural-fingerprint
ORGANIC	To design molecules with required features	https://github.com/aspuru-guzik-group/ORGANIC
PotentialNet	Forecasting the binding affinity of ligands	https://pubs.acs.org/doi/full/10.1021/acscentsci.8b00507

and deep learning algorithms at a less computational cost compared to traditional modeling methodologies [30].

The methods analyzing three-dimensional structures can be used to evaluate more efficiently, including areas like target preparation, identification of the binding site, screening molecular library preparation, ligand docking, the score of binding affinity, MD simulations, etc., by incorporating AI/ML-based techniques [31,32].

From chemical synthesis, virtual screening, poly pharmacology and drug repurposing to almost all major steps in drug design are now revolutionized by the use of AI. In a recent review, the diverse sectors are discussed in detail including the tools employed (Table 8.1) to execute these techniques [28], and the major area can be summed up as shown in Figure 8.6.

8.3 ARTIFICIAL INTELLIGENCE IN DRUG DELIVERY

AI is a hope to replace the traditional trial-and-error approach through efficient delivery techniques in order to minimize dosage and maximize absorption mechanisms which can reduce toxicity, especially for terminal diseases like cancer [33,34] and also infectious diseases [35].

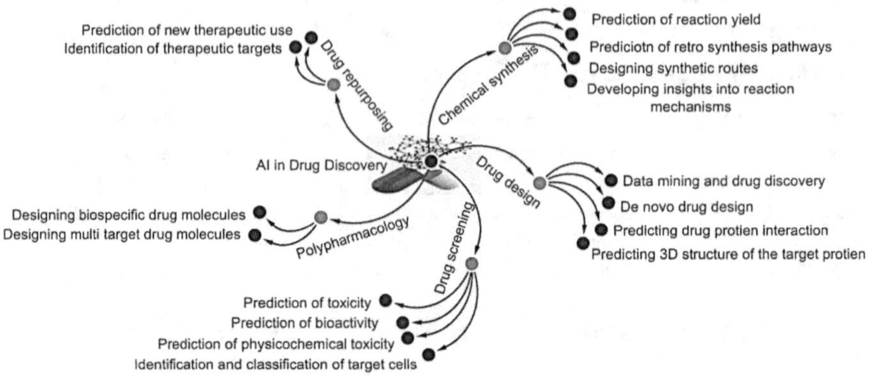

FIGURE 8.6 Role of artificial intelligence in the diverse areas of drug discovery pipeline.

Numerous nanocarriers have been approved for clinical use, starting from diagnosis and/or treatment of several types of cancer to vaccination against SARS-CoV-2 infection. There are different formulations in the pipeline of different stages of clinical trials. Moderna and BioNTech make use of nanocarriers for encapsulating mRNA. Over the last decades, due to the evolution of hundreds of nanocarrier formulations, it has become more difficult to standardize the safety and processing protocols that rule the regulatory permissions of those revolutionary systems. For nanoparticle synthesis, its immediate exploration and optimization, analysis of drug distribution and *in vivo–in vitro* correlation, integration of AI into software-employed lab machinery is considered to be of primary importance. Establishing remote computer access can enable anyone from around the world to take part in experimental procedures and acquire ample research skills. Processing of ever-expanding datasets and recognition of complex patterns are the key elements managed by AI algorithms and are engineered for better design of nanotechnologies for diagnostics as well as treatment. The final stage of nanomedicine formulation relies on the AI-derived prediction of the most suitable interactions of nanoparticles, biological media, and cell membranes with the target drug, in addition to the drug's encapsulation efficiency and release kinetics [36].

- **Designing nanoparticles for improved targeting**

  Theoretical approaches: By utilization of analytical models and molecular simulations, physicochemical properties of small molecules such as solubility and lipophilicity are predicted apart from the structural properties of formulation materials [37]. Physico-chemical parameters help determine promising drug–material pairs by predicting the strength of drug–material interactions based on the knowledge of lipophilicity and hydrophobicity of the molecules, and prediction of retention and permeability through a membrane when a formulation of the drug is done. These theoretical evaluations in nanoparticles include investigation of their structural properties through MD simulation associated with their biological performance (both *in vivo* and *in vitro*), which provides guidance during the designing of potential drug delivery systems [38].

- **AI-based nanorobots for drug delivery**

  Sensors, integrated circuits and secure backup of data, which are secured by computational technologies like AI, are the backbone of nanorobots. Advanced nano/microrobots have the ability to navigate to the targeted location based on physiological conditions, thus refining efficiency and minimizing systemic adverse effects. The progress of implantable nanorobots established for the controlled distribution of drugs and genes needs attention about parameters like dosage, continued release, and regulation in release, and the distribution of the drugs requires automation governed by AI tools. For the automatic release as well as to perceive the location of the implant in the body, microchip implants are utilized [28].

8.4 ARTIFICIAL INTELLIGENCE IN THE DIAGNOSIS OF DISEASES

AI-powered analytics open up a new portal of business analysis in the field of healthcare. With enormous data being generated each day, this AI-based approach can enable better data management and faster and smarter decisions with more confidence.

8.4.1 Biosensors

These days, the arising needs for precise diagnosis and individualized medicine have led to the development of AI-based biosensors which are integrated into smart materials with higher specificity, higher selectivity, faster responsiveness, lower limits of detection, and ease of use. These are being used in developing diagnostics for better prognosis and diagnosis in the existing healthcare system and also to enhance research and development in the field of sustainability and environmental sciences. These are also taking over conventional methods and assays in the fields of industrial biotechnology, chemical engineering, chemistry, pharmaceutical studies, and biophysics [39–42]. These AI-based biosensors interfaced with wireless communication and an intelligent platform like a smartphone provide simplicity in their usage. This wireless technology integration with biosensors increases its cost-effectiveness and reusability.

The AI-based options use ML such as deep learning methods of CNN and RNN for the functioning of these "smart diagnostics". Biosensor networks and multi-biosensor data fusion can be explored for the development of these biosensor systems.

Although nanotechnology has been proven to be a promising technology for sensor applications in various fields, frequent application of nanotechnology in designing nanobiosensors was not devoid of problems like electrical noise,

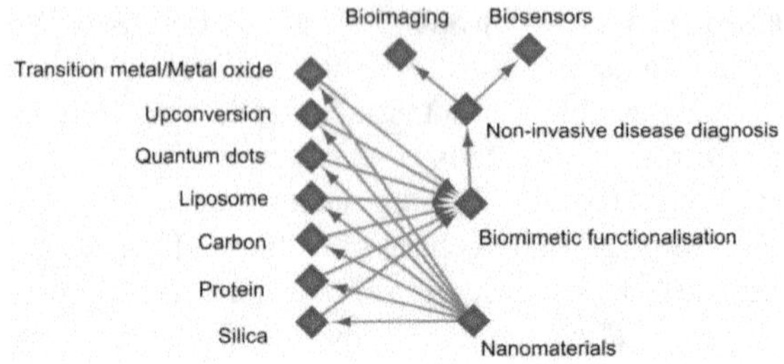

FIGURE 8.7 Nanomaterials employed in a typical nanobiosensor.

random quantum effects, limited specificity, reduced stability, etc. Such limitations are bound to create obstacles against their successful commercialization. Implementation of ML techniques has the potential to mitigate such limitations. A few of the emerging algorithms being applied for data processing and analysis are SVM, random forest, ANNs, Naïve Bayes, CNN and κ-nearest neighbor (κNN), depending on the requirement of level of accuracy, recall, precision and F1 score for a variety of nanobiosensors performance. Figure 8.7 shows the different materials and methodologies employed in a typical nanobiosensor [43]. Detection of biomarkers for multiple diseases simultaneously in very low concentrations (femtomolar) is possible nowadays with the help of nanosensors in liquid biopsies (blood, urine, saliva) and in cell cultures [7].

Nanoparticles of natural or engineered form in variable shapes, sizes and properties and complexed with various chemicals are being used to interact with biomolecules on cell surfaces or inside the cell [44]. Workers of middleware can perform better in diagnostics if they can exploit nanotechnology to effectively design, test and implement new diagnostics that can be utilized in any minimal settings. This will help solve the burden of infectious diseases by leveraging locally available resources along with self-propagating knowledge [45]. The biomimetic nanomaterials can be used in developing promising non-invasive disease-detecting markers, clinical screening of large-scale data, and diagnosis of different diseases, which can pave the way to scaling up of statistical indices denoting better clinical public health globally [46].

First, huge amount of sensing data for complicated matrices or samples can be processed successfully by ML. The ability to derive plausible analytical conclusions from noisy, low-resolution, and sometimes highly overlapping sensing data is another advantage of ML in biosensors. Moreover, proper deployment of ML algorithms can identify hidden connections between sample parameters and sensing signals through data visualization, and eventually mine hidden relations between signals or any biological events. Particularly, ML can be used to assess the raw sensing data from a biosensor in multiple ways. The sensing signals can be categorized into several groups by the algorithms based on the target analyte. Biosensors are inevitably affected by sample matrix and operating conditions, and anomalies must be detected. When biosensors are employed on-site, they can greatly interfere with contamination. Noise is always included in the sensing signals. The signals from biosensors fluctuate over seconds or minutes, whereas signal interference such as electrical noise can occur in the sub-second time frame and must be reduced. It is possible to train ML models to tell the difference between the signal and the noise. Sensing data may be readily and successfully evaluated by finding latent objects and patterns using ML algorithms. For real-time detection and on-site diagnosis, assistance of ML can enable biosensor readout automatically, directly, and accurately making it a smarter tool [11]. The different algorithms used in different biosensors (Figure 8.8) with detailed pros and cons are studied by Feiyun Cui et al., and the advantages are depicted in Figure 8.9.

Surface-enhanced Raman spectroscopy (SERS), electrochemical impedance spectroscopy (EIS), surface plasmon resonance (SPR)-based biosensors, electrical impedance tomography (EIT), cyclic voltammetry (CV), thin-layer chromatography coupled with surface-enhanced Raman spectroscopy (TLC-SERS), electronic nose (E-nose), electronic tongue (E-tongue), and various spectroscopic methodologies use ML algorithms like SVM, CNN, ANN, linear discriminant analysis (LDA), κ-nearest neighbor (κNN), back-propagation neural networks

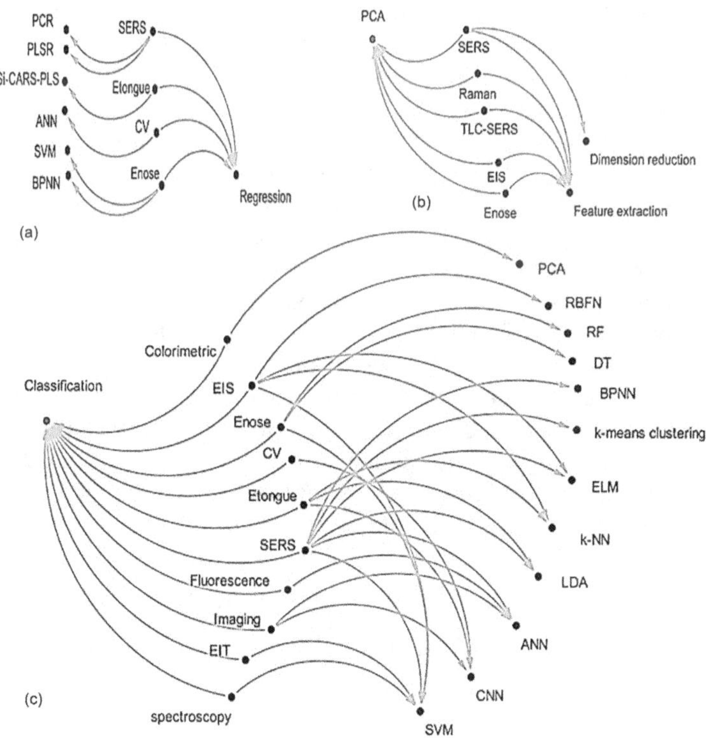

FIGURE 8.8 The biosensing mechanisms and the machine learning algorithm involved in them.

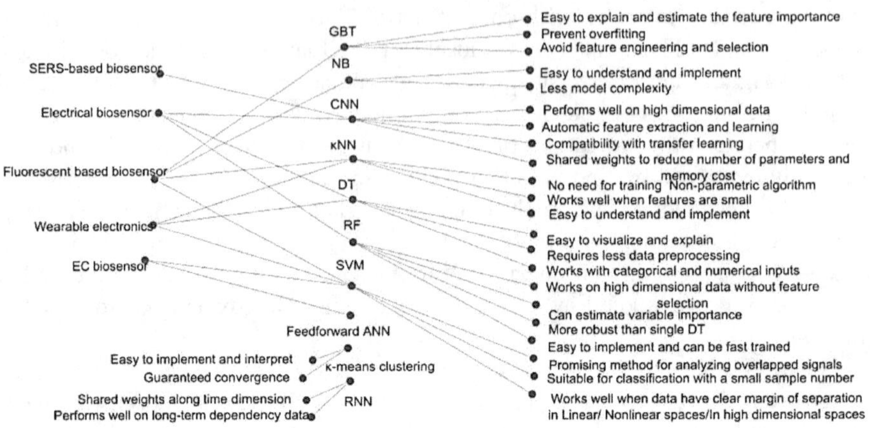

FIGURE 8.9 The different algorithms used in biosensors and their advantages.

(BPNN), DT, random forest (RF), Naïve Bayes (NB), radial basis function networks (RBFN), principal component analysis or regression (PCA or PCR), RNN, gradient-boosted trees (GBT) and partial least-squares discriminant analysis or regression (PLSDA or PLSR).

Gold nanosensor assisted by SERS and CNNs was designed for the detection of oligonucleotide damage [47]. Using binary stochastic filtering techniques, even a very small DNA damage can be detected. AuNPs with similar techniques were used to detect cancerous cells [48]. The first commercialized and most popular glucose oxidase biosensor has been improvised by ML algorithms for comparative analysis [49]. CNN algorithms are frequently used to detect ultralow (<nanomolar) concentrations of Rhodamine 800, microorganisms at the single cellular level, the organic carbon in water, etc. [52,53]. Nanobiosensors assisted by a variety of ML algorithms are reported to catch proteins, bacteria, alcohol, C-reactive protein, amino acids, etc. in various samples [52–59].

Tsutsui et al. employed a rotation forest model for classifying *Escherichia coli* and *Bacillus subtilis* [60]. Zeng et al. illustrated a ML-enabled monitoring method for mental fatigue using epidermal biosensors [61]. Jeong et al. designed a wearable sensor for early detection of COVID-19 symptoms such as high temperature, heart rate and regular coughing patterns [62]. Tatarko et al. developed a quartz crystal microbalance biosensor for precise classification between trypsin and plasmin at low concentrations [63]. Adak et al. used similar sensing techniques to classify five diverse alcohol analytes with the assistance of an artificial bee colony algorithm [64]. Yan et al. used magnetic nanoparticles for the detection of cardiac markers using the SVM technique and improved the performance of nanobiosensor [65].

Researchers have developed ML to bioreceptor-free biosensors to bridge this trade-off gap, improving the limit of detection and specificity [66]. In a sense, ML can be used to take the place of a bioreceptor by reintroducing specificity during the analysis of data. This is made possible by powerful ML techniques capable of detecting subtle patterns in sensor responses. Smith et al. (2021) reported ML modeling through a novel algorithm, "Algorithmically Guided Optical Nano sensor Selector" (AGONS), that could open a biomarker-free detection approach for most challenging biological targets [67–69]. The authors believe that the optical data obtained through a nanosensor array can be selected with much larger and stronger prediction accuracy. The platform is considered highly valuable for medicinal or agricultural automated diagnosis/quality control applications.

8.5 CONCLUSION

With the advancement of the incredible tools and techniques of AI, the goal is to minimize challenges encountered by pharmaceutical companies, in order to strengthen the entire drug development process and enable the current healthcare sector to battle complex threats. Presently, the cost of drugs, treatment modalities and infectious diseases along with the demands from patient society look forward to breakthrough technologies. Augmenting nanotechnology with AI in disease diagnosis, production of pharmaceutical products and targeted delivery of medications with customized doses will lead to the demands for personalized and precision medicine development. AI-based innovations will certainly increase the speed of the entire product development strategies and eventually reach the market. Improved quality and safety of the processes and products will enable the entire system to avail resources efficiently and economically. AI-based technical advancement poses challenges in the implementation, starting from job loss to the ethical concern, and hence, regulations need to formulate and practice for the common good and are a must-have in the agenda of policymakers. AI will be an imperative tool in the pharmaceutical industry and the healthcare sector in the near future.

REFERENCES

1. Askr H, Elgeldawi E, Aboul Ella H, Elshaier YA, Gomaa MM, Hassanien AE. Deep learning in drug discovery: An integrative review and future challenges. *Artificial Intelligence Review.* 2022 Nov 17;56:1–63.
2. Paul D, Sanap G, Shenoy S, Kalyane D, Kalia K, Tekade RK. Artificial intelligence in drug discovery and development. *Drug Discovery Today.* 2021 Jan;26(1):80.
3. Jiang Y, Yu Y, Kong M, Mei Y, Yuan L, Huang Z, Kuang K, Wang Z, Yao H, Zou J, Coley CW. Artificial intelligence for retrosynthesis prediction. *Engineering.* 2022 Aug 20;25:32–50.
4. Patra JK, Das G, Fraceto LF, Campos EV, Rodriguez-Torres MD, Acosta-Torres LS, Diaz-Torres LA, Grillo R, Swamy MK, Sharma S, Habtemariam S. Nano-based drug delivery systems: Recent developments and future prospects. *Journal of Nanobiotechnology.* 2018 Dec;16(1):1–33.
5. Helgaker T, Jorgensen P, Olsen J. *Molecular Electronic-Structure Theory.* New York: John Wiley & Sons; 2013 Feb 18.

6. Keith JA, Vassilev-Galindo V, Cheng B, Chmiela S, Gastegger M, Müller KR, Tkatchenko A. Combining machine learning and computational chemistry for predictive insights into chemical systems. *Chemical Reviews*. 2021 Jul 7;121(16):9816–72.
7. Adir O, Poley M, Chen G, Froim S, Krinsky N, Shklover J, Shainsky-Roitman J, Lammers T, Schroeder A. Integrating artificial intelligence and nanotechnology for precision cancer medicine. *Advanced Materials*. 2020 Apr;32(13):1901989.
8. Witten IH, Frank E, Hall MA, Pal CJ. Data Mining: Practical Machine Learning Tools and Techniques. In *Data Mining* (Vol. 2, No. 4, pp. 403–413). Amsterdam: Elsevier, 2005 Jun.
9. Hansen K. Novel machine learning methods for computational chemistry (Doctoral dissertation, Universitätsbibliothek der Technischen Universität Berlin).
10. Badillo S, Banfai B, Birzele F, Davydov II, Hutchinson L, Kam-Thong T, Siebourg-Polster J, Steiert B, Zhang JD. An introduction to machine learning. *Clinical Pharmacology & Therapeutics*. 2020 Apr;107(4):871–85.
11. Cui F, Yue Y, Zhang Y, Zhang Z, Zhou HS. Advancing biosensors with machine learning. *ACS Sensors*. 2020 Nov 13;5(11):3346–64.
12. Soofi AA, Awan A. Classification techniques in machine learning: Applications and issues. *J. Basic Appl. Sci.* 2017 Aug 29;13:459–65.
13. Kotsiantis SB. Decision trees: A recent overview. *Artificial Intelligence Review*. 2013 Apr;39:261–83.
16. Vapnik V. *The Nature of Statistical Learning Theory*. Berlin: Springer Science & Business Media; 1999 Nov 19.
17. Byvatov E, Schneider G. Support vector machine applications in bioinformatics. *Applied Bioinformatics*. 2003 Jan 1;2(2):67–77.
18. Röttger R. Clustering of biological datasets in the era of big data. *Journal of Integrative Bioinformatics*. 2016 Mar 1;13(1):52–81.
19. Kohonen T. *Self-Organizing Maps*. Berlin: Springer Science & Business Media; 2012 Dec 6.
20. Selzer P, Ertl P. Applications of self-organizing neural networks in virtual screening and diversity selection. *Journal of Chemical Information and Modeling*. 2006 Nov 27;46(6):2319–23.
21. Schneider P, Tanrikulu Y, Schneider G. Self-organizing maps in drug discovery: Compound library design, scaffold-hopping, repurposing. *Current Medicinal Chemistry*. 2009 Jan 1;16(3):258.
22. Dhanalakshmi M, Das K, Pandya M, Shah S, Gadnayak A, Dave S, Das J. Artificial neural network-based study predicts GS-441524 as a potential inhibitor of SARS-CoV-2 activator protein furin: A polypharmacology approach. *Applied Biochemistry and Biotechnology*. 2022 Oct;194(10):4511–29.
23. Parveen R, Nabi M, Memon FA, Zaman S, Ali M. A review and survey of artificial neural network in medical science. *Journal of Advanced Research in Computing and Applications*. 2016;3(1):7–16.
24. Nguyen LH, Holmes S. Ten quick tips for effective dimensionality reduction. *PLoS Computational Biology*. 2019 Jun 20;15(6):e1006907.
25. Jinuraj KR, Rakhila M, Dhanalakshmi M, Sajeev R, Gad A, Jayan K, Muhammed Iqbal P, Manuel AT, Abdul Jaleel UC. Feature optimization in high dimensional chemical space: Statistical and data mining solutions. *BMC Research Notes*. 2018 Dec;11(1):1–7.
26. Vidal R, Ma Y, Sastry SS, Vidal R, Ma Y, Sastry SS. *Principal Component Analysis*. New York: Springer; 2016.
27. Jolliffe IT. *Principal Component Analysis for Special Types of Data*. Springer Series in Statistics. New York: Springer; 2002. https://doi.org/10.1007/0-387-22440-8_13.

28. Mishra V. Artificial intelligence: The beginning of a new era in the pharmacy profession. *Asian Journal of Pharmaceutics (AJP)*. 2018 May 30;12(02):72–6.
29. Paul D, Sanap G, Shenoy S, Kalyane D, Kalia K, Tekade RK. Artificial intelligence in drug discovery and development. *Drug Discovery Today*. 2021 Jan;26(1):80.
30. Zhao L, Ciallella HL, Aleksunes LM, Zhu H. Advancing computer-aided drug discovery (CADD) by big data and data-driven machine learning modeling. *Drug Discovery Today*. 2020;25(9):1624–38.
31. Gupta R, Srivastava D, Sahu M, Tiwari S, Ambasta RK, Kumar P. Artificial intelligence to deep learning: Machine intelligence approach for drug discovery. *Molecular Diversity*. 2021 Aug; 25:1315–60.
32. Pandya M, Shah S, Dhanalakshmi M, Juneja T, Patel A, Gadnayak A, Dave S, Das K, Das J. Unravelling Vitamin B12 as a potential inhibitor against SARS-CoV-2: A computational approach. *Informatics in Medicine Unlocked*. 2022 Jan 1;30:100951.
33. Hassanzadeh P, Atyabi F, Dinarvand R. The significance of artificial intelligence in drug delivery system design. *Advanced Drug Delivery Reviews*. 2019 Nov 1;151:169–90.
34. Adir O, Poley M, Chen G, Froim S, Krinsky N, Shklover J, Shainsky-Roitman J, Lammers T, Schroeder A. Integrating artificial intelligence and nanotechnology for precision cancer medicine. *Advanced Materials*. 2020 Apr;32(13):1901989.
35. He S, Leanse LG, Feng Y. Artificial intelligence and machine learning assisted drug delivery for effective treatment of infectious diseases. *Advanced Drug Delivery Reviews*. 2021 Nov 1;178:113922.
36. Alshawwa SZ, Kassem AA, Farid RM, Mostafa SK, Labib GS. Nanocarrier drug delivery systems: Characterization, limitations, future perspectives and implementation of artificial intelligence. *Pharmaceutics*. 2022 Apr 18;14(4):883.
37. Huynh L, Neale C, Pomès R, Allen C. Computational approaches to the rational design of nanoemulsions, polymeric micelles, and dendrimers for drug delivery. *Nanomedicine: Nanotechnology, Biology and Medicine*. 2012 Jan 1;8(1):20–36.
38. Hui Y, Yi X, Hou F, Wibowo D, Zhang F, Zhao D, Gao H, Zhao CX. Role of nanoparticle mechanical properties in cancer drug delivery. *ACS Nano*. 2019 Jul 9;13(7):7410–24.
39. Shah S, Maharshi A, Pandya M, Dhanalakshmi M, Das K. Nucleic acid based biosensor as a cutting edge tool for point of care diagnosis. In *Biosensors for Emerging and Re-Emerging Infectious Diseases*. 2022 Jan 1 (pp. 265–301). Academic Press. doi: 10.1016/B978-0-323-88464-8.00014-2.
40. Dave S, Kirubavathy SJ. Biosensors based on metal-organic framework (MOF): Paving the way to point-of-care diagnosis. In *Electrochemical Applications of Metal-Organic Frameworks*. 2022 Jan 1 (pp. 255–67). Elsevier. doi: 10.1016/B978-0-323-90784-2.00004-6.
41. Dave S, Dave A, Radhakrishnan S, Das J, Dave S. Biosensors for healthcare: An artificial intelligence approach. In *Biosensors for Emerging and Re-Emerging Infectious Diseases*. 2022 Jan 1 (pp. 365–83). doi: 10.1016/B978-0-323-88464-8.00008-7.
42. Panwar R, Churi H, Dave S. Point-of-care electrochemical biosensors using CRISPR/Cas for RNA analysis. In *Biosensors for Emerging and Re-Emerging Infectious Diseases*. 2022 Jan 1 (pp. 317–33). Academic Press. doi: 10.1016/B978-0-323-88464-8.00003-8.
43. Banerjee A, Maity S, Mastrangelo CH. Nanostructures for biosensing, with a brief overview on cancer detection, IoT, and the role of machine learning in smart biosensors. *Sensors*. 2021 Feb 10;21(4):1253.
44. Laroui H, Rakhya P, Xiao B, Viennois E, Merlin D. Nanotechnology in diagnostics and therapeutics for gastrointestinal disorders. *Digestive and Liver Disease*. 2013 Dec 1;45(12):995–1002.

45. Gomez-Marquez J, Hamad-Schifferli K. Local development of nanotechnology-based diagnostics. *Nature Nanotechnology*. 2021 May;16(5):484–6.
46. Feng Z, Fan H, Cheng L, Zhang H, Fan H, Liu J. Advanced biomimetic nanomaterials for non-invasive disease diagnosis. *Frontiers in Materials*. 2021 Mar 24;8:664795.
47. Guselnikova O, Trelin A, Skvortsova A, Ulbrich P, Postnikov P, Pershina A, Sykora D, Svorcik V, Lyutakov O. Label-free surface-enhanced Raman spectroscopy with artificial neural network technique for recognition photoinduced DNA damage. *Biosensors and Bioelectronics*. 2019 Dec 1;145:111718.
48. Erzina M, Trelin A, Guselnikova O, Dvorankova B, Strnadova K, Perminova A, Ulbrich P, Mares D, Jerabek V, Elashnikov R, Svorcik V. Precise cancer detection via the combination of functionalized SERS surfaces and convolutional neural network with independent inputs. *Sensors and Actuators B: Chemical*. 2020 Apr 1;308:127660.
49. Gonzalez-Navarro FF, Stilianova-Stoytcheva M, Renteria-Gutierrez L, Belanche-Muñoz LA, Flores-Rios BL, Ibarra-Esquer JE. Glucose oxidase biosensor modeling and predictors optimization by machine learning methods. *Sensors*. 2016 Oct 26;16(11):1483.
52. Luo R, Ma G, Bi S, Duan Q, Chen J, Feng Y, Liu F, Lee J. Machine learning for total organic carbon analysis of environmental water samples using high-throughput colorimetric sensors. *Analyst*. 2020;145(6):2197–203.
53. Pandit S, Banerjee T, Srivastava I, Nie S, Pan D. Machine learning-assisted array-based biomolecular sensing using surface-functionalized carbon dots. *ACS Sensors*. 2019 Sep 18;4(10):2730–7.
54. Solmaz ME, Mutlu AY, Alankus G, Kılıç V, Bayram A, Horzum N. Quantifying colorimetric tests using a smartphone app based on machine learning classifiers. *Sensors and Actuators B: Chemical*. 2018 Feb 1;255:1967–73.
55. Gunda NS, Gautam SH, Mitra SK. Artificial intelligence based mobile application for water quality monitoring. *Journal of the Electrochemical Society*. 2019 Mar 9;166(9):B3031.
56. Kim H, Awofeso O, Choi S, Jung Y, Bae E. Colorimetric analysis of saliva-alcohol test strips by smartphone-based instruments using machine-learning algorithms. *Applied Optics*. 2017 Jan 1;56(1):84–92.
57. Ballard ZS, Joung HA, Goncharov A, Liang J, Nugroho K, Di Carlo D, Garner OB, Ozcan A. Deep learning-enabled point-of-care sensing using multiplexed paper-based sensors. *NPJ Digital Medicine*. 2020 May 7;3(1):66.
58. Ali S, Hassan A, Hassan G, Eun CH, Bae J, Lee CH, Kim IJ. Disposable all-printed electronic biosensor for instantaneous detection and classification of pathogens. *Scientific Reports*. 2018 Apr 12;8(1):1.
59. Albrecht T, Slabaugh G, Alonso E, Al-Arif SM. Deep learning for single-molecule science. *Nanotechnology*. 2017 Sep 18;28(42):423001.
60. Tsutsui M, Yoshida T, Yokota K, Yasaki H, Yasui T, Arima A, Tonomura W, Nagashima K, Yanagida T, Kaji N, Taniguchi M. Discriminating single-bacterial shape using low-aspect-ratio pores. *Scientific Reports*. 2017 Dec 12;7(1):17371.
61. Zeng Z, Huang Z, Leng K, Han W, Niu H, Yu Y, Ling Q, Liu J, Wu Z, Zang J. Nonintrusive monitoring of mental fatigue status using epidermal electronic systems and machine-learning algorithms. *ACS Sensors*. 2020 Jan 15;5(5):1305–13.
62. Jeong H, Rogers JA, Xu S. Continuous on-body sensing for the COVID-19 pandemic: Gaps and opportunities. *Science Advances*. 2020 Sep 2;6(36):eabd4794.

63. Tatarko M, Muckley ES, Subjakova V, Goswami M, Sumpter BG, Hianik T, Ivanov IN. Machine learning enabled acoustic detection of sub-nanomolar concentration of trypsin and plasmin in solution. *Sensors and Actuators B: Chemical.* 2018 Nov 1;272:282–8.
64. Adak MF, Lieberzeit P, Jarujamrus P, Yumusak N. Classification of alcohols obtained by QCM sensors with different characteristics using ABC based neural network. *Engineering Science and Technology, an International Journal.* 2020 Jun 1;23(3):463–9.
65. Yan W, Wang K, Xu H, Huo X, Jin Q, Cui D. Machine learning approach to enhance the performance of MNP-labeled lateral flow immunoassay. *Nano-Micro Letters.* 2019 Dec;11:1–5.
66. Schackart III KE, Yoon JY. Machine learning enhances the performance of bioreceptor-free biosensors. *Sensors.* 2021 Aug 17;21(16):5519.
67. Smith CW, Hizir MS, Nandu N, Yigit MV. Algorithmically guided optical nanosensor selector (AGONS): Guiding data acquisition, processing, and discrimination for biological sampling. *Analytical Chemistry.* 2021 Dec 29;94(2):1195–202.
68. Dhanalakshmi M, Pandya M, Sruthi D, Jinuraj KR, Das K, Gadnayak A, Dave S, Andal NM. The artificial neural network selects saccharides from natural sources a promise for potential FimH inhibitor to prevent UTI infections. *In Silico Pharmacology.* 2024;12(1):37.
69. Churi HS, Dave S. Strategic synthesis of diagnostic novel materials against infectious diseases. In *Point-of-Care Biosensors for Infectious Diseases.* 2023 (pp. 209–33). Wiley-VCH GmbH.

9 Artificial Intelligence Driven Nanobiosensors
Virus Detection and Precision Medicine

Aditya Dave

9.1 INTRODUCTION

Nanobiosensors are rapidly evolving as a promising technology for the detection and monitoring of various biological and chemical species. They offer high sensitivity, selectivity, and real-time monitoring capabilities, making them ideal for a wide range of applications in various fields, including healthcare, environmental monitoring, and food safety (Haick and Tang 2021; Rawat et al. 2022a; Serov and Vinogradov 2022).

Artificial intelligence (AI) has the potential to enhance the performance of nanobiosensors by enabling real-time data processing, analysis, and interpretation. AI-enabled nanobiosensors have the ability to improve the accuracy and reliability of data, reduce false positives, and increase the speed of analysis (Kulkarni et al. 2022). In this chapter, we will discuss some of the promising trends in biosensor devices enabled by nanotechnology and AI.

9.2 HISTORY OF ARTIFICIAL INTELLIGENCE IN BRIEF

Here is a brief timeline showing how AI has developed over the last six decades since its inception (Jean 2020; Muthukrishnan et al. 2020; Nakahara 2020) (Figure 9.1).

9.3 ARTIFICIAL INTELLIGENCE (AI) TYPES

Common AI types (Zaza et al. 2019; Mariani et al. 2023) are listed below:

- Purely reactive

  These machines, which specialize on a single line of work, have no memory or data to work with. For instance, when playing chess, the computer watches the moves and chooses the move that will give it the best chance of winning.

DOI: 10.1201/9781003316435-9

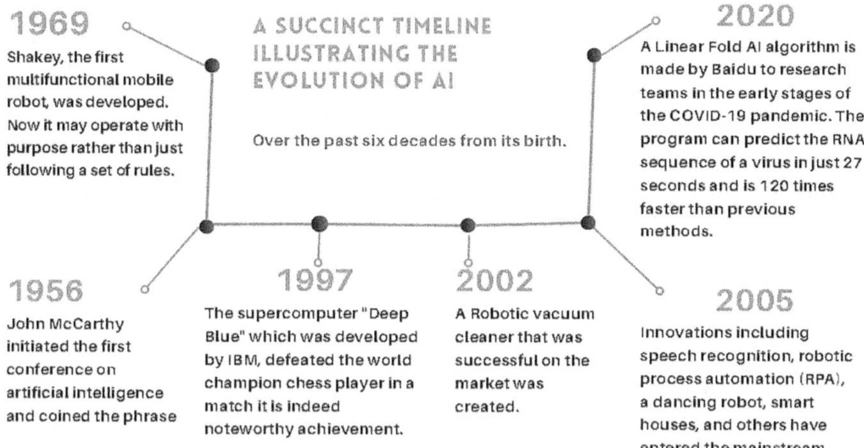

FIGURE 9.1 A brief history of AI.

- Limited memory
  These gadgets collect historical data and keep adding to their memory. They have enough expertise or knowledge to make sensible decisions despite having a poor memory. For instance, this system can suggest a restaurant utilizing the geographic data that has been collected.
- Theory of mind
  This kind of AI is capable of social communication and can understand feelings and thoughts. However, a machine of this kind has not yet been created.
- Self-aware
  Self-aware machines are the future generation of these new technologies. They will be intelligent, sentient, and conscious.

There are various artificial intelligent systems as shown in Figure 9.2.

AI has a wide range of applications across many different fields. Few of the numerous uses of AI are shown in Figure 9.3. It is expected that as AI technology develops, new and creative applications will appear in a variety of industries. Here are some of the possible examples (but not limited to) of AI applications:

- Natural Language Processing (NLP): AI-powered language models can analyze and generate natural language text, speech, and conversation. NLP is used in applications such as chat bots, voice assistants, language translation, and sentiment analysis (Zhou et al. 2020; Houssein et al. 2021; Yuan and Gao 2021; Lauriola et al. 2022).

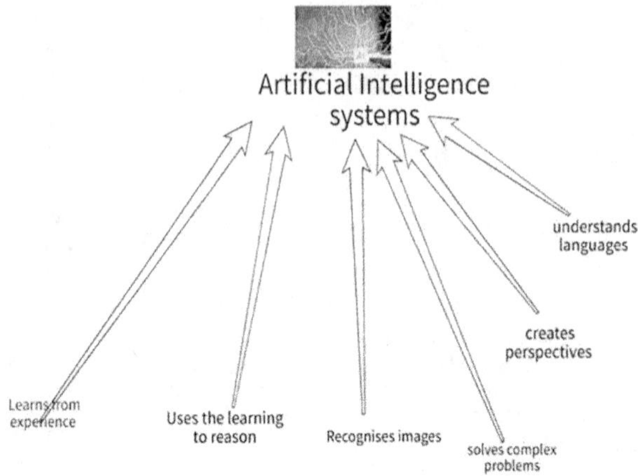

FIGURE 9.2 Various artificial intelligent systems.

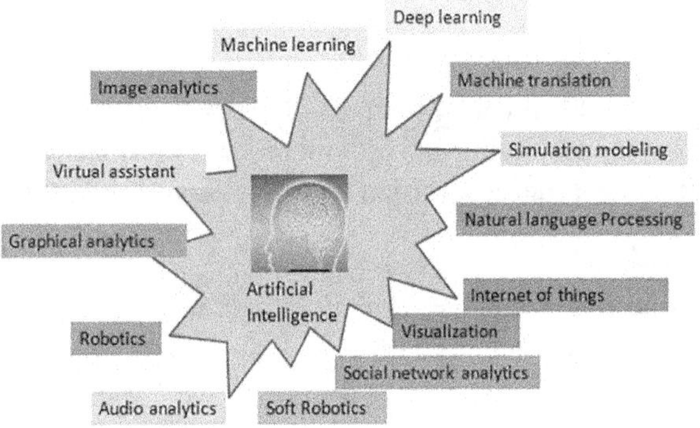

FIGURE 9.3 Applications of AI.

- Computer Vision: AI algorithms can analyze and interpret images and videos, allowing computers to "see" and understand visual data. Computer vision is used in applications such as object recognition, face recognition, autonomous vehicles, and medical image analysis (Kakani et al. 2020; Rhoads 2020; Rakhshan et al. 2022).
- Robotics: AI can be used to control and automate robots, allowing them to perform complex tasks in manufacturing, healthcare, agriculture, and other industries (Mihret 2020; Vrontis et al. 2022).
- Recommendation Systems: AI algorithms can analyze user behavior and preferences to make personalized recommendations for products, services, and content. Recommendation systems are used in applications such as e-commerce, social media, and entertainment (Kim and Lee 2019; Verma and Sharma 2020; Pang 2021).

- Fraud Detection: AI can be used to detect and prevent fraud in financial transactions, insurance claims, and other areas where deception is a risk (Erdogan et al. 2020; Ikhsan et al. 2022).
- Predictive Analytics: AI is capable of analyzing vast volumes of data to find patterns and forecast future events. Applications for predictive analytics include supply chain management, marketing, and stock trading (Schweyer 2018; Chong et al. 2020; Galaz et al. 2021).
- Healthcare: AI can be used to diagnose diseases, monitor patient health, and personalize treatment plans. AI is also used in drug discovery and medical research (Yu et al. 2018; Joshi and Sabharwal 2022; Dicuonzo et al. 2023).
- Education: AI can be used to personalize learning for students, modify the curriculum to suit their requirements, and grade student work (Chen et al. 2020; Ouyang and Jiao 2021; Levin et al. 2022).
- Cyber Security: AI can detect and prevent cyber-attacks, as well as identify vulnerabilities in computer systems (Li 2018; Sedjelmaci et al. 2020; Sivasankar 2022).
- Agriculture: AI can be used to forecast weather patterns, manage pests and crop diseases, and maximize crop yields (Jha et al. 2019; CTA 2020; Subeesh and Mehta 2021; Vazquez et al. 2021).

AI and machine learning (ML) are two related concepts that have gained a lot of attention in recent years due to their potential to transform many industries. Although often used interchangeably, AI and ML are not the same thing. There is a relationship between AI, ML, and deep learning as described in Figure 9.4.

Artificial Intelligence (AI): It describes a system's capacity to carry out operations that ordinarily require human intelligence, such as speech recognition, decision-making, and NLP. Either rule-based or learning-based AI systems are possible. While learning-based systems use algorithms and statistical models to

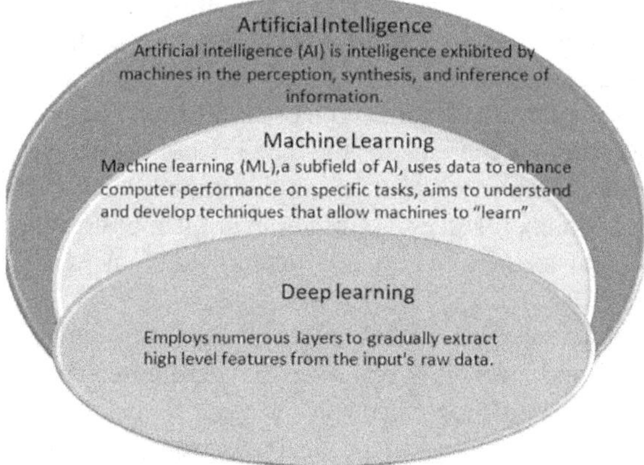

FIGURE 9.4 Relationship curves.

learn from data and improve their performance over time, rule-based systems rely on predefined rules to make decisions.

A branch of AI called machine learning (ML) focuses on precisely teaching computers to learn from data. It entails the automatic detection of patterns in data using algorithms and statistical models, followed by the application of those patterns to generate predictions or take action. Supervised, unsupervised, or semi-supervised ML algorithms are all possible (Jadhav et al. 2022). Unsupervised learning makes use of unlabeled data to find patterns, whereas supervised learning uses labeled data to train the model. In semi-supervised learning, both methods are used (Janiesch et al. 2021; Sarker 2021; Zhou et al. 2022).

The ability of AI and ML to swiftly and accurately handle and analyses enormous amounts of data is one of its main advantages. Because of this, they are especially helpful in sectors like healthcare, finance, and marketing, where a lot of data are produced every day. Many repetitive jobs can be automated using AI and ML, freeing up human labor for more difficult and imaginative tasks.

Machine Learning: Creating algorithms that let machines learn from data and get better over time without explicit programming is a subset of AI. It uses methods like support vector machines, decision trees, and neural networks (Raschka et al. 2020).

A branch of AI, ML includes creating statistical models and algorithms that let machines pick up new skills and improve their performance on a given activity without having to be explicitly programmed.

In ML, the computer is taught to recognize patterns in a huge dataset and to anticipate outcomes using the data it has seen. The more the data a computer has been trained on, the better the performance of the computer (Zhou 2022).

ML algorithms are classified into three main types:

i. Supervised Learning: In this type of algorithm, the machine is trained on labeled data, which means the data are already labeled with the correct answers. The machine learns to make predictions based on the patterns it recognizes in the labeled data. Common examples of supervised learning include image recognition and speech recognition (Wang et al. 2022; Zhang et al. 2022b).
ii. Unsupervised Learning: In this type of algorithm, the machine is trained on unlabeled data, which means the data are not labeled with the correct answers. The machine learns to recognize patterns in the data and group similar data points together. Common examples of unsupervised learning include clustering and anomaly detection (Wang et al. 2022; Zhang et al. 2022b).
iii. Reinforcement Learning: In this type of algorithm, the machine learns through trial and error. It is rewarded for making correct decisions and penalized for making incorrect decisions. Over time, the machine learns to make better decisions based on the feedback it receives. Common examples of reinforcement learning include game playing and robotics (Kormushev et al. 2013; Goldwaser and Thielscher 2020; Zhang et al. 2022b).

Image identification, NLP, fraud detection, recommendation systems, and predictive maintenance are just a few of the many uses of ML. The discipline of ML is expanding quickly, and new tools and applications are continuously being created.

Natural Language Processing: It is the capacity of computers to comprehend and translate human language. It uses methods including speech recognition, sentiment analysis, and machine translation. The interaction between human language and computers is the focus of the computer science and AI field known as natural language processing (NLP). It entails instructing computers to comprehend, decode, and produce spoken and written human language (Zhou et al. 2020; Yuan and Gao 2021; Lauriola et al. 2022).

Machine translation, sentiment analysis, text summarization, speech recognition, and chat bots are just a few of the many uses for NLP. It is heavily utilized in the creation of virtual and voice assistants like Siri and Alexa, as well as in a wide range of other fields like healthcare, banking, and customer service.

Robotics: It includes the progress of machines that can perform physical tasks and interact with the environment. It includes techniques such as computer vision, motion planning, and control systems. The study of robotics encompasses the creation, advancement, and use of robots. A robot is a mechanism or technology that can carry out a task without much assistance from humans. Robots can be controlled by a human operator or can be programmed to perform tasks automatically (Mihret 2020; Rabinovich et al. 2020; Hussain et al. 2021; Sarker et al. 2021).

Robotics combines various disciplines including mechanical engineering, electrical engineering, computer science, and AI. It involves designing and building robots that can sense their environment, make decisions, and take actions to achieve a specific goal. Robotics also involves developing algorithms and software that enable robots to perceive their surroundings, interact with humans and other robots, and learn from their experiences.

Robots are used in a wide range of industries, including manufacturing, healthcare, transportation, and entertainment. They can perform repetitive and dangerous tasks, such as welding or inspecting hazardous environments. Robotics is also used in research and exploration, such as in space exploration or in the study of underwater environments.

Expert Systems: It involves developing systems that can perform tasks that typically require human expertise, such as medical diagnosis, financial analysis, and legal reasoning. It involves techniques such as rule-based systems and knowledge representation (Fischer 1985; Horvitz et al. 1988).

Expert systems are computer-based tools that employ AI to simulate human decision-making in a given field. These systems are designed to provide intelligent advice or recommendations to users, based on a set of rules, heuristics, and knowledge base.

Expert systems use a knowledge representation technique to capture and store domain-specific knowledge in the form of rules or facts. The knowledge base is created by experts in the domain who encode their knowledge and expertise into the system. The system then uses this knowledge to reason about problems, make decisions, and provide recommendations to users (Waller et al. 1988; Bae 2013; Sutton et al. 2016).

Expert systems are used in a variety of fields including medicine, finance, engineering, and law to provide advice or support decision-making. They are particularly useful in situations where there is a large amount of complex and specialized knowledge that needs to be considered and where a human expert may not be available or accessible (Horvitz et al. 1988; Waller et al. 1988). A common benefit of expert systems is that they can provide consistent, reliable, and accurate advice or recommendations, as they are not subject to the same biases or errors that can affect human experts. They can also be used to train or educate novice users by providing explanations and justifications for their recommendations. However, expert systems also have limitations, such as their inability to handle new or unexpected situations, and their dependence on accurate and complete knowledge base. As a result, they are often used in combination with other AI techniques, such as ML, to enhance their capabilities and overcome their limitations.

1. Neural Networks: It is a kind of ML algorithm that is based on how the human brain works and is structured. It involves creating layers of interconnected nodes that can learn and adapt to new data. Neural networks are a subset of AI and ML that are designed to mimic the structure and function of the human brain. They are composed of interconnected nodes, or neurons, that process and transmit information. Neural networks are trained using large amounts of data, where the network learns to recognize patterns and relationships within the data. This process is called supervised learning, where the network is provided with labeled data and adjusts its connections based on the feedback it receives. There are several types of neural networks, including feedforward neural networks, convolutional neural networks (CNNs), and recurrent neural networks (RNNs) (Kumar and Thakur 2012; Liimatainen et al. 2021; Qiao et al. 2023). Each type of network is designed to perform specific tasks, such as image recognition, speech recognition, or NLP. NLP, robotics, autonomous vehicles, and picture and speech recognition are just a few of the many uses of neural networks. Due to their ability to learn and adapt to new situations based on the data they are trained on, they are especially helpful in situations where traditional rule-based programming may not be effective. One of the main advantages of neural networks is its capacity to spot patterns and relationships in data, even when those patterns aren't clearly stated. However, they also have limitations, such as their dependence on large amounts of labeled data for training, and their inability to explain their decisions or predictions in a way that is easily understood by humans (Intelligence 2010; Öztürk and Şahin 2018; Ugurlu 2022).

9.4 AN OVERVIEW OF NANOBIOSENSORS

Nanotechnology and biosensors, in general, are where nanobiosensors have their roots. These are typically sensors made from nanomaterials, which is fascinating because they are not specifically designed to identify activities and measurements in the nano range. Nanotechnology has given humans the unique ability to create nanomaterials with essential physiochemical properties that are very different from the identical nanostructures generated at a bulk size. Here, nanomaterials effectively aid the biosensing technology's detection mechanism (Kulkarni et al. 2022). Microelectromechanical systems (MEMS), which are in charge of providing the means of transducers, are also created when nanomaterial devices are integrated with electrical components. Many nanomaterials have recently been investigated for their potential use in improved biological signal processing through the use of electrical and mechanical properties. Several widely used nanomaterials in sensing applications include crystalline thin films, nanowires, nanotubes, and nanorods. Quantum dots (QDs) can be used as fluorescent agents for binding detection, amperometric devices for enzyme-based glucose sensing, and even bioconjugated nanomaterials for focused biomolecular detection. These include colloidal nanoparticles that can be combined with antibodies to be used in immunosensing and immunolabeling applications. These chemicals can also be used to enhance electron microscope detections. Additionally, electronic and optical applications benefit greatly from the use of metal-based nanomaterials. They can be effectively employed to find nucleic acid sequences by utilizing their optoelectronic properties. In order to better understand their characteristics and potential uses in biosensors, several nanomaterials have been reported (Ra et al. 2012; Azimzadeh et al. 2017; Tavakkoli Yaraki and Tan 2020; Naresh and Lee 2021; Sheervalilou et al. 2021; Luciano et al. 2022).

Response time, selectivity, sensitivity, and linearity are among the characteristics of biosensors that make it more effective.

Research studies show a persistent increase in implementing either transducer or receptor operation on numerous nanomaterials to increase their multi-detection sensitivity and capability. Additionally, these nanomaterials include nanoparticles, nanotubes, QDs, and other biological nanomaterials. These might aid the bio-recognition element, the transducer, or both. Nanosensors, nanoprobes, and other nanodevices have revolutionized biochemical and biological inquiry fields by making it possible to quickly examine a wide range of compounds *in vivo*. Recent years have seen the emergence of a wide variety of nanomaterials with varied properties, such as tiny size, quick speeds, shorter distances for electrons to travel, reduced power consumption, and lower voltages (Bhalla et al. 2018; Özmen et al. 2021; Sellappan et al. 2021; Sharifianjazi et al. 2022; Yaraki et al. 2022; Dam et al. 2023).

As a result of significant developments in the field of nanotechnology, nanomaterials such as metal nanoparticles, oxide nanoparticles, magnetic nanomaterials, carbon materials, and QDs are now utilized to improve the electrochemical signals of biocatalytic processes that occur at the electrode and electrolyte interference.

For application in biosensors, functional nanomaterials joined to biological molecules like proteins, peptides, and DNA have been created. The top-to-bottom approach involves micro-/nanomachining macroscopic materials down to the appropriate nanoscale environment using chemical (isotropic) and physical (anisotropic) processes (Kumar and Panda 2021). This procedure combines lithography, chemical etching, ion milling, laser ablation, and lithography. On the other hand, with a bottom-up approach, a material is added to and built upon after the initial production of a critical mass. Additional techniques used in bottom-up nanofabrication include molecular beam epitaxy, evaporation, physical or chemical vapor deposition, and protein–polymer nanocomposites.

QDs, graphene, gold, and silver nanoparticles, among other forms of nanomaterials, have lately been employed in the construction of sensors. Nanobiosensors are a common name for biosensors created using nanoscale materials. These biosensors based on nanotechnology can be roughly categorized into four types: electrochemical, optical, thermal, and piezoelectric. Further advancements in detecting sensitivity and specificity have been made possible by fluorescent nanocluster biosensors, electrochemical nanobiosensors, and microfluidic nanomaterials (Abu-Salah et al. 2015; Chamorro-Garcia and Merkoçi 2016; Srivastava et al. 2018; Sharifi et al. 2021). For a variety of applications, microfluidics, nanotechnology, and biosensors are currently being integrated.

The connection of AI for health care monitoring-based biosensors for the point of care (POC) diagnostics applications offers an important area for health care devices and helpful hierarchical procedures for scientific decision-making (More 2021; Dave et al. 2022b).

The combination of AI and nanotechnology has opened up new possibilities for the development of sensors that are more sensitive, faster, and more accurate than traditional sensors. These sensors are capable of detecting and analyzing complex chemical and biological signals that are difficult to detect using traditional sensors. In this chapter, we will explore the concept of AI- and nanotechnology-based sensors and their potential applications (More 2021; Sharma et al. 2022).

9.5 ARTIFICIAL INTELLIGENCE AND NANOTECHNOLOGY

AI and nanotechnology are two rapidly advancing fields of technology that are changing the world we live in. The simulation of human intelligence processes by computer systems is known as AI. It entails the creation of algorithms that can absorb knowledge from data and generate predictions or judgments based on that knowledge.

Nanotechnology, on the other hand, is the manipulation of matter at the atomic and molecular level. It involves the use of nanoscale materials and devices to create new products and technologies. Nanotechnology has many applications, including the development of sensors.

The combination of AI and nanotechnology has led to the development of sensors that can detect and analyze complex signals. These sensors are capable of detecting and analyzing chemical and biological signals that are difficult to detect using traditional sensors (Adir et al. 2020; Egorov et al. 2021; Hayat et al. 2021; Ahmad et al. 2022; Naaz and Asghar 2022; Serov and Vinogradov 2022; Tan et al. 2023).

AI- and nanotechnology-based sensors are designed to be more sensitive, faster, and more accurate than traditional sensors. They are capable of detecting and analyzing complex chemical and biological signals that are difficult to detect using traditional sensors. One example of an AI- and nanotechnology-based sensors is the nano-electrochemical sensor. This sensor is based on the use of nanoscale electrodes that can detect and measure the concentration of specific molecules in a solution. The sensor uses AI algorithms to analyze the data and make predictions or decisions based on that data. Another example of an AI- and nanotechnology-based sensors is the biosensor. Biosensors are devices that use biological molecules to detect and measure specific substances. The use of nanoscale materials and devices has made biosensors more sensitive and more accurate than traditional biosensors (Hayat et al. 2021; Tan et al. 2023).

AI- and nanotechnology-based sensors have many potential applications, including:

a. Medical Diagnostics: AI and nanotechnology-based sensors can be used to detect and diagnose diseases at an early stage. These sensors can detect and analyze biological signals that are indicative of disease, such as the presence of specific proteins or DNA (Roy et al. 2022).
b. Environmental Monitoring: AI- and nanotechnology-based sensors can be used to monitor the environment for the presence of pollutants and other contaminants. These sensors can detect and analyze chemical signals in the air, water, and soil (Stetter and Li 2008; Dewan et al. 2016; Hairom et al. 2021).
c. Food Safety: AI- and nanotechnology-based sensors can be used to detect and monitor foodborne pathogens and other contaminants in food. These sensors can detect and analyze biological signals in food samples (Kumar et al. 2020b;Vijayakumar et al. 2023).
d. Homeland Security: AI- and nanotechnology-based sensors can be used for homeland security applications, such as detecting and identifying chemical and biological agents (Denecke and Baudoin 2022; Hemmati and Rahmani 2022).
e. Industrial Process Monitoring: AI- and nanotechnology-based sensors can be used to monitor industrial processes, such as chemical reactions and manufacturing processes. These sensors can detect and analyze chemical signals in real time, allowing for the optimization of the process.

9.6 APPLICATION OF AI IN DISEASE DETECTION

ML algorithms can be used to analyze large datasets generated by nanobiosensors to identify patterns and correlations that are indicative of specific biological or chemical species. These algorithms can then be used to predict the presence or concentration of these species in real time. For example, a nanobiosensor integrated with ML can be used to detect biomarkers in blood samples for early diagnosis of diseases such as cancer. The ML algorithm can analyze the data generated by the nanobiosensor to identify patterns that are indicative of the presence of cancer biomarkers. Wearable nanobiosensors are emerging as a promising technology for real-time monitoring of various physiological parameters such as glucose levels, blood pressure, and heart rate. These devices can be worn on the skin or integrated into clothing and offer continuous monitoring capabilities. AI can be used to analyze the data generated by wearable nanobiosensors to identify patterns and correlations that are indicative of changes in physiological parameters. For example, AI can be used to predict the onset of hypoglycemia in diabetic patients based on continuous monitoring of glucose levels using a wearable nanobiosensor (Chandra 2016; Advances in Materials Science and Engineering 2022). Internet of Things (IoT) devices can be used to connect nanobiosensors to the cloud, enabling real-time data processing, analysis, and interpretation. AI algorithms can be used to analyze the data generated by nanobiosensors connected to IoT devices to identify patterns and correlations that are indicative of specific biological or chemical species. For example, an IoT-enabled nanobiosensor can be used to monitor air quality in a city. The data generated by the nanobiosensor can be transmitted to an IoT device that analyzes the data using AI algorithms to identify patterns that are indicative of specific pollutants. The integration of nanobiosensors with AI has the potential to revolutionize the field of biosensors by enabling real-time data processing, analysis, and interpretation. AI-enabled nanobiosensors offer high sensitivity, selectivity, and real-time monitoring capabilities, making them ideal for a wide range of applications in various fields. The promising trends in nanotechnology- and AI-enabled sensor devices discussed in this chapter offer a glimpse of the potential of this technology to transform healthcare, environmental monitoring, and food safety. The integration of AI with biosensors is leading to the development of more advanced and sophisticated sensing devices. Some of the emerging trends in this field include the following.

9.6.1 Point of Care (POC) Devices

The objective of a real POC diagnostics is to speed up and improve the diagnosis process at the precise location and time that events occur (Montenegro-López 2020; Dulmage et al. 2021; Li et al. 2021; Lu et al. 2021). Along with improvements in multidisciplinary sensing technologies, such as nanotechnologies, microfluidics, and advanced materials, it is anticipated that POC diagnostics will greatly profit from a closer relationship with AI. Indeed, AI and ML can be used to create methods for integrating, analyzing, and comprehending multimedia data from a variety of different devices. The results are tailored to the patient's individual background in accordance with a more individualized and adaptable approach to care, favoring an accurate prediction of future status (Mejía-Salazar et al. 2020; Ilhan et al. 2021). The patient's current status and prior history can be correlated using multivariate techniques. AI is being used to develop compact and portable biosensors for real-time diagnosis and monitoring of various medical conditions. In order to do this, it is necessary to investigate many areas of AI and POC diagnostics research. On the one hand, AI models can be integrated into proof-of-concept testing devices, expanding their functionality and enabling studies that would not otherwise be feasible, such as those involving image analysis. As a result, pervasive computing and POC diagnostics may converge (Onweni et al. 2021; Zhang et al. 2023). Distributed AI can also be used to create networks of local devices, allowing wearable sensors and portable devices to connect with one another and analyze data in a cumulative and coherent manner. Finally, it is possible to decentralize AI by using a cloud-based strategy and expanding the capabilities of POC diagnostics across the entire computing spectrum. For example, a timely decentralized survey may enable the discovery of anomalies that, once combined with previously gathered data and anamnesis, with the additional goal of a quality check to employ accurate data, can be classified by AI systems. The user and his caretakers can then be immediately informed by the system.

Additionally, particular aid networks can ensure control and rescue over the area. Even though POC devices are expensive, they save lives and reduce costs.

9.6.2 Lab-on-a-Chip (LOC) Devices

AI is being used to develop microfluidic devices that integrate multiple biosensors on a single chip, allowing for high-throughput analysis and on-demand testing. Continuous monitoring: AI-powered biosensors are being developed for continuous monitoring of various biological parameters, including glucose levels, blood pressure, and other vital signs. Deep learning algorithms: AI algorithms, such as deep learning, are being used to improve the accuracy and precision of biosensors by enabling real-time analysis and decision-making based on sensor readings. The integration of AI in biosensors is transforming the way biological samples are analyzed and providing new opportunities for disease diagnosis, monitoring, and treatment (Mejía-Salazar et al. 2020).

Infectious diseases are a major global health problem, causing significant morbidity and mortality worldwide. Early and accurate diagnosis of infectious diseases is critical for effective treatment and prevention of transmission (Sharma et al. 2022). Traditional diagnostic methods, such as culture-based methods, are time-consuming and require specialized equipment and trained personnel. In recent years, there has been significant interest in the development of POC diagnostic tests for infectious diseases that can be used in resource-limited settings. The combination of AI and nanotechnology has the potential to revolutionize POC diagnostics by enabling the development of highly sensitive and specific sensors (Cui et al. 2020).

AI- and nanotechnology-based sensors for infectious diseases are designed to be highly sensitive and specific, allowing for early and accurate diagnosis of infections. These sensors are capable of detecting and analyzing complex biological signals that are indicative of infectious agents (Dave et al. 2022b; Dhanalakshmi et al. 2022).

One example of an AI- and nanotechnology-based sensor for infectious diseases is the use of gold nanoparticles as a biosensor. Gold nanoparticles are functionalized with antibodies or aptamers that bind to specific biomolecules, such as antigens or nucleic acids, associated with infectious agents. The binding of the biomolecule to the gold nanoparticle results in a change in the optical properties of the nanoparticle that can be detected using a simple handheld device. AI algorithms can be used to analyze the data and make predictions or decisions based on that data (Das et al. 2022; Dave et al. 2022a; Dave and Jone Kirubavathy 2022).

Another example of an AI- and nanotechnology-based sensor for infectious diseases is the use of microfluidic chips. Microfluidic chips are small, portable devices that use nanoscale materials and devices to detect and analyze biological signals. These chips can be functionalized with specific antibodies or nucleic acid probes to detect infectious agents. AI algorithms can be used to analyze the data and make predictions or decisions based on that data (Sahoo et al. 2022).

Integration with existing healthcare systems: AI- and nanotechnology-based sensors must be integrated with existing healthcare systems to ensure proper diagnosis and treatment. Regulatory approval: AI- and nanotechnology-based sensors must undergo regulatory approval before they can be used in clinical settings. Despite these challenges, the potential benefits of AI- and nanotechnology-based sensors for infectious diseases are significant. The development of highly sensitive and specific POC diagnostic tests has the potential to revolutionize the diagnosis and treatment of infectious diseases.

The IoT is a fast developing interdisciplinary field that connects physical items, both living and non-living, with computer hardware, software, and other electronic devices through a network. There are many IoT-enabled technologies being tested in the healthcare industry that connect patients to healthcare facilities remotely (Panwar et al. 2022). The Internet of Medical Things (IoMT), a fast developing IoT network, allows patients and physicians to communicate with one another via a variety of wirelessly connected medical equipment. One of the most important steps in identifying the signs and symptoms of an infection disease, even though its effects were not immediately apparent, is a quick and accurate screening of health issues (Venkata Sateesh Yadav and Vishwanth 2018; Acharya and Patil 2020; Jayakumar et al. 2021).

However, due to their lengthy reaction times, requirement for qualified staff, and high cost per study, traditional healthcare settings find it difficult and expensive to manage the real-time identification of viral infections. In light of this, the healthcare sector is working to increase the precision, dependability, and productivity of POC devices based on biosensors (Montenegro-López 2020). The ability to control epidemic outbreaks is the main benefit of these diagnostic tools that are combined with IoMT capabilities. They can aid in screening, offer effective medical care, and help in outbreak control.

Due to their widespread use, portability, flexibility, and wireless communication technology, smartphones have a wide range of applications for biosensors that allow for the collection and sharing of data for medical investigation. Researchers are also drawn to smartphone-based biosensors because they enable real-time qualitative and quantitative analyses of the sample with ease. This is possible by using a smartphone application that can measure colorimetric, fluorescent, reflection-based, current, and turbidity signals (Chayalakshmi 2016; Jadczyk et al. 2021). They are equipped with the ability to manage the recognition process, receive recognition data via a variety of interfaces (including Bluetooth, a camera, an audio connection, and a micro-USB port), and show recognition results. As a result, these characteristics make smartphone-based devices perfect for creating viral detection tests that can be carried out outside of clinical laboratories.

9.6.3 Precision Medicine

Each patient is different. We have distinct molecular signatures in addition to our obvious variations, such as age, gender, height, eye color, and blood type. Patient phenotypic alterations and medication reactions are consequently variable. Patient diversity is particularly noticeable in several cancer forms, where an accumulation of driver mutations causes intratumor and interpatient heterogeneities that make diagnosis and treatment more difficult. Precision medicine strives to individually adapt a patient treatment plan by taking into account a variety of genetic and epigenetic traits. Nanomaterials have helped precision medicine advance at every level of the medical process. In order to maintain genetic context, new omics collection methods, such single-molecule nanopore sequencing, offer quick and sensitive single-molecule detection together with larger sequence read lengths (Roberti et al. 2019; Adir et al. 2020; Yang et al. 2021a; Alghamdi et al. 2022; Chen et al. 2022; Zhang et al. 2022a; Tan et al. 2023). Nanosensor-based diagnostic tests are enabled by biomarkers. Liquid biopsies can simultaneously scan for several disease biomarkers and identify them at femtomolar quantities as well as in cell cultures (blood, urine, and saliva). Over the past few decades, nanomedicine-based cancer treatments have evolved from a population-wide approach that focused primarily on increasing efficacy and minimizing adverse effects to localized systems that provide information about drug activity within the patient body. The logical design of targeted therapeutic approaches utilizing endogenous and external triggers for enhanced drug distribution was encouraged by advancements in nanomedicine fabrication techniques and a better understanding of cancer biology. Theranostic nanomedicines (Kumar et al. 2020a; Ladju et al. 2022), which combine a drug and an imaging agent to further assess the effectiveness of treatment inside the patient body, were also made possible by these developments. Nonetheless, the clinical translation of contemporary nanosensors and focused nanomedicine in the field of cancer has been hampered. Precision medicine's objective—tailoring the optimum course of treatment for each cancer patient—can be realized thanks in large part to two scientific fields: AI and nanotechnology. Recent integration of these two sectors is making things better, one is collection of patient data and the other is enhanced nanomaterial design for precise cancer treatment. A patient's unique disease profile is put together using diagnostic nanomaterials, and it is then used in conjunction with a number of therapeutic nanotechnologies to enhance the effectiveness of treatment. High intratumor and interpatient heterogeneities, however, make it extremely challenging to create sensible diagnostic and treatment platforms and analyze their results. Utilizing pattern analysis and classification algorithms for increased diagnostic and treatment accuracy, the integration of AI techniques can bridge this gap. The use of AI in nanomedicine design also has benefits by maximizing material (Marshall et al. 2022; Shen et al. 2022).

Improved design of nanotechnologies for diagnosis and therapy can be achieved by taking advantage of AI algorithms' capacity to process massive datasets and recognize complicated patterns. Formulations for nanomedicine can be made more effective by predicting how nanoparticles will interact with the target drug, biological medium, and cell membranes as well as with drug absorption and release kinetics. Algorithms for pattern identification and classification can also be used to distinguish between healthy and sick individuals and to foretell a patient's response to a treatment. The enormous complexity of cancer makes these analysis capabilities all the more important. Here, we explain how nanomaterials are being used to create omics, diagnostics, and therapy technologies for precision cancer medicine, highlighting the role that AI plays in the data analysis and design of nanomedicine (Khandker et al. 2020).

Diabetes is a chronic metabolic disorder that affects millions of people worldwide. It is characterized by high levels of glucose in the blood, which can lead to serious complications such as heart disease, kidney failure, and blindness. Early and accurate diagnosis of diabetes is critical for effective management and prevention of complications. Nanosensors and ML have the potential to revolutionize diabetes diagnosis and management by enabling the development of highly sensitive and specific sensors (Singla et al. 2019; Vettoretti et al. 2020; Vu et al. 2020; Gautier et al. 2021).

Nanosensors for diabetes diagnosis (Venkadesh et al. 2021) and management are designed to be highly sensitive and specific, allowing for early and accurate diagnosis and monitoring of glucose levels. These sensors are capable of detecting and analyzing complex biological signals that are indicative of glucose levels. One example of nanosensors for diabetes diagnosis and management is the use of nanowires. Nanowires are small, nanoscale wires that are functionalized with glucose oxidase, an enzyme that catalyzes the oxidation of glucose. The oxidation of glucose results in a change in the electrical properties of the nanowire that can be detected using a simple electrical circuit. This change in electrical properties is proportional to the glucose concentration in the sample, allowing for accurate measurement of glucose levels. Another example of a nanosensor for diabetes diagnosis and management is the use of carbon nanotubes. Carbon nanotubes are small, cylindrical structures that are functionalized with glucose-binding proteins. When glucose binds to the protein, it induces a change in the electrical properties of the nanotube that can be detected using an electrical circuit. This change in electrical properties is proportional to the glucose concentration in the sample, allowing for accurate measurement of glucose levels. ML for diabetes diagnosis and management involves the use of algorithms and statistical models to analyze large datasets and make predictions or decisions based on that data (Sun and Zhang 2019; Granillo and Goldsztein 2022; Rawat et al. 2022b). ML can be used to analyze data from nanosensors and other sources to improve diabetes diagnosis and management. One example of ML for diabetes diagnosis and management is the use of predictive algorithms to analyze data from continuous glucose monitors (CGMs) (Jones 2019; Jacobs et al. 2020; Arya et al. 2022). CGMs are wearable devices that continuously monitor glucose levels in real time. ML algorithms can be used to analyze the data from CGMs to predict future glucose levels and provide personalized recommendations for diabetes management. Another example of ML for diabetes diagnosis and management is the use of decision support systems. Decision support systems are computer programs that use algorithms and statistical models to provide recommendations for diabetes management based on patient data. These systems can be used to analyze data from nanosensors, CGMs, and other sources to provide personalized recommendations for diabetes management.

Cancer is a complex and heterogeneous disease that affects millions of people worldwide. Early and accurate diagnosis of cancer is critical for effective treatment and prevention of complications. ML has the potential to revolutionize cancer diagnosis and management by enabling the development of highly sensitive and specific diagnostic tools (Hornbrook et al. 2017; Suarez-Ibarrola et al. 2020; Jin et al. 2023).

ML algorithms can be used to analyze complex datasets, including medical images, genomic data, and clinical data, to improve cancer diagnosis. For example, ML algorithms can be trained on large datasets of medical images to identify patterns and features that are indicative of cancer. These algorithms can then be used to analyze new images and make predictions about whether a patient has cancer or not. Another example of ML for cancer diagnosis is the use of genomic data. Genomic data contain information about a patient's genetic makeup and can be used to identify mutations and genetic markers that are associated with cancer. ML algorithms can be used to analyze genomic data and make predictions about a patient's risk of developing cancer or whether a patient has a specific type of cancer (Santhamoorthy et al. 2023). ML algorithms can also be used to improve cancer treatment by enabling personalized medicine. Personalized medicine involves tailoring treatment to individual patients based on their unique characteristics, such as their genetic makeup and clinical history. ML algorithms can be used to analyze these characteristics and make predictions about which treatments are likely to be most effective for individual patients.

For example, ML algorithms can be used to analyze genomic data to identify mutations and genetic markers that are associated with specific types of cancer. This information can then be used to identify targeted therapies that are designed to specifically target these mutations. ML algorithms can also be used to analyze clinical data to identify patient subgroups that are likely to respond differently to certain treatments (Karplus 2022; Nauta et al. 2022; Rasool et al. 2022).

ML and nanomaterials are two promising technologies that have shown great potential for cancer detection. By combining these two technologies, researchers have been able to develop highly sensitive and accurate cancer detection systems.

Nanomaterials, which are materials with dimensions less than 100 nm, have unique physical and chemical properties that make them ideal for use in biosensors. These materials can be engineered to interact specifically with cancer biomarkers, enabling highly sensitive detection of cancer cells or molecules (Xiong et al. 2019; Gong et al. 2021; Zhang and Lyu 2021; Han et al. 2022).

ML, on the other hand, is a subset of AI that allows computer systems to learn from data without being explicitly programmed. In the context of cancer detection, ML algorithms can be trained on large datasets of cancer-related data to identify patterns and predict outcomes.

One example of the use of nanomaterials and ML in cancer detection is the development of a nanosensor-based system for detecting early-stage pancreatic cancer (Wang et al. 2020; Yang et al. 2021b). Researchers have developed a nanosensor that can detect minute levels of mesothelin, a protein that is overexpressed in pancreatic cancer cells. The nanosensor is coated with antibodies that specifically bind to mesothelin, enabling highly sensitive detection of the protein in blood samples.

To improve the accuracy of the nanosensor-based system, ML algorithms have been used to analyze large datasets of pancreatic cancer–related data, such as gene expression profiles and clinical data. By training these algorithms on these datasets, researchers have been able to identify patterns and biomarkers associated with early-stage pancreatic cancer, which can be used to develop more accurate and sensitive detection systems (Wang et al. 2020).

Another example is the use of ML to analyze imaging data from cancer patients. Researchers have developed ML algorithms that can analyze imaging data, such as computed tomography (CT) scans and magnetic resonance imaging (MRI) scans, to predict patient outcomes and detect cancer at an early stage (Alafeef et al. 2020; Hayat et al. 2021; Hassan 2022).

In addition to improving cancer detection, ML and nanomaterials can also be used to develop personalized cancer treatments. By analyzing large datasets of patient data, ML algorithms can identify genetic mutations and other biomarkers associated with specific types of cancer. This information can then be used to develop personalized treatment plans that target the specific genetic mutations and biomarkers present in each patient's cancer cells (Alafeef et al. 2020).

The combination of ML and nanomaterials has the potential to revolutionize cancer detection and treatment. These technologies offer highly sensitive and accurate detection systems that can detect cancer at an early stage and provide personalized treatment plans. While there are still challenges to be addressed, such as the validation of results and the ethical implications of collecting and analyzing large amounts of personal data, the potential benefits of these technologies are significant and warrant further exploration (Na et al. 2012; Zhou et al. 2019; Xu et al. 2020).

9.7 CHALLENGES AND FUTURE PERSPECTIVES

AI- and nanotechnology-based sensors face several challenges, including sensitivity, selectivity, durability, and cost. The sensitivity of AI- and nanotechnology-based sensors is critical for their success. These sensors must be capable of detecting and analyzing signals that are present in very low concentrations. AI- and nanotechnology-based sensors must be able to differentiate between similar signals. For example, a biosensor must be able to differentiate between different strains of bacteria. AI- and nanotechnology-based sensors must be able to withstand harsh environments and continue to operate reliably and should be affordable.

REFERENCES

Abu-Salah KM, Zourob MM, Mouffouk F, Alrokayan SA, Alaamery MA, Ansari AA (2015) DNA-based nanobiosensors as an emerging platform for detection of disease. *Sensors (Switzerland)* 15, 14539.

Acharya AD, Patil SN (2020) IoT based health care monitoring kit. In: *Proceedings of the 4th International Conference on Computing Methodologies and Communication, ICCMC 2020*, Erode, India.

Adir O, Poley M, Chen G, Froim S, Krinsky N, Shklover J, Shainsky-Roitman J, Lammers T, Schroeder A (2020) Integrating artificial intelligence and nanotechnology for precision cancer medicine. *Adv Mater.* 32, e1901989.

Advances in Materials Science and Engineering (2022) Retracted: Monitoring of sports health indicators based on wearable nanobiosensors. *Adv Mater Sci Eng.* https://doi.org/10.1155/2022/9758123.

Ahmad T, Zhu H, Zhang D, Tariq R, Bassam A, Ullah F, AlGhamdi AS, Alshamrani SS (2022) Energetics systems and artificial intelligence: Applications of industry 4.0. *Energy Reports* 8, 334–361.

Alafeef M, Srivastava I, Pan D (2020) Machine learning for precision breast cancer diagnosis and prediction of the nanoparticle cellular internalization. *ACS Sensors.* https://doi.org/10.1021/acssensors.0c00329.

Alghamdi MA, Fallica AN, Virzì N, Kesharwani P, Pittalà V, Greish K (2022) The promise of nanotechnology in personalized medicine. *J Pers Med.* 12, 673.

Arya M, Sastry G H, Motwani A, Kumar S, Zaguia A (2022) A novel extra tree ensemble optimized DL framework (ETEODL) for early detection of diabetes. *Front Public Heal.* https://doi.org/10.3389/fpubh.2021.797877.

Azimzadeh M, Rahaie M, Nasirizadeh N, Daneshpour M, Naderi-Manesh H (2017) Electrochemical miRNA biosensors: The benefits of nanotechnology. *Nanomed Res J.* https://doi.org/10.22034/NMRJ.2017.23336.

Bae J (2013) Development and application of a web-based expert system using artificial intelligence for management of mental health by Korean emigrants. *J Korean Acad Nurs.* https://doi.org/10.4040/jkan.2013.43.2.203.

Bhalla N, Chiang HJ, Shen AQ (2018) Cell biology at the interface of nanobiosensors and microfluidics. In: *Methods in Cell Biology*. https://doi.org/10.1016/bs.mcb.2018.09.009.

Chayalakshmi C L (2016) Smart phone for personal health care monitoring system. *Int J Instrum Control Syst.* https://doi.org/10.5121/ijics.2016.6401.

Chamorro-Garcia A, Merkoçi A (2016) Nanobiosensors in diagnostics. *Nanobiomedicine.* https://doi.org/10.1177/1849543516663574.

Chandra P (2016) *Nanobiosensors for Personalized and Onsite Biomedical Diagnosis.* doi: https://doi.org/10.1049/PBHE001E.

Chen J, Fu S, Zhang C, Liu H, Su X (2022) DNA logic circuits for cancer theranostics. *Small*, 18, e2108008.

Chen L, Chen P, Lin Z (2020) Artificial intelligence in education: A review. *IEEE Access.* https://doi.org/10.1109/ACCESS.2020.2988510.

Chong LR, Tsai KT, Lee LL, Foo SG, Chang PC (2020) Artificial intelligence predictive analytics in the management of outpatient MRI appointment no-shows. *Am J Roentgenol.* https://doi.org/10.2214/AJR.19.22594.

CTA (2020) *Smart Farming: Transforming Agriculture with Artificial Intelligence*. Spore, Wageningen.

Cui F, Yue Y, Zhang Y, Zhang Z, Zhou HS (2020) Advancing biosensors with machine learning. *ACS Sensors*. https://doi.org/10.1021/acssensors.0c01424.

Dam P, Paret ML, Mondal R, Mandal AK (2023) Advancement of noble metallic nanoparticles in agriculture: A promising future. *Pedosphere*. https://doi.org/10.1016/j.pedsph.2022.06.026.

Das J, Dave S, Radhakrishnan S, Mohanty P (2022) *Biosensors for Emerging and Re-emerging Infectious Diseases*. https://doi.org/10.1016/C2020-0-03552-8.

Dave S, Das J, Ghosh S (2022a) *Advanced Nanomaterials for Point of Care Diagnosis and Therapy*. https://doi.org/10.1016/C2020-0-02584-3.

Dave S, Dave A, Radhakrishnan S, Das J, Dave S (2022b) Biosensors for healthcare: An artificial intelligence approach. In: *Biosensors for Emerging and Re-emerging Infectious Diseases*. https://doi.org/10.1016/C2020-0-03552-8.

Dave S, Jone Kirubavathy S (2022) Biosensors based on metal-organic framework (MOF): Paving the way to point-of-care diagnosis. In: *Electrochemical Applications of Metal-Organic Frameworks: Advances and Future Potential*. https://doi.org/10.1016/B978-0-323-90784-2.00004-6.

Denecke K, Baudoin CR (2022) A review of artificial intelligence and robotics in transformed health ecosystems. *Front Med*. https://doi.org/10.3389/fmed.2022.795957.

Dewan N, Ahmed P, Chowdhury G, Pandit S, Dasgupta D (2016) Nanotechnology based biosensors and its application. *Pharma Innov.* 5, 18–25.

Dhanalakshmi M, Das K, Pandya M, Shah S, Gadnayak A, Dave S, Das J (2022) Artificial neural network-based study predicts GS-441524 as a potential inhibitor of SARS-CoV-2 activator protein furin: A polypharmacology approach. *Appl Biochem Biotechnol*. https://doi.org/10.1007/s12010-022-03928-2.

Dicuonzo G, Donofrio F, Fusco A, Shini M (2023) Healthcare system: Moving forward with artificial intelligence. *Technovation*. https://doi.org/10.1016/j.technovation.2022.102510.

Dulmage B, Tegtmeyer K, Zhang MZ, Colavincenzo M, Xu S (2021) A point-of-care, real-time artificial intelligence system to support clinician diagnosis of a wide range of skin diseases. *J Invest Dermatol*. https://doi.org/10.1016/j.jid.2020.08.027.

Egorov E, Pieters C, Korach-Rechtman H, Shklover J, Schroeder A (2021) Robotics, microfluidics, nanotechnology and AI in the synthesis and evaluation of liposomes and polymeric drug delivery systems. *Drug Deliv Transl Res*. 11. https://doi.org/10.1007/s13346-021-00929-2.

Erdogan I, Kurto O, Kurt A, Bahtiyar S (2020) A new approach for fraud detection with artificial intelligence | Yapay Zeka Ile Sahtekarlik Tespitine Yonelik Yeni Bir Yaklasim. In: *2020 28th Signal Processing and Communications Applications Conference, SIU 2020- Proceedings*, Gaziantep, Turkey.

Fischer CH (1985) Expert systems and artificial intelligence. *Iron Steel Eng*. https://doi.org/10.1300/j025v04n02_05.

Galaz V, Centeno MA, Callahan PW, Causevic A, Patterson T, Brass I, Baum S, Farber D, Fischer J, Garcia D, McPhearson T, Jimenez D, King B, Larcey P, Levy K (2021) Artificial intelligence, systemic risks, and sustainability. *Technol Soc*. https://doi.org/10.1016/j.techsoc.2021.101741.

Gautier T, Ziegler LB, Gerber MS, Campos-Náñez E, Patek SD (2021) Artificial intelligence and diabetes technology: A review. *Metabolism*. https://doi.org/10.1016/j.metabol.2021.154872.

Goldwaser A, Thielscher M (2020) Deep reinforcement learning for general game playing. In: *AAAI 2020-34th AAAI Conference on Artificial Intelligence.*

Gong N, Sheppard NC, Billingsley MM, June CH, Mitchell MJ (2021) Nanomaterials for T-cell cancer immunotherapy. *Nat Nanotechnol.* https://doi.org/10.1038/s41565-020-00822-y.

Granillo Y, Goldsztein GH (2022) Machine learning as a tool to the diagnosis of diabetes. *J Student Res.* https://doi.org/10.47611/jsrhs.v11i1.2513.

Haick H, Tang N (2021) Artificial intelligence in medical sensors for clinical decisions. *ACS Nano* 15. https://doi.org/10.1021/acsnano.1c00085.

Hairom NHH, Soon CF, Mohamed RMSR, Morsin M, Zainal N, Nayan N, Zulkifli CZ, Harun NH (2021) A review of nanotechnological applications to detect and control surface water pollution. *Environ Technol Innov.* https://doi.org/10.1016/j.eti.2021.102032.

Han B, Song Y, Park J, Doh J (2022) Nanomaterials to improve cancer immunotherapy based on ex vivo engineered T cells and NK cells. *J Control Release.* 343, 379–391.

Hassan RYA (2022) Advances in electrochemical nano-biosensors for biomedical and environmental applications: From current work to future perspectives. *Sensors.* 22, 7539.

Hayat H, Nukala A, Nyamira A, Fan J, Wang P (2021) A concise review: The synergy between artificial intelligence and biomedical nanomaterials that empowers nanomedicine. *Biomed. Mater.* https://doi.org/10.1088/1748-605X/ac15b2.

Hemmati A, Rahmani AM (2022) The Internet of Autonomous Things applications: A taxonomy, technologies, and future directions. *Internet of Things (Netherlands).* https://doi.org/10.1016/j.iot.2022.100635.

Hornbrook MC, Goshen R, Choman E, O'Keeffe-Rosetti M, Kinar Y, Liles EG, Rust KC (2017) Early colorectal cancer detected by machine learning model using gender, age, and complete blood count data. *Dig Dis Sci.* https://doi.org/10.1007/s10620-017-4722-8.

Horvitz EJ, Breese JS, Henrion M (1988) Decision theory in expert systems and artificial intelligence. *Int J Approx Reason.* https://doi.org/10.1016/0888-613X(88)90120-X.

Houssein EH, Mohamed RE, Ali AA (2021) Machine learning techniques for biomedical natural language processing: A comprehensive review. *IEEE Access.* https://doi.org/10.1109/ACCESS.2021.3119621.

Huggins W, Piyush Patil, Bradley Mitchell, Birgitta Whaley K, Miles Stoudenmire E (2019) Towards quantum machine learning with tensor networks. *Quantum Sci Technol.* 4(2), 024001.

Hussain K, Wang X, Omar Z, Elnour M, Ming Y (2021) Robotics and artificial intelligence applications in manage and control of COVID-19 pandemic. In: *2021 International Conference on Computer, Control and Robotics, ICCCR 2021.*

Ikhsan WM, Ednoer EH, Kridantika WS, Firmansyah A (2022) Fraud detection automation through data analytics and artificial intelligence. *Riset.* https://doi.org/10.37641/riset.v4i2.166.

Ilhan B, Guneri P, Wilder-Smith P (2021) The contribution of artificial intelligence to reducing the diagnostic delay in oral cancer. *Oral Oncol.* https://doi.org/10.1016/j.oraloncology.2021.105254.

Intelligence A (2010) Fundamentals of Neural Networks Artificial Intelligence Fundamentals of Neural Networks Artificial Intelligence. Fundam Neural Networks AI Course Lect 37-38, notes, slides

Jacobs P, Li Z, Young G, Calhoun P, Gal R, Beck R, Castle J, Clements M, Dassau E, Doyle F, et al. (2020) Predictive factors contributing to glucose changes during aerobic, resistance, and high intensity interval training in type 1 diabetes. *Diabetes Technol Ther.* 22, A59-A59.

Jadczyk T, Wojakowski W, Tendera M, Henry TD, Egnaczyk G, Shreenivas S (2021) Artificial intelligence can improve patient management at the time of a pandemic: The role of voice technology. *J Med Internet Res*. 23, e22959.

Jadhav B V, Mujumdar G S, Jadhav N A (2022) Applications of artificial intelligence in machine learning: Review. *Int J Adv Res Sci Commun Technol*. https://doi.org/10.48175/ijarsct-5104.

Janiesch C, Zschech P, Heinrich K (2021) Machine learning and deep learning. *Electron Mark*. https://doi.org/10.1007/s12525-021-00475-2.

Jayakumar S, Ranjith Kumar R, Tejswini R, Kavil S (2021) IoT based health monitoring system. *Adv Parallel Comput*. https://doi.org/10.3233/APC210140.

Jean A (2020) A brief history of artificial intelligence. *Medecine/Sciences* 36, 1059–1067.

Jha K, Doshi A, Patel P, Shah M (2019) A comprehensive review on automation in agriculture using artificial intelligence. *Artif Intell Agric*. 2, 1–12.

Jin J, Zhang L, Leng E, Metzger GJ, Koopmeiners JS (2023) Multi-resolution super learner for voxel-wise classification of prostate cancer using multi-parametric MRI. *J Appl Stat*. https://doi.org/10.1080/02664763.2021.2017411

Jones RW (2019) A smart body area network for diabetes management. In: *FUSION 2019-22nd International Conference on Information Fusion*. Ottawa, ON, Canada

Joshi D, Sabharwal A (2022) Artificial intelligence in healthcare. In: *The Internet of Medical Things: Enabling Technologies and Emerging Applications*. ISBN: 9781839532733 IEEE.

Kakani V, Nguyen VH, Kumar BP, Kim H, Pasupuleti VR (2020) A critical review on computer vision and artificial intelligence in food industry. *J Agric Food Res*. 2, 100033.

Karplus A (2022) Machine Learning Algorithms for Cancer Diagnosis. Santa Cruz County Science Fair.

Khandker SS, Shakil MS, Hossen MS (2020) Gold nanoparticles; potential nanotheranostic agent in breast cancer: A comprehensive review with systematic search strategy. *Curr Drug Metab*. https://doi.org/10.2174/1389200221666200610173724.

Kim HS, Lee S (2019) Multi-purpose hybrid recommendation system on artificial intelligence to improve telemarketing performance. *Asia Pacific J Inf Syst*. https://doi.org/10.14329/apjis.2019.29.4.752.

Kormushev P, Calinon S, Caldwell DG (2013) Reinforcement learning in robotics: Applications and real-world challenges. *Robotics*. https://doi.org/10.3390/robotics2030122.

Kulkarni MB, Ayachit NH, Aminabhavi TM (2022) Recent advancements in nanobiosensors: Current trends, challenges, applications, and future scope. *Biosensors* 12, 892.

Kumar A, Chaudhary RK, Singh R, Singh SP, Wang SY, Hoe ZY, Pan CT, Shiue YL, Wei DQ, Kaushik AC, Dai X (2020a) Nanotheranostic applications for detection and targeting neurodegenerative diseases. *Front Neurosci*. 14, 305.

Kumar A, Panda U (2021) Microfluidics-based devices and their role on point-of-care testing. In: *Biosensor Based Advanced Cancer Diagnostics: From Lab to Clinics*. https://doi.org/10.1016/B978-0-12-823424-2.00011-9.

Kumar H, Kuča K, Bhatia SK, Saini K, Kaushal A, Verma R, Bhalla TC, Kumar D (2020b) Applications of nanotechnology in biosensor-based detection of foodborne pathogens. *Sensors (Switzerland)* 20, 1966.

Kumar K, Thakur GSM (2012) Advanced applications of neural networks and artificial intelligence: A review. *Int J Inf Technol Comput Sci*. https://doi.org/10.5815/ijitcs.2012.06.08.

Ladju RB, Ulhaq ZS, Soraya GV (2022) Nanotheranostics: A powerful next-generation solution to tackle hepatocellular carcinoma. *World J Gastroenterol*. 28, 176–187.

Lauriola I, Lavelli A, Aiolli F (2022) An introduction to deep learning in natural language processing: Models, techniques, and tools. *Neurocomputing*. https://doi.org/10.1016/j.neucom.2021.05.103.

Levin BA, Piskunov AA, Poliakov VY, Savin A V. (2022) Artificial intelligence in engineering education. *Vyss Obraz v Ross*. https://doi.org/10.31992/0869-3617-2022-31-7-79-95.

Li J (2018) Cyber security meets artificial intelligence: A survey. *Front Inf Technol Electron Eng*. 19, 1462–1474.

Li LR, Du B, Liu HQ, Chen C (2021) Artificial intelligence for personalized medicine in thyroid cancer: Current status and future perspectives. *Front Oncol*. 10, 604051.

Liimatainen K, Huttunen R, Latonen L, Ruusuvuori P (2021) Convolutional neural network-based artificial intelligence for classification of protein localization patterns. *Biomolecules*. https://doi.org/10.3390/biom11020264.

Lu Z, Qian P, Bi D, Ye Z, He X, Zhao Y, Su L, Li S, Zhu Z (2021) Application of AI and IoT in clinical medicine: Summary and challenges. *Curr Med Sci*. https://doi.org/10.1007/s11596-021-2486-z.

Luciano K, Wang X, Liu Y, Eyler G, Qin Z, Xia X (2022) Noble metal nanoparticles for point-of-care testing: Recent advancements and social impacts. *Bioengineering*. 9, 666.

Mariani MM, Machado I, Nambisan S (2023) Types of innovation and artificial intelligence: A systematic quantitative literature review and research agenda. *J Bus Res*. 155. https://doi.org/10.1016/j.jbusres.2022.113364.

Marshall SK, Angsantikul P, Pang Z, Nasongkla N, Hussen RSD, Thamphiwatana SD (2022) Biomimetic targeted theranostic nanoparticles for breast cancer treatment. *Molecules*. https://doi.org/10.3390/molecules27196473.

Mejía-Salazar JR, Cruz KR, Vásques EMM, de Oliveira ON (2020) Microfluidic point-of-care devices: New trends and future prospects for ehealth diagnostics. *Sensors (Switzerland)*. https://doi.org/10.3390/s20071951.

Mihret ET (2020) Robotics and artificial intelligence. *Int J Artif Intell Mach Learn*. https://doi.org/10.4018/ijaiml.2020070104.

Montenegro-López D (2020) Use of point-of-care technologies for the management of the COVID-19 pandemic in Colombia. *Rev Panam Salud Publica/Pan Am J Public Heal*. https://doi.org/10.26633/RPSP.2020.97.

More P (2021) Technological tools and Biosensors for detection and diagnosis of COVID-19. *Res J Biotechnol*. 16, 163–170.

Muthukrishnan N, Maleki F, Ovens K, Reinhold C, Forghani B, Forghani R (2020) Brief history of artificial intelligence. *Neuroimaging Clin N Am*. 30, 393–399.

Naaz S, Asghar A (2022) Artificial intelligence, nano-technology and genomic medicine: The future of anaesthesia. *J Anaesthesiol Clin Pharmacol*. 38, 11–17.

Nakahara R (2020) The history of artificial intelligence. *Okayama Igakkai Zasshi (Journal Okayama Med Assoc*. https://doi.org/10.4044/joma.132.144.

Naresh V, Lee N (2021) A review on biosensors and recent development of nanostructured materials-enabled biosensors. *Sensors (Switzerland)* 21, 1109.

Nauta M, Walsh R, Dubowski A, Seifert C (2022) Uncovering and correcting shortcut learning in machine learning models for skin cancer diagnosis. *Diagnostics*. https://doi.org/10.3390/diagnostics12010040.

Onweni CL, Venegas-Borsellino CP, Treece J, Turnbull MT, Ritchie C, Freeman WD (2021) The power of mobile health. *Mayo Clin Proc Innov Qual Outcomes*. https://doi.org/10.1016/j.mayocpiqo.2021.01.001.

Ouyang F, Jiao P (2021) Artificial intelligence in education: The three paradigms. *Comput Educ Artif Intell*. https://doi.org/10.1016/j.caeai.2021.100020.

Özmen EN, Kartal E, Turan MB, Yazıcıoğlu A, Niazi JH, Qureshi A (2021) Graphene and carbon nanotubes interfaced electrochemical nanobiosensors for the detection of SARS-CoV-2 (COVID-19) and other respiratory viral infections: A review. *Mater Sci Eng C*. 129, 112356.

Öztürk K, Şahin ME (2018) A general view of artificial neural networks and artificial intelligence. Tak Vekayi.

Pang L (2021) Library book intelligent recommendation system based on artificial intelligence. *J Intell Fuzzy Syst*. https://doi.org/10.3233/jifs-189934.

Panwar R, Churi H, Dave S (2022) Point-of-care electrochemical biosensors using CRISPR/Cas for RNA analysis. In: *Biosensors for Emerging and Re-emerging Infectious Diseases*. https://doi.org/10.1016/B978-0-323-88464-8.00003-8.

Qiao D, Yao J, Yang Z, Chu Y, Chen X, Li X (2023) Research on environmental planning method based on neural network and artificial intelligence technology. *Phys Chem Earth*. https://doi.org/10.1016/j.pce.2023.103370.

Ra M, Gade A, Gaikwad S, Marcato PD, Durán N (2012) Biomedical applications of nanobiosensors: The state-of-the-art. *J Braz Chem Soc*. https://doi.org/10.1590/S0103-50532012000100004.

Rabinovich EP, Capek S, Kumar JS, Park MS (2020) Tele-robotics and artificial-intelligence in stroke care. *J Clin Neurosci*. https://doi.org/10.1016/j.jocn.2020.04.125.

Rakhshan V, Okano AH, Huang Z, Castelnuovo G, Baptista AF (2022) Biomedical applications of computer vision using artificial intelligence. *Comput Intell Neurosci*. 2022, 9843574.

Raschka S, Patterson J, Nolet C (2020) Machine learning in python: Main developments and technology trends in data science, machine learning, and artificial intelligence. *Information*. 11, 193.

Rasool A, Bunterngchit C, Tiejian L, Islam MR, Qu Q, Jiang Q (2022) Improved machine learning-based predictive models for breast cancer diagnosis. *Int J Environ Res Public Health*. https://doi.org/10.3390/ijerph19063211.

Rawat B, Bist AS, Supriyanti D, Elmanda V, Sari SN (2022a) AI and nanotechnology for healthcare: A survey. *APTISI Trans Manag*. 7. https://doi.org/10.33050/atm.v7i1.1819.

Rawat V, Joshi S, Gupta S, Singh DP, Singh N (2022b) Machine learning algorithms for early diagnosis of diabetes mellitus: A comparative study. *Mater Today Proc*. https://doi.org/10.1016/j.matpr.2022.02.172.

Rhoads DD (2020) Computer vision and artificial intelligence are emerging diagnostic tools for the clinical microbiologist. *J. Clin. Microbiol*. https://doi.org/10.1128/jcm.00511-20.

Roberti A, Valdes AF, Torrecillas R, Fraga MF, Fernandez AF (2019) Epigenetics in cancer therapy and nanomedicine. *Clin. Epigenetics*. 11, 81.

Roy S, Meena T, Lim SJ (2022) Demystifying supervised learning in healthcare 4.0: A new reality of transforming diagnostic medicine. *Diagnostics*. 12, 2549.

Sahoo S, Nayak A, Gadnayak A, Sahoo M, Dave S, Mohanty P, Mohanty JN, Das J (2022) Quantum dots enabled point-of-care diagnostics: A new dimension to the nanodiagnosis. In: *Advanced Nanomaterials for Point of Care Diagnosis and Therapy*. https://doi.org/10.1016/B978-0-323-85725-3.00005-2.

Santhamoorthy M, Thirupathi K, Krishnan S, Guganathan L, Dave S, Phan TTV, Kim S-C (2023) Preparation of magnetic iron oxide incorporated mesoporous silica hybrid composites for pH and temperature-sensitive drug delivery. *Magnetochemistry*. https://doi.org/10.3390/magnetochemistry9030081.

Sarker IH (2021) Machine learning: Algorithms, real-world applications and research directions. *SN Comput Sci.* 2, 160.

Sarker S, Jamal L, Ahmed SF, Irtisam N (2021) Robotics and artificial intelligence in healthcare during COVID-19 pandemic: A systematic review. *Rob Auton Syst.* 146, 103902.

Schweyer A (2018) Predictive analytics and artificial intelligence in people management. *Incent Res Found.* 1–18.

Sedjelmaci H, Guenab F, Senouci SM, Moustafa H, Liu J, Han S (2020) Cyber security based on artificial intelligence for cyber-physical systems. *IEEE Netw.* 34, 6–7.

Sellappan L, Manoharan S, Sanmugam A, Anh NT (2021) Role of nanobiosensors and biosensors for plant virus detection. In: *Nanosensors for Smart Agriculture* https://doi.org/10.1016/B978-0-12-824554-5.00004-5.

Serov N, Vinogradov V (2022) Artificial intelligence to bring nanomedicine to life. *Adv Drug Deliv Rev.* 184, 114194.

Sharifi M, Hasan A, Haghighat S, Taghizadeh A, Attar F, Bloukh SH, Edis Z, Xue M, Khan S, Falahati M (2021) Rapid diagnostics of coronavirus disease 2019 in early stages using nanobiosensors: Challenges and opportunities. *Talanta* 223, 121704.

Sharifianjazi F, Jafari Rad A, Bakhtiari A, Niazvand F, Esmaeilkhanian A, Bazli L, Abniki M, Irani M, Moghanian A (2022) Biosensors and nanotechnology for cancer diagnosis (lung and bronchus, breast, prostate, and colon): A systematic review. *Biomed Mater.* https://doi.org/10.1088/1748-605X/ac41fd.

Sharma P, Suleman S, Farooqui A, Ali W, Narang J, Malode SJ, Shetti NP (2022) Analytical methods for Ebola virus detection. *Microchem J.* 178, 107333.

Sheervalilou R, Shirvaliloo M, Sargazi S, Shirvalilou S, Shahraki O, Pilehvar-Soltanahmadi Y, Sarhadi A, Nazarlou Z, Ghaznavi H, Khoei S (2021) Application of nanobiotechnology for early diagnosis of SARS-CoV-2 infection in the COVID-19 pandemic. *Appl Microbiol Biotechnol.* 105, 2615–2624.

Shen CL, Liu HR, Lou Q, Wang F, Liu KK, Dong L, Shan CX (2022) Recent progress of carbon dots in targeted bioimaging and cancer therapy. *Theranostics* 12, 2860–2893.

Singla R, Singla A, Gupta Y, Kalra S (2019) Artificial intelligence/machine learning in diabetes care. *Indian J Endocrinol Metab.* https://doi.org/10.4103/ijem.IJEM_228_19.

Sivasankar G A (2022) The review of artificial intelligence in cyber security. *Int J Res Appl Sci Eng Technol.* https://doi.org/10.22214/ijraset.2022.40072.

Srivastava AK, Dev A, Karmakar S (2018) Nanosensors and nanobiosensors in food and agriculture. *Environ Chem Lett.* 16, 161–182.

Stetter JR, Li J (2008) Amperometric gas sensors - A review. *Chem Rev.* 108, 352–366.

Suarez-Ibarrola R, Hein S, Reis G, Gratzke C, Miernik A (2020) Current and future applications of machine and deep learning in urology: A review of the literature on urolithiasis, renal cell carcinoma, and bladder and prostate cancer. *World J Urol.* 38, 2329–2347.

Subeesh A, Mehta CR (2021) Automation and digitization of agriculture using artificial intelligence and internet of things. *Artif Intell Agric.* 5, 278–291.

Sun YL, Zhang DL (2019) Machine learning techniques for screening and diagnosis of diabetes: A survey. *Teh Vjesn.* 26, 872–880.

Sutton SG, Holt M, Arnold V (2016) "The reports of my death are greatly exaggerated"-Artificial intelligence research in accounting. *Int J Account Inf Syst.* https://doi.org/10.1016/j.accinf.2016.07.005.

Tan P, Chen X, Zhang H, Wei Q, Luo K (2023) Artificial intelligence aids in development of nanomedicines for cancer management. *Semin Cancer Biol.* 89, 61–75.

Tavakkoli Yaraki M, Tan YN (2020) Recent advances in metallic nanobiosensors development: Colorimetric, dynamic light scattering and fluorescence detection. *Sensors Int.* 1, 100049.

Ugurlu M (2022) Performance of a convolutional neural network- based artificial intelligence algorithm for automatic cephalometric landmark detection. *Turkish J Orthod.* https://doi.org/10.5152/turkjorthod.2022.22026.

Vazquez JPG, Torres RS, Perez DBP (2021) Scientometric analysis of the application of artificial intelligence in agriculture. *J Scientometr Res.* https://doi.org/10.5530/JSCIRES.10.1.7.

Venkadesh A, Mathiyarasu J, Dave S, Radhakrishnan S (2021) Amine mediated synthesis of nickel oxide nanoparticles and their superior electrochemical sensing performance for glucose detection. *Inorg Chem Commun.* https://doi.org/10.1016/j.inoche.2021.108779.

Venkata Sateesh Yadav K, Vishwanth M (2018) IoT based health care monitoring system. *J Adv Res Dyn Control Syst.* https://doi.org/10.22214/ijraset.2019.6171.

Verma P, Sharma S (2020) Artificial intelligence based recommendation system. In: *Proceedings - IEEE 2020 2nd International Conference on Advances in Computing, Communication Control and Networking*, ICACCCN 2020

Vettoretti M, Cappon G, Facchinetti A, Sparacino G (2020) Advanced diabetes management using artificial intelligence and continuous glucose monitoring sensors. *Sensors (Switzerland)* 20, 3870.

Vijayakumar G, Venkatesan SA, Kannan VA, Perumal S (2023) Detection of food toxins, pathogens, and microorganisms using nanotechnology-based sensors. In: *Nanotechnology Applications for Food Safety and Quality Monitoring.* https://doi.org/10.1016/B978-0-323-85791-8.00022-7.

Vrontis D, Christofi M, Pereira V, Tarba S, Makrides A, Trichina E (2022) Artificial intelligence, robotics, advanced technologies and human resource management: A systematic review. *Int J Hum Resour Manag.* https://doi.org/10.1080/09585192.2020.1871398.

Vu GT, Tran BX, McIntyre RS, Pham HQ, Phan HT, Ha GH, Gwee KK, Latkin CA, Ho RCM, Ho CSH (2020) Modeling the research landscapes of artificial intelligence applications in diabetes (GAPresearch). *Int J Environ Res Public Health.* https://doi.org/10.3390/ijerph17061982.

Waller P, Sol HG, Takkenberg CAT, Robbe PFDV (1988) Expert systems and artificial intelligence in decision support systems. *The Statistician.* https://doi.org/10.2307/2348181.

Wang C, Wu Y, Chen S, Liu S, Li J, Qian Y, Yang Z (2022) Improving self-supervised learning for speech recognition with intermediate layer supervision. In: *ICASSP, IEEE International Conference on Acoustics, Speech and Signal Processing – Proceedings*, Singapore.

Wang J, He Z-W, Jiang J-X (2020) Nanomaterials: Applications in the diagnosis and treatment of pancreatic cancer. *World J Gastrointest Pharmacol Ther.* https://doi.org/10.4292/wjgpt.v11.i1.1.

Xiong Z, Shen M, Shi X (2019) Zwitterionic modification of nanomaterials for improved diagnosis of cancer cells. *Bioconjug Chem.* 30, 2519–2527.

Xu Y, WANG D, Kuang T, Wu W, Xu X, Jin D, Zhang H, Zhong S, Wang Y, Lou W (2020) Nanomaterials augmented LDI-TOF-MS for pancreatic ductal adenocarcinoma diagnosis and classification. *J Clin Oncol.* https://doi.org/10.1200/jco.2020.38.15_suppl.e16761.

Yang J, Jia C, Yang J (2021a) Designing nanoparticle-based drug delivery systems for precision medicine. *Int J Med Sci.* https://doi.org/10.7150/IJMS.60874.

Yang J, Xu R, Wang C, Qiu J, Ren B, You L (2021b) Early screening and diagnosis strategies of pancreatic cancer: A comprehensive review. *Cancer Commun.* 41, 1257–1274.

Yaraki MT, Zahed Nasab S, Zare I, Dahri M, Moein Sadeghi M, Koohi M, Tan YN (2022) Biomimetic metallic nanostructures for biomedical applications, catalysis, and beyond. *Ind Eng Chem Res.* 61, 7547–7593.

Yu KH, Beam AL, Kohane IS (2018) Artificial intelligence in healthcare. *Nat Biomed Eng.* 2, 719–731.

Yuan A, Gao L (2021) Research on the application of NLP artificial intelligence tools in university natural language processing. In: *IOP Conference Series: Earth and Environmental Science.*

Zaza I, Harfouche A, Greer T (2019) Types of Artificial Intelligence and Decision Making in Organizations.

Zhang Y, Hu Y, Jiang N, Yetisen AK (2023) Wearable artificial intelligence biosensor networks. *Biosens Bioelectron.* 219, 114825.

Zhang Y, Lyu H (2021) Application of biosensors based on nanomaterials in cancer cell detection. *J Phys Conf Ser.* https://doi.org/10.1088/1742-6596/1948/1/012149.

Zhang Y, Yang H, Yu Y, Zhang Y (2022a) Application of nanomaterials in proteomics-driven precision medicine. *Theranostics* 12, 2674–2686.

Zhang Z, Ma S, Yang Z, Xiong Z, Kang J, Wu Y, Zhang K, Niyato D (2022b) Robust semi-supervised federated learning for images automatic recognition in internet of drones. *IEEE Internet Things J.* https://doi.org/10.1109/JIOT.2022.3151945.

Zhou J, Liu W, Zhao L, Jiang J, Lu Y, Hu J, Zhang H, Bai J, Li X (2019) Nanomaterials augmented LDI-TOF-MS for hepatocellular carcinoma diagnosis and classification. *Ann Oncol.* https://doi.org/10.1093/annonc/mdz257.027.

Zhou L, Song Y, Ji W, Wei H (2022) Machine learning for combustion. *Energy AI.* https://doi.org/10.1016/j.egyai.2021.100128.

Zhou M, Duan N, Liu S, Shum HY (2020) Progress in neural NLP: Modeling, learning, and reasoning. *Engineering.* 6, 275–290.

Zhou ZH (2022) Open-environment machine learning. *Natl Sci Rev.* https://doi.org/10.1093/nsr/nwac123.

10 Advanced Nanomaterials for Diabetes Monitoring and Therapeutics

Shimaa M. Ali, Khadijah M. Emran, and Rawda M. Okasha

10.1 INTRODUCTION TO NANOMATERIALS-BASED GLUCOSE SENSORS

Diabetes and hyperglycemia are diseases caused by the metabolic disorders of glucose in human body. Hence, the determination of glucose content is very important in clinic diagnosing. Diabetes is considered to be a globally prevalent metabolic illness, which causes the blood glucose level to increase to 126 mg/dL (6.9 mmol/L) or higher. According to the American Diabetes Association, a fasting blood sugar level less than 100 mg/dL (5.6 mmol/L) is normal [1,2]. Actually, frequent monitoring of blood glucose levels provides patients and physicians with an understanding of diabetes progression [3]. Unfortunately, lag times, lack of precision and difficulty with patient use remain major challenges. A number of technologies are currently available that facilitate outpatient self-administered blood glucose testing (SMBG). One of them is continuous glucose monitoring (CGM). This practice is becoming more widely established as evidence supporting its use has accumulated. The data available through CGM can permit significantly more fine-tuned adjustments in insulin dosing and other therapies than the data provided by spot testing from self-monitoring of blood glucose (SMBG) [4].

Biosensing devices offer important opportunities for research, especially for clinical diagnosis, due to their numerous advantages (ease of use, portability, unprocessed samples, rapid result and small sample volume) [5,6]. In general, the key components of sensing devices are a detector that measures blood glucose concentrations, a transducer that converts measurements into output signals, and finally, a reporter that processes the generated signal into data that can then be interpreted. The three main classes of glucose-sensing molecules that are used to engineer nanoparticle-based glucose sensors are glucose oxidase, glucose-binding proteins and glucose-binding small molecules. When these partials are coupled with nanoparticles and engineered as transducers, these glucose-specific

 DOI: 10.1201/9781003316435-10

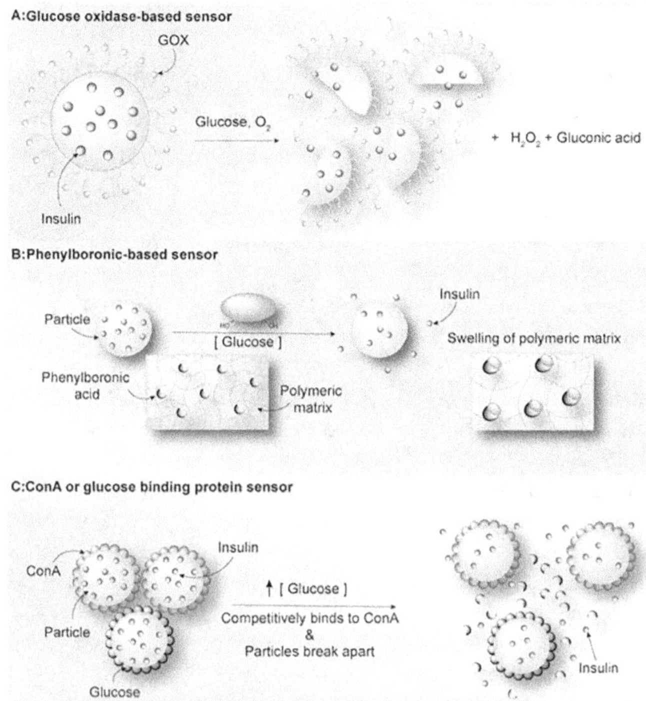

FIGURE 10.1 Particle-based glucose sensors: (a) glucose oxidase, (b) phenylboronic acids, and (c) concanavilin-A, natural protein [9]. (Reproduced with permission from R. Primavera, Nanomaterials; published by MDPI, 2020.)

detecting molecules are enabling the design of new types of sensors that have the potential to be more patient-friendly, provide rapid measurements and improve precision [7–9] (Figure 10.1). A biosensor consists of four parts, namely, a bioreceptor, a transducer, a signal processor for converting electronic signal to a desired signal, and an interface to display. A variety of samples such as body fluids, food samples, and cell cultures can be explored to analyze using biosensors [6,10].

Nanomaterials are currently undergoing rapid development due to their potential applications in the field of catalysis, nanoelectronics, magnetic data storage, structural components, biomaterials, and biosensors [10]. The use of nanoparticles (NPs), nanotubes (NTs), nanowires (NWs), etc. in biosensor diagnostic devices is being explored. The dimensions of nanomaterials at the nanoscale level, one of their major advantages, let the development of new biodevices (smart biosensors) that can detect minute concentration of a desired analyte. Nanomaterials are generally used as transducer materials that are an important part for biosensor development [6,11–16].

The application of nanotechnology to medicine holds many possible advantages, such as access to small and clinically relevant areas of cells and analysis of small volumes of analytes. This technology has the potential to enable the

TABLE 10.1
A Summary of Nanotechnology-Enabled Glucose-Sensing Technologies [18]

Type	Detection Principle	Response Time	Detection Limit	Reference
Optical	Nanotube near-IR emission	~1 minute	34.7 μM	[21]
	Nanotube fluorescence enhancement	~1 minute	2.5 mM	[22]
	Fluorescence enhancement and AuNP growth	30–60 minutes	0.01 mM (QDs); 0.1 mM (AuNPs)	[23]
	Graphene catalytic activity	1 hour	1 μM	[24]
	Nanotube fluorescence enhancement	~1 minute	5 mM	[25]
	Raman spectroscopy	~10 minute	0.5 μM	[26]
	Hydrogel-mediated Bragg diffraction	5 minutes	90 μM	[27]
	Protein FRET signal	~1 minute	25 μM	[28]
Electrical	Nanotube conductance modulation	~20 seconds	0.1 mM	[29]
	Hydrogen peroxide catalysis via nanotubes	<20 seconds	0.08 mM	[30]
	Hydrogen peroxide catalysis	<5 seconds	1.5 μM	[31]
	Hydrogen peroxide catalysis via AuNPs	<30 seconds	180 μM	[32]
	Nanomaterial-enhanced conductance modulation	<20 seconds	0.5 μM; 5 μM	[33]

development of improved sensors and the fabrication of a wide variety of nanomaterials, and has introduced an excess of selective and highly responsive glucose sensors [17–20] (Table 10.1).

The initiative for biosensors dates back to the 1960s with the revolutionary study of Clark and Lyons, followed by the work of the first enzyme-based glucose sensor by Updike and Hicks in 1967 [2,34,35]. Generally, glucose sensors can be broadly divided into GOx-based sensing (i.e., enzymatic glucose sensing) and nonenzymatic glucose sensing.

10.1.1 Enzymatic Glucose Sensing

Due to their increasing demand in the medical and pharmaceutical industry, more attention has been paid to develop glucose sensors with low price, high sensitivity and high stability [36–38]. Although the three generations of enzymatic glucose sensors have high sensitivity and high selectivity, they always suffer from the performance variation due to environmental factors (such as change in temperature, pH values, humidity, and toxic chemicals) and the degradation of enzyme activity [39,40]. Enzymatic glucose detection involves the presence of GOx enzyme, that is, oxidation for glucose (redox-active enzyme). This oxidation agent has been extensively utilized for constructing several sensors for glucose detection, mainly because of their high sensitivity and high selectivity to glucose. The immobilization of enzymes on a suitable matrix along with their stability for the fabrication of these sensors is critical.

Many sensitive and selective electrochemical biosensors have been developed to monitor blood glucose levels, which involve immobilization of GOx onto different nanomaterials. Tang et al. [33] utilized the multiwalled carbon nanotubes (MWCNTs)-CHIT (enzyme electrode is chitosan-CHIT) hybrid, and before the immobilization of glucose oxidase (GOx), Pt-NPs were electro-deposited to modify the surface of Pt electrodes for the first time. Then, MWCNT-CHIT/GOx/Pt and CHIT/GOx/Pt-NPs/Pt electrodes were used as gate electrodes of the PEDOT:PSS-based OECTs [organic thin-film transistors (OTFT), organic electrochemical transistors (OECT), conducting polymer (PEDOT:PSS)]. This electrode shows high sensitivity with low cost. The detection limit of the CHIT/GOx/Pt-NPs/Pt modified with Pt nanoparticles on the gate electrode is about 5 nM, which is three orders of magnitude better than a device without the nanoparticles, MWCNT-CHIT/GOx/Pt. This improvement of the device performance can be attributed to the excellent electrocatalytic properties of the nanomaterials (Pt-NPs) and more effective immobilization of enzyme on the gate electrodes. A novel AuNPs-decorated MoS_2 nanocomposite was explored to develop an electrochemical glucose biosensor [41]. It was found that use of the AuNPs-decorated MoS_2 nanocomposite accelerates the electron transfer from electrode (the conductivity) to the immobilized enzyme. The AuNPs@MoS_2 nanocomposite film can provide a favorable microenvironment for GOx to realize direct electrochemistry. Glucose can be detected in the concentration range from 10 to 300 μM, and down to levels as low as 2.8 μM. Additionally, this biosensor displays good reproducibility and long-term stability. In the same field, Darabdhara and co-workers [42] demonstrated the synthesis of Cu-Pd nanoparticles on 2D sheets, namely, reduced graphene oxide (rGO), g-C_3N_4 and MoS_2 demonstrating enzymatic peroxidase- and oxidase-like behaviors. Compared to Cu-Pd/g-C_3N_4 and Cu-Pd/MoS_2 nanocomposites, the Cu-Pd/rGO nanocomposite demonstrated the best peroxidase- and oxidase-mimicking activity. This nanocomposite used for a glucose oxidase (GOx)–based glucose sensor is based on the enzymatic formation of H_2O_2 and the Cu-Pd NPs–assisted oxidation of tetramethylbenzidine by H_2O_2 to give a blue-green coloration with absorption maxima at 652 nm. The assay has a 0.29 μM detection limit and a detection range that extends from 0.2 to 50 μM. The need for flexible biosensors has increased because of their potential applications for point of care diagnosis for glucose measuring. Yoon et al. [43] developed a flexible electrochemical enzyme biosensor by immobilizing an enzyme (*Aspergillus niger* and myoglobin (Mb)) on the flexible polymer (Kapton® polyimide film) electrode modified with a gold/MoS_2/gold nanofilm. The electrode shows more sensitivity (the detection limit for glucose was estimated to be 10 nM) as compared with a previously reported flexible glucose sensor which was due to the facilitation of electron transfer by MoS_2 nanoparticle. Additionally, when there was when there was presence of GOx on gold/MoS_2/gold nanofilm, the biosensor showed an increased electrochemical signal, with a 389.9 μA average reduction peak current as compared with the result of 125.8 μA at GOx on the gold-deposited polymer electrode. Derya Bal Altuntaş and FilizKuralay [44] proposed a MoS_2/chitosan composite–modified pencil graphite electrode (MoS_2/Chitosan/PGE) and its use as glucose biosensor after the modified electrode was immobilized with (GOx)-gelatin (MoS_2/Chitosan/GOx-Gelatin/PGE). Compared to the unmodified electrode, this electrode shows superior electrochemical responses, including good electroactivity and sensitive glucose biosensing. A linear glucose concentration range was obtained from 10 to 800 μM with MoS_2/Chitosan/GOx-Gelatin–modified PGE electrode. When this biosensor was tested in the presence of dopamine and ascorbic acid, the results presented the high selectivity of this novel MoS_2/Chitosan/GOx-Gelatin–modified PGE as a glucose biosensor. Other enzyme-functionalized nanobiosensor platforms have been demonstrated recently, for example, portable glucose biosensor based on polynorepinephrine@magnetite nanomaterial integrated with a smartphone analyzer for glucose measurement [45]. Covering the magnetite nanoparticles (Fe_3O_4) surface with the biomimetic polymer polynorepinephrine significantly increased the effectiveness of enzyme immobilization which was 38.40 mg/g, compared with 17.30 mg/g on the bare surface of magnetite. This biosensor (Fe_3O_4@PNE-Gox) displayed a broad range of linearity (0.2–24 mM), a low detection limit (6.1 μM), and good sensitivity (97.34 μA/mM cm^2). Moreover, it exhibited a fast electrocatalytic response (8 seconds) and long-term stability (up to 20 weeks). It was used to detect glucose in real samples such as human serum, human blood, infusion fluid, and commercial glucose solutions.

10.1.2 Nonenzymatic Glucose Sensing

In recent years, nonenzymatic electrochemical glucose sensors based on the oxidation of glucose to gluconolactone on electrode surface arise as a promising candidate for the detection of glucose concentrations [46,47]. Many nonenzymatic electrode materials have been developed including noble metal nanomaterials [48)] and their alloys [49–51], and transition metals and their alloys [52–54]. A novel nonenzymatic glucose sensor based on porous AuNPs-CS membranes and platinum hollow nanoparticle chains (Pt HNPCs) was developed by Li et al. [55]. The glassy carbon electrode (GCE) was modified by porous AuNPs-CS membranes which greatly increased the effective electrode surface for Pt HNPCs immobilizing and made the redox process more accessible to the electrode surface. The Pt HNPCs display excellent redox electrochemical activity and as good catalytic efficiency for the oxidation of both hydrogen peroxide and glucose, high stability, and a large surface for immobilization of the Pt HNPCs. In addition, in order to improve the anti-interferent ability of fabricated glucose sensor, Nafion (Nf) was coated on the top of the as-prepared electrode. The resulting glucose nanostructured porous AuNPs-CS sensor has a linear response toward glucose over the concentration range from 3.0 to 7.7 mM, with a detection limit of 1.0 μM.

In a similar study, a nonenzymatic glucose sensor based on 3D Ni/MnO_2 nanocomposite–modified GCE was researched by Wang et al. [56]. The electrochemical investigation of Ni/MnO_2 sensor indicated that it possessed an excellent electrocatalytic property for glucose and could be applied to the quantification of glucose with a linear range from 2.5×10^{-7} to 3.5×10^{-3} M, with a sensitivity of 1.04 mA/mM cm^2 and a detection limit of 1×10^{-7}M (S/N=3). The proposed sensor also presented long-term stability. Also, from $NiMoO_4$ nanomaterials with α and β phases (α-$NiMoO_4$ nanoparticles to β-$NiMoO_4$ nanosheets), Kusha Kumar Naik and his team [57] built a glucose sensor. It is observed that the α-$NiMoO_4$ exhibits a sensitivity of 0.208 μA/μM cm^2 compared to the sensitivity of 1.057 μA/μM cm^2 achieved by β-$NiMoO_4$. According to that, it is confirmed that β-$NiMoO_4$ nanosheets show five times higher glucose-sensing performance as compared to α-$NiMoO_4$ nanoparticles. The monodispersed PtNi nanoparticles (NPs) were placed on a glassy electrode which then displayed a superior response to glucose due to a large number of exposed atoms on the surface, which promotes the catalytic activity of PtNi NPs for glucose electro-oxidation [51]. Best operated at a potential of 0.43 V (vs. saturated calomel electrode (SCE)), the electrode has a wide linear range (from 0.5 to 40 mM), rapid response (<1 second), a low detection limit (0.35 μM) and a sensitivity of 40.17 μA/mM cm^2. The NP sensor also is fairly selective over ascorbic acid, uric acid and fructose. The sensor has repeatability and durability for up to 30 days after its manufacture. The most important reasons for its desirable features are the improved particle distribution and rich exposed atoms on the corners. Pt Ni NPs have a large electrochemically active surface area (ECSA) and the adjustments in Ni to Pt. A new type of glucose sensor was developed consisting of vertically aligned ZnO nanotubes (NTs) grown on low-cost printed circuit board substrates, which are developed as sensitive fluorescent glucose sensor [58]. The sensor function is based on the photoluminescence (PL) quenching of ZnO NTs treated with different concentrations of glucose. The UV emission decreases linearly with increasing glucose concentration. The most advantage of this sensor is that it exhibits a sensitivity of $3.5\% \cdot mM^{-1}$ (defined as the percentage change of PL peak intensity per mM) and a lower limit of detection (LOD) of 70 μM. Severally, a sensitive and selective glucose sensor was fabricated using molybdenum trioxide (α-MoO_3) nanomaterials via sol–gel method [59]. The synthesized molybdenum trioxide was modified with the capping molecule poly-(vinylpyrrolidone) (PVP) (wt%=2, 4 and 6). The fabricated PVP-modified MoO_3 nanocomposites show a magnificent performance toward the detection of glucose. This is owing to enhancement effect as well as mesoporous nature of MoO_3/(6%) PVP nanocomposite. The sensor demonstrates a low detection limit of 0.022 μM with a sensitivity of 86.42 μA/mM cm^2 with good selectivity, stability and simplicity for the rapid detection of glucose. In the same field, Malhotra et al. [60] fabricated first time a novel and simple nonenzymatic glucose sensor by immobilization of platinum (Pt) particles on polyvinylferrocene-coated Pt electrode (Pt/PVF/Pt). The Pt/PVF/Pt sensor showed a fast response time of less than 3 s with linear glucose concentration range from 0.1 to 11.0 mM (R^2=0.996). The sensitivity of the sensor was 327 μA/mM cm^2 with a low detection limit of 0.026 mM. Additionally, this new sensor showed good stability and reproducibility along with excellent anti-interference properties to ascorbic acid, uric acid, sucrose, and fructose. Palladium/nickel nanoparticles decorated on functionalized multiwalled carbon nanotube Pd–Ni@*f*-MWCNT are synthesized and applied as a sensitive nonenzymatic electrochemical glucose sensor [61]. The prepared electrode exhibits high electrocatalytic activity for the oxidation of glucose into gluconolactone and shows an extended linear range of from 0.01 to 1.4 mM, very low detection limit of 0.026 μM, very high sensitivity of 71 μA/mM cm^2, good reproducibility, high stability and applicability in the real-sample analysis. In another study, nickel was used as nickel sulfide nanoworm (Ni_3S_2 NW). Ni_3S_2 NW was directly grown on the poly(3,4-ethylenedioxythiophene)-reduced graphene oxide hybrid films (PEDOT-rGO HFs) modified on GCE for high-performance nonenzymatic glucose monitoring [62]. The enhanced electrocatalytic activity of the sensor toward glucose oxidation was attributed to the particular morphology, satisfying hydrophilic nature, due to a strong combination of Ni_3S_2 NWs, PEDOT-rGO, and bare GCE. This sensor has many advantages such as the satisfactory sensitivity (2,123 μA/mM cm^2), wide linear range (15~9105 μM), low detection limit (0.48 μM), and rapid response time (<1.5 seconds) at a potential of 0.5 V (vs. SCE) in 0.1 M NaOH. It possessed good selectivity, reproducibility, and stability. Moreover, it can be used for assaying glucose in human serum samples without dilution, indicating potential for clinical diagnostic applications. In other work, poly(caffeic acid)(PCA)@multi-walled carbon nanotubes (MWCNT) was decorated with CuO nanoparticles [63]. The decorated PCA@MWCNT-CuO electrode showed a high sensitivity of 2,412 μA/mM cm^2. The electrode exhibited a broad linear range of 2 μM to 9 mM and a low LOD of 0.43 μM (relative standard deviation, RSD = 2.3%) at +0.45 V vs Ag/AgCl. The excellent properties obtained for glucose detection were most likely due to the synergistic effect of the combination of individual components: poly(caffeic acid), MWCNTs, and CuO. Also, Ag/Ni@MWCNT nanocomposites with different Ag/Ni ratios have been prepared by Tariq and his team [64]. Due to a greater number of active sites provided by support material (MWCNTs) and synergistic effect present among the atoms of Ag and Ni, the Ag–Ni@MWCNT nanocomposites show better electrocatalytic activity toward glucose oxidation. The optimized Ag1–Ni9@MWCNT catalyst displayed high sensitivity (1,485 μA/mM cm^2), wide linear range (4 mM) and low LOD (7 μM) toward glucose sensing. In a recent study, palladium (Pd) nanoparticles were deposited onto Co_3O_4 nanostructures to build an enzyme-free glucose sensor [65]. The proposed Pd–Co_3O_4 nanostructures showed excellent electrochemical activity for the quantitative detection of glucose with a linear response over the range of 1–6.0 mM glucose, with an LOD of 0.01 mM. Importantly, this sensor shows high selectivity toward glucose detection in the presence of different interfering substances and highly stable.

10.2 NANOCARRIERS FOR INSULIN DELIVERY

Drug delivery and release is one of the vastly and thoroughly explored premises in medicinal research for the treatment of chronic diseases. A particularly demanding instance of chronic illnesses is diabetes, which is characterized by the loss of euglycemic regulation and is a consequence of either diminished insulin cell secretion or a reduced binding affinity to the receptors on cell surfaces [66,67]. Diabetes has been cataloged into two distinctive varieties: Type 1, which encompasses the failure in production and extreme deficiency of insulin resulting from the demolition of insulin-inducing cells in the pancreas, and Type 2, which incorporates two distinguishable markers of resistance and deficient release of insulin resulting from deformities of cell surface receptors. An additional form of diabetes besides the preceding is gestational diabetes, arising from anomalous hormonal manufacture in pregnant women and an elevated sensitivity to insulin which yields hyperglycemia (high levels of blood sugar).

Current remedial and therapeutic approaches regarding diabetes require an extensive process of observing glycemia, controlling blood glucose levels *via* personalized glucose consumption, and insulin ingestion (subcutaneous administration) to achieve normoglycemia [67]. This form of insulin therapy (subcutaneous administration) is a hormone regulatory methodology, which modulates glycemia, and is administered to patients with Type 1 diabetes. However, this subcutaneous treatment exhibits a myriad of drawbacks, including insulin's deficient physicochemical stability due to its brief plasma half-life, its aggregation and precipitation at the frequent site of injection (a hindrance on prolonged administration), its low pH and minimal protease hydrolysis, its significant molecular mass and hydrophilic temperament (which impedes the absorptive aptitude of insulin through the intestinal tract), and its transportation throughout the circulatory system [66]. Additionally, several adverse effects arise alongside this manner of administration, which sporadically yield hypoglycemia, insulin neuropathy, insulin presbyopia, lipoatrophy, lipohyperatrophy, obesity, and peripheral hyperinsulinemia [67]. Thus, the identification of alternate administration approaches is a constructive and critical foundation to address the preceding setbacks. A prosperous and feasible route is the oral administration of insulin, which is transmitted through the liver and incorporates itself in the systematic physiological circulation of insulin. This therapeutic mechanism is particularly favorable as it mimics the inherent biological behavior of insulin emission. However, oral insulin ingestion exhibits several enzymatic and physical complications upon entry within the gastrointestinal tract, as insulin experiences severe degradation upon contact with gastric and intestinal enzymes and inadequate insulin absorptive efficacy (bioavailability) of the cell membranes of intestinal epithelium [67]. A promising resolution of these restrictions is the encapsulation of oral insulin within polymeric-matrices nanocarriers.

10.2.1 Polylactide-co-Glycolide (PLGA) Nanoparticles

An early attempt of encapsulated insulin incorporates the engagement of a microsphere polymeric scaffold. A pH-responsive polymer (poly-methacrylic-g-ethylene glycol hydrogel) has been utilized as an efficacious insulin carrier for oral treatment, which sustained the reduction of hyperglycemia in Wistar rats, according to the obtained dose [68]. The size of the particles has a significant impact on the intracellular uptake of the encapsulated insulin [69]. This phenomenon has been demonstrated with the exploitation of nano-sized insulin drug delivery vehicles that enhance the release and uptake of insulin dosage [70,71]. Additionally, several studies addressed the development of pH-responsive nanopolymers as oral drug delivery vehicles for insulin. Polymers such as dextran sulfate [72–75], hydroxypropyl methylcellulose phthalate (HPMCP(HP55)) [73], and poly-γ-glutamic acid [76,77] have been reported as potential candidates for orally diabetic treatments, which stimulate a drop in blood glucose levels.

In literature, it is notorious that the oral dosage of insulin is preferably absorbed in the upper intestinal area to prevent its loss through the intestinal tract. Encapsulation of the insulin within an excellent pH-sensitive polymeric matrix assists in achieving this goal. The biodegradable poly(lactide-co-glycolide (PLGA))/HP55 nanoparticles loaded with insulin have been scrutinized for this purpose, which is attained *via* the modified multiple emulsion-solvent evaporation (MESE) methodology and demonstrated tremendous proficiency in insulin loading and release with a maximal effect up to 8 hours [78].

Despite the remarkable biodegradability and biocompatibility of poly-(lactic-co-glycolic) acid (PLGA) nano scaffold, its hydrophobic feature restrained the combination with the hydrophilic insulin molecule [79–81]. However, the self-assembly functionalization of insulin with amphiphilic lipid moieties defeats this obstacle and enhances the insulin-loading performance into the PLGA nanoscale matrix. García-Díaz et al. reported the self-assembly of insulin molecule with soybean phosphatidylcholine or sodium caprate, prior to its coordination with the PGLA matrix [81] (Figure 10.2). This process was achieved utilizing double emulsion-solvent evaporation method and resulted in a substantial upsurge of the insulin-loading capacity up to 90%. Another advantageous feature of this protocol is that the insulin is solely released, while the lipid moiety remains intact within the nanoparticles scaffold. Another modified PLGA insulin carrier has been reported by Malathi and co-workers [66]. In this report, PLGA-co-PEG has been successfully synthesized and employed as an insulin delivery vehicle with the assistance of d-α-tocopherol poly(ethylene glycol) 1000 succinate (TPGS) as an emulsifier.

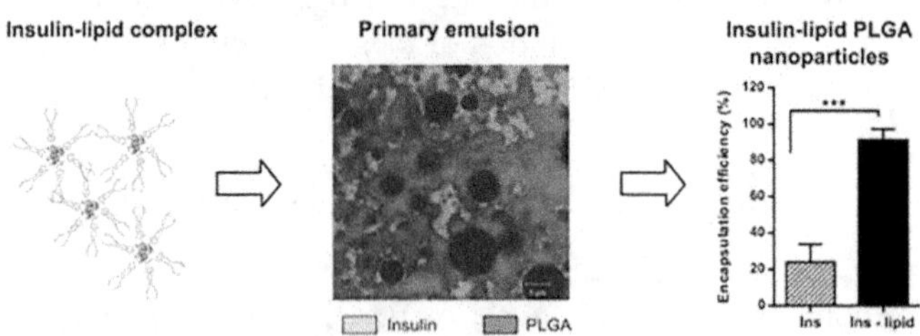

FIGURE 10.2 Insulin loading in poly(lactic-co-glycolic) acid (PLGA) nanoparticles upon self-assembly with lipids [81].

The copolymerization of PLGA with polyethylene glycol (PEG) has a crucial impact in escalating the biostability of the carrier system as well as its penetration through the mucosal surfaces [82–84]. Meanwhile, the presence of TPGS improved the loading capacity of the insulin and eliminated the aggregation effect of the enzyme [66]. The new insulin nanoparticles oral delivery system displayed a distinctive reduction of the blood glucose level up to 12 hours in diabetic rats and depleted the level of cholesterol, urea, creatinine, and ALT as well. Furthermore, the synthesis of a microsphere system of PLGA-loaded insulin capped with multialternating layers of polyvinyl alcohol (PVA) and poly(acrylamide phenyl boronic acid-co-N–vinylcaprolactam) (p(AAPBA-co-NVCL)) has been reported. The amorphous porous particles exhibited high efficiency to trap and release insulin molecules, which is in synchronous with the blood glucose level [85].

10.2.2 Chitosan Nanoparticles

Delivery of insulin, a protein drug, to the blood stream is subjected to various physicochemical barriers. The layer of columnar epithelial cells connected with tight complex junctions can constitute a barrier for the insulin absorption, physical barrier. While pH inactivation and enzymatic degradation represent chemical barriers [86]. Chitosan- and modified-chitosan-based nanoparticles are the most important polymeric scaffolds that can overcome these barriers for the oral insulin delivery. The oral delivery of insulin is retarded by the unstable protein and peptide structure in the highly acidic environment of the stomach [87]. Chitosan nanoparticles, as well as hydrogels, microspheres, and natural or synthetic polymers/chitosan, can offer excellent protein carriers that are non-toxic, biocompatible, cheap, easily prepared and characterized [70]. When recall the requirements for effective carriers used for oral protein delivery, it should be selective, reversible, biocompatible, and pH sensitive and have a specific and controlled site release. Therefore, chitosan can be considered an excellent component for oral drug delivery with many interesting biomedical applications. Chitosan as a mucoadhesive polymer can open tight junctions between epithelial cells, leading to excellent protein absorption. Nanomedicine is the use of nano- or microparticles for drug delivery. These small particles can encapsulate protein drugs, such as insulin, and protect them from degradation, thus providing a stable drug structure in physiological fluids. Nanoparticles can also enhance the transportation of drugs into the blood stream, thus increasing their bioavailability and therapeutic efficacy. The synthesis of nanoparticles can be performed by a variety of methods such as gelation, microemulsion, coprecipitation, complex coacervation, solvent evaporation and self-assembly [88], as shown in Figure 10.3. Reported chitosan-based nanoparticles have a size range of 100–500 nm and insulin association efficiency of about 85% [89]. Smaller particles can be prepared by the self-assembled method, in the size of ~100 nm, with an average zeta potential value of 25 mV, with a good stability, homogeneous particle distribution, and high efficiency [90–92].

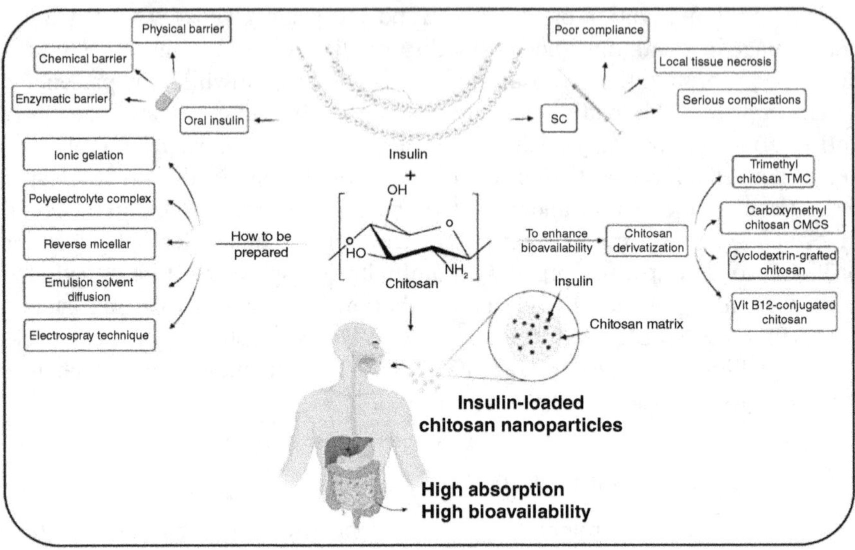

FIGURE 10.3 Chitosan and its derivatives as nanocarriers for the oral insulin delivery [86].

Chitosan-insulin nanoparticles synthesized by ionic gelation method using tripolyphosphate sodium or poly(acrylic acid) showed long residence time and enhanced permeation of insulin to the blood stream [93]. The mechanism was studied by transmission electron microscope, and it was shown that chitosan can reversibly open tight junctions between epithelial cells [76]. However, these particles can dissociate in the acidic medium of the environment, releasing insulin, and in turn resulting in a low bioavailability. This problem can be overcome by the synthesis of magnetite nanoparticles inside chitosan/alginate matrix by coprecipitation method [94] or by combining nanoencapsulation and lipid emulsion [95]. The oral insulin delivery can also be enhanced by insulin encapsulation in carboxylated chitosan-grafted poly(methyl methacrylated) nanoparticles. This pH-sensitive shell showed a slow release at acidic conditions and a quick release in neutral/slight alkaline medium [96]. The isoelectric point of insulin is 5.9, and thus, the release is expected to be reduced at this pH value. Polyelectrolyte complexes can be formed by the electrostatic interactions between the positively charged amino group (chitosan) and the negatively charged insulin molecules, and they stabilize insulin at high temperatures up to 50°C for several hours [97]. These pH-dependent polyelectrolyte complexes can minimize the insulin release at acidic conditions due to the electrostatic repulsion [98]. By using of anonic polymers such as alginate and pectin, polyelectrolyte complexes are stable at low pH (stomach condition) and undergo swelling under alkaline conditions, thus protecting insulin and overcoming pH release carrier [99]. Proteolytic enzymes of the stomach can also degrade insulin, if not protected. The protection can be achieved by incorporating protease inhibitors within the polymeric insulin formulations, such as trypsin and bacitracin. On the other hand, chitosan–EDTA conjugates can inhibit metallo-peptidases [100]. Chitosan is a mucoadhesive polymer that can open tight junctions in the mucosal cell membrane. Moreover, a long contact between the drug and the intestine arises from the electrostatic interaction between the positively charged chitosan and the negatively charged mucin, thus promoting drug adsorption [101]. It was reported that chitosan nanoparticles could be successively used for the oral insulin delivery due to the enhanced intestinal absorption of insulin [102]. Moreover, thiolated chitosan can offer a better delivery, since thiol groups are efficient mucoadhesion agents to the intestinal walls. It was reported that chitosan/glutathione provides bioavailability of insulin three times higher than the unmodified chitosan [103]. The limited solubility of chitosan at neutral conditions can be overcome by using positively charged qaternized derivatives of chitosan for the oral insulin delivery. Dimethylethyl chitosan and triethyl chitosan were nanoparticles showed a drug release of 44% and 47%, respectively, at neutral pH [89]. Therefore, a specific interaction occurs between tight junction and cationic nanoparticles, enhancing the permeation and drug transport. Controlled insulin release can be achieved by using succinyl chitosan, which has a pH-sensitive swelling property. The insulin release is enhanced compared to the native insulin due to the swelling of the negatively charged carboxylate groups at neutral pH conditions. While 60% of insulin was released after 8 hours, 90% is released from native chitosan nanoparticles [104]. Insulin-loaded chitosan succinate microspheres, in the presence of glutathione as a permeation mediator, showed a controlled release of insulin, about 140 μmol, due to the enhanced mucoadhesion and permeation ability [105].

10.2.3 Dextran Nanoparticles

Dextran is a neutral polysaccharide containing α-1,6 glycosidic linkages between glucose molecules. Besides the natural fermentation process, dextran can be synthesized by chemical methods such as cationic polymerization of leyoglucosan and pyrolysis of polyglucans [106]. Delivery systems based on dextran and its derivatives can be designed in forms of nanoparticles, nanoemulusions, micelles, and self-assembly. These systems offer excellent nanocarriers for many drugs such as insulin, due to the biodegradability, biocompatibility, nontoxicity, and so on [107,108]. Fabrication of dextran-based delivery systems can be done via different strategies such as self-assembly, emulsification, and coprecipitation. In the self-assembly, the amphiphilic dextran polymers are formed by electrostatic and hydrophobic interactions, as well as hydrogen bonding. These polymers can be self-assembled as spherical micelles in aqueous solution and can be further chemically modified to exhibit outstanding properties such as stability, unusual rheology, and enhanced accumulation in target sites [109–112]. pH-sensitive micelles of an average size of 110 nm was self-assembled from deoxycholic acid–conjugated dextran esters by chemically coupling [113]. The photosensitive glycopolymers can be prepared by grafting azido-poly(o-nitrobenzyl acrylate) onto alkynated dextran [114]. On the other hand, nanoemulsions can be used to improve the delivery of unstable drugs of low solubility and therapeutic efficacy. A delivery system based on acetalated dextran–based nanoemulsion was prepared by oil/water single emulsion method [115]. Dextran-coated magnetic iron oxide can be prepared by coprecipitation, which promotes safety and biocompatibility of biomedical applications [116–118]. Potential applications of different dextran-based delivery systems fabricated by various strategies are shown in Table 10.2.

Dextran-based nanoparticles are promising biopolymer-based nanocarriers for insulin oral delivery based on the biocompatibility and biodegradability.

TABLE 10.2
Potential Applications of Different Dextran-Based Delivery Systems Fabricated by Various Strategies [119]

Dex/Dex Derivatives	Types of Delivery System	Therapeutic Agents	Applications
Succinate-Dex		DOX	Chemotherapeutics
Succinic anhydride-Dex		DOX, silybin, paclitaxel	Chemotherapeutics
Benzimidazole-Dex		DOX	Chemotherapeutics
Dex-poly (ε-caprolactone)		DOX	Chemotherapeutics
Oxidized Dex		DOX, bortezomib	Chemotherapeutics
Reduced graphene oxide-Dex	Self-assembled micelles	DOX	Chemotherapeutics
D-poly(o-nitrobenzyl acrylate)		N/A	Photodegradable surfactant
Deoxycholic acid-Dex		DOX	Chemotherapeutics
Carboxymethyl-Dex		DOX	Chemotherapeutics
Stearic acid-Dex		Rapamycin	Chemotherapeutics
Acetalated-Dex		Asiatic acid	Chemotherapeutics
Polyacrylic acid-Dex		DOX	Chemotherapeutics
Oxidized Dex	Nanogels	DOX	Chemotherapeutics
Pristine Dex		siRNA/paclitaxel	Chemotherapeutics
Dex-PLGA	Nanopolymersomes	Insulin	Insulin oral delivery
Oxidized Dex		siRNA	Gene silencing in tumor cells
Dex-methacrylate	Self-assembled nanoparticles	Tn antigen mimetic	Anticancer vaccine
Naproxen-Dex		Naproxen	Anti-inflammatory drug delivery
Acryloyl Dex	Nanoparticles prepared by solvent evaporation method	Insulin	Insulin oral delivery
Phenoxy-modified Dex	Miniemulsions	N/A	Stabilizer
Acetalated-Dex		CHIR99021, SB203580	Myocardial infarction treatment

(*Continued*)

TABLE 10.2 (*Continued*)
Potential Applications of Different Dextran-Based Delivery Systems Fabricated by Various Strategies [119]

Dex/Dex Derivatives	Types of Delivery System	Therapeutic Agents	Applications
Acetal-modified Dex	Nanoemulsions	siRNA, tetraphenylporphyrin	Liver macrophages targeting delivery, photodynamic therapy
Dex	Dex-coated iron oxide nanoparticles	N/A	Lymph node imaging, contract agent for MRI
Carboxymethylated Dex		N/A	Protein A adsorbents
Dex-methacrylate	Hydrogels	Biocide	Biocide delivery system for antibiofilm treatment
Dex		Dexamethasone, indomethacin	Electro-responsive drug delivery system
Aldehyde Dex	Microgels	DOX	Drug delivery system
Dex		N/A	Drug delivery system
Dex	Dry powder inhaler	Rifampicin	Deep lung delivery system

In vitro experiment showed a sustained insulin release by using dextran-poly(lactide-co-glycolic acid) nanocarrier [120]. pH-sensitive insulin delivery system was fabricated from dextran-based glucose nanocarrier [121]. Hydrolysis of glucose to gluconic acid by the glucose oxidase, immobilized on the surface of dextran nanoparticles, occurred. Degradation of the nanostructure was noticed at low pH, resulting in the release of insulin. However, a more rapid insulin release profile was obtained at neutral conditions. A novel reverse microemulsion glucose-responsive dextran crosslinked with glucose-binding protein, Concanavalin A, was reported for controlled insulin delivery [122]. Concanavalin A released polymeric glucose to bind with free glucose, leading to disintegration of hydrogel. Oppositely charged dextran sulfate and polyethylenimine were proposed as dextran-based insulin delivery to achieve stable insulin formulation. Vitamin B12–dextran nanoparticles, coupled with insulin, were used as an oral delivery system to protect insulin from gut proteases and to accelerate its release [123]. A multilayered system of sodium alginate and dextran sulfate was reported to enhance the residence time of insulin at the absorption sites. Further stabilization can be done by chitosan to protect insulin from enzymatic degradation [75,124].

10.2.4 Solid Lipid Nanoparticles (SLN)

Solid lipid nanoparticles (SLN) can be substituted to polymeric nanoparticles as drug carriers. SLN are solid particles of submicron size (50–1,000 nm) that made of triacylglycerols, acylglycerol or waxes, dispersed in water or aqueous surfactant solution [125]. SLN offer advantages of biodegradability, tolerability, and large-scale production. It was reported that insulin encapsulated in SLN has high bioavailability, long residence time in blood and modified distribution [126]. The rate of degradation of SLN, by the lipolytic enzyme pancreatic lipase, and therefore the controlled drug release are affected by the lipid composition and the type of the stabilizing surfactant [127]. The wax cetyl palmitate is highly recommended for the synthesis of SLN due to its low *in vivo* toxicity and high *in vitro* degradation rate, where poloxamer 407 is a stabilizing surfactant [128].

Insulin nanocarriers are developed from cetyl palmitate containing poloxamer 407 as a surfactant [129]. Carriers have spherical shape with a size of 361 nm and a zeta potential value of –3.4 mV. The calculated bioavailability was 5.1%, suggesting a promising SLN-insulin carrier. Another insulin nanocarrier based on stearic acid, lecithin, and poloxamer 188 was constructed [130]. The binding to the cell surface was increased by incorporating wheat germ agglutinin-N-glutaryl-phosphatidylethanolamine into nanoparticles. This modification increased the particle size from 64.5 to 75.3 nm and changed the zeta potential to a less negative value. By using the same insulin dose, the decrease in the glucose level in blood was 70% after 1 hour, while for modified SLN, the decrease was 45%. The bioavailability was increased from 4.46% to 6.08% via modification. SLN were made of stearic acid, soybean phospholipids, poloxamer 188, and octaarginine as a cell penetration enhancer [131]. Incorporation of the enhancer resulted in an increase in size from 126 to 151 nm and a higher decrease in the glucose level resulted. The bioavailability was also doubled from 5.66% to 10.39%. Different types of SLN, cetyl palmitate, glyceryl tripalmitate, or glyceryl palmitostearate were prepared with conjugation with lecithin and polyoxyl 15 hydroxystearate [132]. All SLN are spherical with different sizes and zeta potential, and the maximum decreases in the glucose level were 15%, 20%, and 25% for cetyl palmitate, glyceryl tripalmitate, and glyceryl palmitostearate nanoparticles, respectively, and the bioavailability were 2.92%, 3.44%, and 4.53%, respectively.

10.2.5 Polyalkylcyanoacrylated (PACA) Nanoparticles

Polyalkylcyanoacrylated (PACA) nanoparticles have been notorious for their stability and biodegradability, which tolerates its utilization as a surgery tissue glue [133,134]. The pioneering instance of biodegradable PACA as a drug delivery vehicle was instigated by Patrick Couvreur, which has attained stage III of clinical examinations [135]. Couvreur's contributions not only extended to the encapsulation of insulin within the PACA polymer matrix but also incorporated the endeavor to innovate a biodegradable nano drug carrier vehicle that conforms with an assortment of drugs. Among the miscellaneous varieties of nano polymeric carriers, PACA disclosed several advantageous features, including feasibility in development, drug versatility, and biocompatibility [136]. Moreover, this polymeric scaffold performs a critical role in the inference of the nanoparticle structure and offers diverse methodologies of administration (*via* injections and/or oral intake). Subsequently, Damge et al. reported the development of insulin-encapsulated PACA nanospheres [137]; however, despite the intermediate encapsulation rate of insulin, the glycemic levels were diminished for an extended period of time in diabetic rats. This behavior is ascribed to the protective layering the polymeric shells provide to the entrapped insulin, which prevents or severely hinders the degradation of insulin. Lately, PACA has been merged in the drug delivery approach as a one of the most remarkable drug delivery vehicles for insulin molecule. MacDowell et al. reported the *in situ* polymerization and combination of PACA with insulin which substantiated by MALDI ionization–coupled tandem time-of-flight mass spectrometry [138]. The modification of PACA's micro-porosity encompasses the manipulation of the utilized microstructure moieties such as caprylocaproyl macrogolglycerides, isopropyl myristate, and polyglyceryl oleate in order to ameliorate the insulin entrapment and release from the microemulsion scaffold [139]. The affinity of insulin molecules to coordinate with the polymeric platform was addressed by Vauthier et al. The study encompasses the interfacial polymerization of isobutyl cyanoacrylate to elucidate the behavior of the insulin toward the polymeric cavity wall [140]. This report revealed the absence of any chemical reactions between the polymeric matrix and the insulin; in fact, the polymerization process has been initiated through the employment of an ethanol solvent. The superior efficacy of insulin entrapment within the polymeric cavity could be attributable to the tendency of the insulin hormone to the oily scaffold of nanospheres.

The stepwise dispersion polymerization is a successful strategy for the assembly of controlled molecular architecture of n-butyl cyanoacrylate nanodomains [141]. In this class of polymerization, insulin molecules operate as initiators and encapsulated drugs. The efficiency of loading the insulin moieties was up to 72% in the acidic media and ambient temperature. The degradation of the polymeric shell and the release of insulin have been established via an enzymatic hydrolyzed procedure with an optimized time and varying esterase levels. Up to date, there are several challenges encountered in the oral administration of insulin including its stability, mucus penetration, and retention in the gastrointestinal area. Recently, Mao and co-workers explored the influence of insulin's release rate from the polymeric framework regarding the *in vitro* and *in vivo* treatments upon manipulating the previous obstacles [142]. The polymeric scaffold was accomplished through the self-polymerization of n-butyl cyanoacrylate alongside the entrapment of the insulin hormone. The new particles demonstrated adequate stability in the gastric fluids and regulated release throughout the intestine, which is adjusted accordingly to the insulin incorporating polymer proportions, as illustrated in Figure 10.4.

10.3 CONCLUSION

The nonenzymatic glucose sensing, however, has greater sensitivity, a larger linear range, a low operating potential, and superior selectivity. Contrarily, this class of applications make it easier to administer insulin orally, which is preferable to

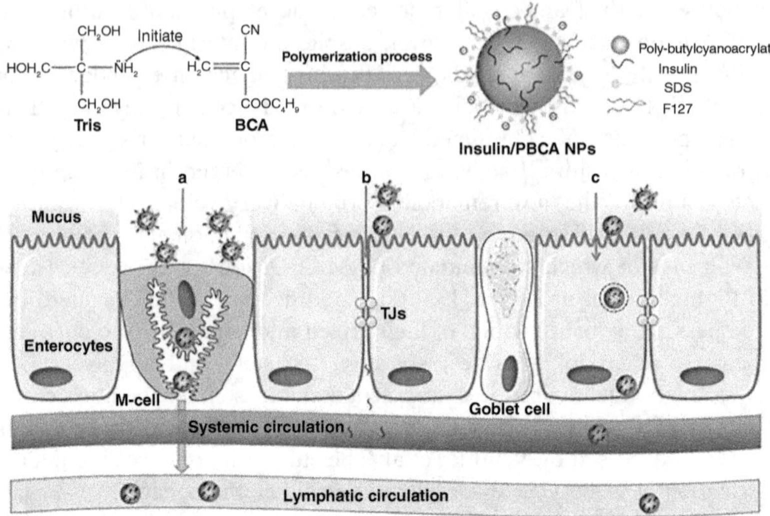

FIGURE 10.4 Schematic diagram of insulin/PBCA NPs preparation and mechanism of absorption in the intestine: (a) macropinocytosis, (b) paracellular transport, and (c) clathrin/caveolae-mediated endocytosis [142].

the conventional method of administering insulin through injection. Nevertheless, this therapy has run into a number of challenges, including low stability/degradation, pH sensitivity, and low biostability. The development of nanomaterials including polymeric matrices that are used in diabetic diagnosis and oral/pulmonary treatment is the subject of the research reports in future.

REFERENCES

1. Henry P., Thomas F., Benetos A., Guize L. Impaired fasting glucose, blood pressure and cardiovascular disease mortality. *Hypertension* 2002; 40:458–463.
2. Senthamizhan A., Balusamy B., Uyar T. Glucose sensors based on electrospun nanofibers: A review. *Anal. Bioanal. Chem.* 2016; 408:1285–1306.
3. Mauras N., Fox L., Englert K., Beck R.W. Continuous glucose monitoring in type 1 diabetes. *Endocrinology* 2013; 43:41–50.
4. Reddy N., Verma N., Dungan K. Monitoring technologies-continuous glucose monitoring, mobile technology, biomarkers of glycemic control. In: Feingold, K. R., Anawalt, B., Boyce, A., et al., editors. *Endotext.* South Dartmouth (MA): MDText.com, Inc. 2020.
5. Srinivasan B., Tung S. Development and applications of portable biosensors. *J. Lab. Autom.* 2019; 20:365–389.
6. Malhotra B., Ali M. Nanomaterials in Biosensors: Fundamentals and Applications 2018. doi: 10.1016/B978-0-323-44923-6.00001-7.
7. Scognamiglio V. Nanotechnology in glucose monitoring: Advances and challenges in the last 10 years. *Biosens. and Bioelectron.* 2013; 47C:12–25.
8. Veiseh O., Tang B.C., Whitehead K.A., Langer D.G., Robert A. Managing diabetes with nanomedicine: Challenges and opportunities. *Nat. Rev.* 2015; 41:45–57.

9. Primavera R., Kevadiya B.D., Swaminathan G., Wilson R.J., Pascale A.D., Decuzzi P., Thakor A.S. Emerging nano- and micro-technologies used in the treatment of type-1 diabetes. *Nanomater.* 2020; 10:789.
10. Cao G. *Nanostructures and Nanomaterials. Synthesis, Properties and Applications.* Imperial College Press, London. 2004.
11. Dave S., Dave A., Radhakrishnan S., Das J., Dave S. Biosensors for healthcare: An artificial intelligence approach. In: *Biosensors for Emerging and Re-Emerging Infectious Diseases* 2022; 365–383. doi: 10.1016/B978-0-323-88464-8.00008-7.
12. Dave S., Kirubavathy S.J. Biosensors based on metal-organic framework (MOF): Paving the way to point-of-care diagnosis. In: *Electrochemical Applications of Metal-Organic Frameworks* 2022; 255–267. doi: 10.1016/B978-0-323-90784-2.00004-6.
13. Panwar R., Churi H., Dave S. Point-of-care electrochemical biosensors using CRISPR/Cas for RNA analysis. In: *Biosensors for Emerging and Re-Emerging Infectious Diseases* 2022; 317–333. doi: 10.1016/B978-0-323-88464-8.00003-8.
14. Radhakrishnan S., Kim B.S., Dave S. Surface modification with nanomaterials for electrochemical biosensing application. In: *Advanced Nanomaterials for Point of Care Diagnosis and Therapy* 2022; 101–120. doi: 10.1016/B978-0-323-85725-3.00002-7.
15. Sahoo M., Gadnayak A., Nayak A., Sahoo S., Dave S., Mohanty P. Advantages of silicon nanowire-based biosensors as wireless technology for infectious disease diagnosis. In: *Biosensors for Emerging and Re-Emerging Infectious Diseases* 2022; 407–417. doi: 10.1016/B978-0-323-88464-8.00019-1.
16. Venkadesh A., Mathiyarasu J., Dave S., Radhakrishnan S. Amine mediated synthesis of nickel oxide nanoparticles and their superior electrochemical sensing performance for glucose detection. *Inorg. Chem. Commun.* 2021; 131:108779.
17. Victor S.U., José Roberto V.B., Rodolfo G.P. The new field of the nanomedicine. *Int. J. Appl. Sci. Eng.* 2015; 5:79–88.
18. DiSanto R.M., Subramanian V., Gu Z. Recent advances in nanotechnology for diabetes treatment. *WIREs Nanomed. Nanobiotechnol.* 2015; 74:548–564.
19. Hovancová J., Ivana Š., Ori R., Ori A. Nanomaterial-based electrochemical sensors for detection of glucose and insulin. *J. Solid State Electrochem.* 2017; 21:2147–2166.
20. Wang T., Huang X., Huang H., Luo P., Qing L. Nanomaterial-based optical- and electrochemical-biosensors for urine glucose detection: A comprehensive review. *Adv. Energy Mater.* 2022; 1:100016.
21. Barone P., Baik S., Heller D., Strano M. Near-infrared optical sensors based on single-walled carbon nanotubes. *Nat. Mater.* 2005; 4:86–92.
22. Yoon H., Ahn J., Barone P., Yum K., Sharma R., Boghossian A., et al. Periplasmic binding proteins as optical modulators of single-walled carbon nanotube fluorescence: Amplifying a nanoscale actuator. *Angew. Chem.* 2011; 123:1868–1871.
23. Bahshi L., Freeman R., Gill R., Willner I. Optical detection of glucose by means of metal nanoparticles or semiconductor quantum dots. *Small* 2009; 5:676–680.
24. Song Y., Qu K., Zhao C., Ren J., Qu X. Graphene oxide: Intrinsic peroxidase catalytic activity and its application to glucose detection. *Adv. Mater.* 2010; 22:2206–2210.
25. Yum K., Ahn J., McNicholas T., Barone P., Mu B., Kim J., et al. Boronic acid library for selective, reversible near-infrared fluorescence quenching of surfactant suspended single-walled carbon nanotubes in response to glucose. *ACS Nano* 2011; 6:819–830.
26. Bratlie K., York R., Invernale M., Langer R., Anderson D. Materials for diabetes therapeutics. *Adv. Healthc. Mater.* 2012; 1:267–284.

27. Yetisen A.K., Montelongo Y., Vasconcellos F.C., Martinez-Hurtado J.L., Neupane S., Butt H., et al. Reusable, robust, and accurate laser-generated photonic nanosensor. *Nano Lett.* 2014; 14:3587–3593.
28. Veetil J., Jin S., Ye K. A glucose sensor protein for continuous glucose monitoring. *Biosens. Bioelectron.* 2010; 26:1650–1655.
29. Besteman K., Lee J.O., Wiertz F., Heering H., Dekker C. Enzyme-coated carbon nanotubes as single-molecule biosensors. *Nano Lett.* 2003; 3:727–730.
30. Lin Y., Lu F., Tu Y., Ren Z. Glucose biosensors based on carbon nanotube nanoelectrode ensembles. *Nano Lett.* 2003; 4:191–195.
31. Zeng X., Li X., Xing L., Liu X., Luo S., Wei W., et al. Electrodeposition of chitosan-ionic liquid-glucose oxidase biocomposite onto nano-gold electrode for amperometric glucose sensing. *Biosens. Bioelectron.* 2009; 24:2898–2903.
32. Shan C., Yang H., Han D., Zhang Q., Ivaska A., Niu L. Graphene/AuNPs/chitosan nanocomposites film for glucose biosensing. *Biosens. and Bioelectron.* 2010; 25:1070–1074.
33. Tang H., Yan F., Lin P., Xu J., Chan H.L.W. Highly sensitive glucose biosensors based on organic electrochemical transistors using platinum gate electrodes modified with enzyme and nanomaterials. *Adv. Funct. Mater.* 2011; 21:2264–2272.
34. Clark Jr. C.L., Lyons C. Electrode systems for continuous monitoring in cardiovascular surgery. *Ann. N. Y. Acad. Sci.* 1962; 102:29–45.
35. Updike S., Hicks G. The enzyme electrode. *Nature* 1967; 214:986–988.
36. Yoo E.H., Lee S.Y. Glucose biosensors: An overview of use in clinical practice. *Sens.* 2010; 10:4558–4576.
37. Tian K., Prestgard M., Ashutosh T. A review of recent advances in nonenzymatic glucose sensors. *Mater. Sci. Eng.* 2014; C 41:100–118.
38. Galant A.L., Kaufman R.C., Wilson J.D. Glucose: Detection and analysis. *Food Chem.* 2015; 188:149–160.
39. Katakis I., Dominguez E. Characterization and stabilization of enzymebiosensors. *TrAC Trends Analyt Chem.* 1995; 14:310–319.
40. Toghill K.E., Compton R.G. Electrochemical non-enzymatic glucose sensors: A perspective and an evaluation. *Int. J. Electrochem. Sci.* 2010; 5:1246–1301.
41. Su S., Sun H., Xu F., Yuwen L., Fan C., Wang L. Direct electrochemistry of glucose oxidase and a biosensor for glucose based on a glass carbon electrode modified with MoS2 nanosheets decorated with gold nanoparticles. *Microchim. Acta* 2014; 181:1497–1503.
42. Darabdhara G., Boruah P.K., Das M.R. Colorimetric determination of glucose in solution and via the use of a paper strip by exploiting the peroxidase and oxidase mimicking activity of bimetallic Cu-Pd nanoparticles deposited on reduced graphene oxide, graphitic carbon nitride, or MoS2 nanoshe. *Microchim. Acta* 2019; 186:13.
43. Yoon J., Lee S.N., Shi M.K., Kim H.W., Choi H.K., Lee T., et al. Flexible electrochemical glucose biosensor based on GOx/gold/MoS_2/gold nanofilm on the polymer electrode, *Biosens. Bioelectron.* 2019; 140:111343.
44. Altuntaş D., Kuralay F. MoS_2/Chitosan/GOx-Gelatin modified graphite surface: Preparation, characterization and its use for glucose determination. *Mater. Sci. Eng. B* 2021; 270:115215.
45. Jędrzak A., Kuznowicz M., Rębiś T., Jesionowski T. Portable glucose biosensor based on polynorepinephrine @ magnetite nanomaterial integrated with a smartphone analyzer for point-of-care application. *Bioelectrochemistry* 2022; 145:108071.

46. Lu L., Zhang L., Qu F., Lu H., Zhang X., Wu Z., et al. A nano-Ni based ultrasensitive nonenzymatic electrochemical sensor for glucose: Enhancing sensitivity through a nanowire array strategy. *Biosens. Bioelectron.* 2009; 25:218–223.
47. Wang G., Lu X., Zhai T., Ling Y., Wang H., Tong Y., et al. Free-standing nickel oxide nanoflake arrays: Synthesis and application for highly sensitive non-enzymatic glucose sensors. *Nanoscale* 2012; 4:3123–3127.
48. Jena B.K., Raj C.R. Enzyme-free amperometric sensingof glucose by using gold nanoparticles. *Chemistry* 2006; 12:2702–2708.
49. Sun Y., Yang H., Yu X., Meng H., Xu X. A novel nonenzymatic amperometric glucose sensor based on a hollow Pt-Ni alloy nanotube array electrode with enhanced sensitivity. *RSC Advances* 2015; 5:70387–70394.
50. Wang L., Zhu W., Lu W., Qin X., Xu X. Surface plasmon aided high sensitive non-enzymatic glucose sensor using Au/NiAu multilayered nanowire arrays. *Biosens. Bioelectron.* 2018; 111:41–46.
51. Wang R., Liang X., Liu H., Cui L., Zhang X., Liu C. Non-enzymatic electrochemical glucose sensor based on monodispersed stone-like PtNi alloy nanoparticles. *Microchim. Acta* 2018; 185:339.
52. Jafarian M., Forouzandeh F., Danaee I., Gobal F., Mahjani M.G. Electrocatalytic oxidation of glucose on Ni and NiCu alloymodified glassy carbon electrode. *J. Solid State Electrochem.* 2008; 13:1171–1179.
53. Mu Y., Jia D., He Y., Miao Y., Wu H.L. Nano nickel oxide modified non-enzymatic glucose sensors with enhanced sensitivity through an electrochemical process strategy at high potential. *Biosens. Bioelectron.* 2011; 26:2948–2952.
54. Liu X., Yang W., Chen L., Jia J. Three-dimensional copper foam supported CuO nanowire arrays: An efficient non-enzymatic glucose sensor. *Electrochim. Acta* 2017; 235:519–526.
55. Li J., Yuan R., Chai Y., Che X., Li W., Zhong X. Nonenzymatic glucose sensor based on a glassy carbon electrode modified with chains of platinum hollow nanoparticles and porous gold nanoparticles in a chitosan membrane. *Microchim. Acta* 2011; 172:163–169.
56. Wang Y., Bai W., Nie F., Zheng J. A non-enzymatic glucose sensor based on Ni/MnO_2 nanocomposite modified glassy carbon electrode. *Electroanal.* 2015; 27:2399–2405.
57. Naik K.K., Ratha S., Rout C.S. Phase and shape dependent non-enzymatic glucose sensing properties of nickel molybdate. *Chemistry Select* 2016; 1:5187–5195.
58. Mai H.H., Tran D.H., Janssens E. Non-enzymatic fluorescent glucose sensor using vertically aligned ZnO nanotubes grown by a one-step, seedless hydrothermal method. *Microchim. Acta* 2019; 186:245.
59. Azharudeen A.M., Karthiga M., Rajarajan A., Suganthi A. Selective enhancement of non-enzymatic glucose sensor by used PVP modified on α-MoO_3 nanomaterials. *Microchem. J.* 2020; 157:105006.
60. Malhotra S., Pradeep Y.T., Varshney K. Fabrication of highly sensitive nonenzymatic sensor based on Pt/PVF modified Pt electrode for detection of glucose. *J. Iran. Chem. Soc.* 2020; 17:521–531.
61. Maleh H.K., Cellat K., Arıkan K., Savk A., Karimi F., Şen F. Palladium-Nickel nanoparticles decorated on Functionalized-MWCNT for high precision nonenzymatic glucose sensing. *Mater. Chem. Phys.* 2020; 250:123042.
62. Meng A., Hong X., Zhang H., Tian W., Li Z., Sheng L., et al. Nickel sulfide nanoworm network architecture as a binder-free high-performance non-enzymatic glucose sensor. *Microchim. Acta* 2021; 188:1–9.

63. Kuznowicz M., Rębiś T., Jędrzak A., Nowaczyk G., Szybowicz M. Glucose determination using amperometric non - enzymatic sensor based on electroactive poly(caffeic acid)@ MWCNT decorated with CuO nanoparticles. *Microchim. Acta* 2022; 189:1–14.
64. Akbar F., Tariq M., Khan H.U., Khan J., Uddin M.K., Ahmed S.S., et al. Development of Ag-Ni NPs loaded on MWCNTs for highly sensitive, selective and reproducible non-enzymatic electrochemical detection of glucose. *J. Mater. Sci. Mater. Electron.* 2021; 32:16166–16181.
65. Chang A.S., Tahira A., Ali Z., Solangi A.G., Ibupoto M.H., Chang F., et al. Pd-Co_3O_4-based nanostructures for the development of enzyme-free glucose sensor. *Bull. Mater. Sci.* 2022; 45:62.
66. Malathi S., Nandhakumar P., Pandiyan V., Webster T.J., Balasubramanian S. Novel PLGA-based nanoparticles for the oral delivery of insulin. *Int. J. Nanomed.* 2015; 10:2207–2218.
67. Sharma G., Sharma A.R., Nam J.S., Doss G.P.C., Lee S.S., Chakraborty C. Nanoparticle based insulin delivery: The next generation efficient therapy for Type 1 diabetes. *J. Nanobiotech.* 2015; 13:74.
68. Lowman A.M., Morishita M., Kajita M., Nagai T., Peppas N.A. Oral delivery of insulin using pH-responsive complexation gels. *J. Pharm. Sci.* 1999; 88:933–937.
69. Woitiski C.B., Carvalho R.A., Ribeiro A.J., Neufeld R.J., Veiga F. Strategies toward the improved oral delivery of insulin nanoparticles via gastrointestinal uptake and translocation. *Bio Drugs* 2008; 22:223–237.
70. des Rieux A., Fievez V., Garinot M., Schneider Y.J., Préat V. Nanoparticles as potential oral delivery systems of proteins and vaccines: A mechanistic approach. *J. Control. Release* 2006; 116:1–27.
71. Damge C., Reis C.P., Maincent P. Nanoparticle strategies for the oral delivery of insulin. *Expert Opin Drug Deliv.* 2008; 5:45–68.
72. Martins S., Sarmento B., Souto E.B., Ferreira D.C. Insulin-loaded alginate microspheres for oral delivery-effect of polysaccharide reinforcement on physicochemical properties and release profile. *Carbohydr. Polym.* 2007; 69:725–731.
73. Reis C., Ribeiro A., Houng S., Veiga F., Neufeld R. Nanoparticulate delivery system for insulin: Design, characterization and in vitro/in vivo bioactivity. *Eur. J. Pharm. Sci.* 2007; 30:392–397.
74. Sarmento B., Martins S., Ferreira D., Souto E.B. Oral insulin delivery by means of solid lipid nanoparticles. *Int. J. Nanomed.* 2007; 2:743–749.
75. Woitiski C.B., Neufeld R.J., Veiga F., Carvalho R.A., Figueiredo I.V. Pharmacological effect of orally delivered insulin facilitated by multilayered stable nanoparticles. *European J. Pharm. Sci.* 2010; 41:556–563.
76. Lin Y.H., Chen C.T., Liang H.F., Kulkarni A.R., Lee P.W., Chen C.H., et al. Novel nanoparticles for oral insulin delivery via the paracellular pathway. *Nanotechnology* 2007; 18:105102.
77. Sonaje K., Lin Y.H., Juang J.H., Wey S.P., Chen C.T., Sung H.W. In vivo evaluation of safety and efficacy of self-assembled nanoparticles for oral insulin delivery. *Biomater.* 2009; 30:2329–2339.
78. Wu Z.M., Ling L., Zhou L.Y., Guo X.D., Jiang W., Qian Y., et al. Novel preparation of PLGA/HP55 nanoparticles for oral insulin delivery. *Nanoscale Res. Lett.* 2012; 7:299.
79. Gentile P., Chiono V., Carmagnola I., Hatton P. An overview of poly(lactic-co-glycolic) acid (PLGA)-based biomaterials for bone tissue engineering. *Int. J. Mol. Sci.* 2014; 15:3640–3659.

80. Danhier F., Ansorena E., Silva J.M., Coco R., Le Breton A., Préat V. PLGA-based nanoparticles: An overview of biomedical applications. *J. Control. Release* 2012; 161:505–522.
81. García-Díaz M., Foged C., Nielsen H.M. Improved insulin loading in poly(lactic-co-glycolic) acid (PLGA) nanoparticles upon self-assembly with lipids. *Int. J. Pharm.* 2015; 482:84–91.
82. Bazile D., Prudhomme C., Bassoullet M.T., Marlard M., Spenlehauer G., Veillard M. Stealth Me.PEG-PLA nanoparticles avoid uptake by the mononuclear phagocytes system. *J. Pharm. Sci.* 1995; 84:493–498.
83. Reix N., Parat A., Seyfritz E., Van der Werf R., Epure V., Ebel N., et al. In vitro uptake evaluation in Caco-2 cells and in vivo results in diabetic rats of insulin-loaded PLGA nano- particles. *Int. J. Pharm.* 2012; 437:213–220.
84. De Campos A., Sanchex A., Gref R., Clavo P., Alonso M.J. The effect of a PEG versus a chitosan coating on the interaction of drug colloidal carriers with the ocular mucosa. *Eur. J. Pharm. Sci.* 2003, 20:73–81.
85. Wu J.Z., Williams G.R., Li H.Y., Wang D.X., Li S.D., Zhu L.M. Insulin-loaded PLGA microspheres for glucose-responsive release. *Drug Deliv.* 2017; 24:1513–1525.
86. Mukhopadhyay G., Mishra R., Rana D., Kundua P.P. Strategies for effective oral insulin delivery with modified chitosan nanoparticles: A review. *Prog. Polym. Sci.* 2012; 37:1457–1475.
87. Sonaje K., Lin K.J., Wey S.P., Lin C.K., Yeh T.H., Nguyen H.N., et al. Biodistribution, pharmacodynamics and pharmacokinetics of insulin analogues in a rat model: Oral delivery using pH-responsive nanoparticles vs. subcutaneous injection. *Biomater.* 2010; 31:6849–6858.
88. Nagpal K., Singh S.K., Mishra D.N. Chitosan nanoparticles: A promising system in novel drug delivery. *Chem. Pharm. Bull.* 2010; 58:1423–1430.
89. Mi F.L., Wu Y.Y., Lin Y.H., Sonaje K., Ho Y.C., Chen C.T., et al. Oral delivery of peptide drugs using nanoparticles self-assembled by poly(gamma-glutamic acid) and a chitosan derivative functionalized by trimethylation. *Bioconjug. Chem.* 2008; 19:1248–1255.
90. Sandri G., Bonferoni M.C., Rossi S., Ferrari F., Boselli C., Caramella C. Insulin-loaded nanoparticles based on N-trimethyl chitosan: In vitro (Caco-2 model) and ex vivo (excised rat jejunum, duodenum, and ileum) evaluation of penetration enhancement properties. *AAPS Pharm. Sci. Tech.* 2010; 11:362–371.
91. Avadi M.R., Sadeghi A.M., Mohammadpour N., Abedin S., Atyabi F., Dinarvand R., et al. Preparation and characterization of insulin nanoparticles using chitosan and Arabic gum with ionic gelation method. *Nanomed.* 2010; 6:58–63.
92. Shelma R., Paul W., Sharma C.P. Development and characterization of self-aggregated nanoparticles from anacardoylated chitosan as a carrier for insulin. *Carbohyd. Polym.* 2010; 80:285–290.
93. Ma Z., Lim T.M., Lim L.Y. Pharmacological activity of peroral chitosaninsulin nanoparticles in diabetic rats. *Int. J. Pharm.* 2005; 293:271–280.
94. Finotelli P.V., Da Silva D., Sola-Penna M., Rossi A.M., Farina M., Andrade L.R., et al. Microcapsules of alginate/chitosan containing magnetic nanoparticles for controlled release of insulin. *Colloids Surf. B.* 2010; 81:206–211.
95. Li X., Qi J., Xie Y., Zhang X., Hu S., Xu Y., et al. Nanoemulsions coated with alginate/chitosan as oral insulin delivery systems: Preparation, characterization, and hypoglycemic effect in rats. *Int. J. Nanomed.* 2013; 8:23–32.
96. Cui F., Qian F., Zhao Z., Yin L., Tang C., Yin C. Preparation, characterization, and oral delivery of insulin loaded carboxylated chitosan grafted poly(methyl methacrylate) nanoparticles. *Biomacromolecules.* 2009; 10:1253–1258.

97. Mao S., Bakowsky U., Jintapattanakit A., Kissel T. Self-assembled polyelectrolyte nanocomplexes between chitosan derivatives and insulin. *J. Pharm. Sci.* 2006; 95:1035–1048.
98. Mao S., Germershaus O., Fischer D., Linn T., Schnepf R., Kissel T. Uptake and transport of PEG-graft-trimethyl-chitosan copolymer-insulin nanocomplexes by epithelial cells. *Pharm. Res.* 2005; 22:2058–2068.
99. Kumar T.M., Paul W., Sharma C.P., Kuriachan M.A. Bioadhesive, pH responsive micromatrix for oral delivery of insulin. *Trends Biomater. Artif. Organs.* 2005; 18:198–202.
100. Bernkop-Schnürch A. Chitosan and its derivatives: Potential excipients for peroral peptide delivery systems. *Int. J. Pharm.* 2000; 194:1–13.
101. Narayani R. Oral delivery of insulin making needles needless. *Trends Biomater. Artif. Organs.* 2001; 15:12–16.
102. Pan Y., Li Y.J., Zhao H.Y., Zheng J.M., Xu H., Wei G., et al. Bioadhesive polysaccharide in protein delivery system: Chitosan nanoparticles improve the intestinal absorption of insulin in vivo. *Int. J. Pharm.* 2002; 249:139–147.
103. Bernkop-Schnürch A., Guggi D., Pinter Y. Thiolatedchitosans: Development and in vitro evaluation of a mucoadhesive, permeation enhancing oral drug delivery system. *J. Control. Release* 2004; 94:177–186.
104. Rekha M.R., Sharma C.P. pH sensitive succinyl chitosan microparticles: A preliminary investigation towards oral insulin delivery. *Trends Biomater. Artif. Organs.* 2008; 21:107–115.
105. Ubaidulla U., Khar R.K., Ahmad F.J., Sultana Y., Panda A.K. Development and characterization of chitosan succinate microspheres for the improved oral bioavailability of insulin. *J. Pharm. Sci.* 2007; 96:3010–3023.
106. Longley C.J., Fung D.P. Potential applications and markets for biomass-derived levoglucosan. In *Advances in Thermochemical Biomass Conversion.* Springer 1993; 1484–1494. doi: 10.1007/978-94-011-1336-6_120.
107. Hu Q., Luo Y. Chitosan-based nanocarriers for encapsulation and delivery of curcumin: A review. *Int. J. Biol. Macromol.* 2021; 179:125–135.
108. Qin Y., Xiong L., Li M., Liu J., Wu H., Qiu H., et al. Preparation of bioactive polysaccharide nanoparticles with enhanced radical scavenging activity and antimicrobial activity. *J. Agric. Food Chem.* 2018; 66:4373–4383.
109. Chen C., Wang Z., Zhang J., Fan X., Xu L., Tang X. Dextran-conjugated caged siRNA nanoparticles for photochemical regulation of RNAi-induced gene silencing in cells and mice. *Bioconjug. Chem.* 2019; 30:1459–1465.
110. Fang Y., Wang H., Dou H.J., Fan X., Fei X.C., Wang L., et al. Doxorubicin-loaded dextran-based nano-carriers for highly efficient inhibition of lymphoma cell growth and synchronous reduction of cardiac toxicity. *Int. J. Nanomed.* 2018; 13:5673–5683.
111. Hu Y., He L., Ding J., Sun D., Chen L., Chen X. One-pot synthesis of dextran decorated reduced graphene oxide nanoparticles for targeted photo-chemotherapy. *Carbohydr. Polym.* 2016; 144:223–229.
112. Wannasarit S., Wang S., Figueiredo P., Trujillo C., Eburnea F., Simón-Gracia L., et al. A virus-mimicking pH-Responsive acetalated dextran-based membrane-active polymeric nanoparticle for intracellular delivery of antitumor therapeutics. *Adv. Funct. Mater.* 2019; 29:1905352.
113. Jin R., Guo X., Dong L., Xie E., Cao A. Amphipathic dextran-doxorubicin prodrug micelles for solid tumor therapy. *Colloids Surf. B: Biointerfaces* 2017; 158:47–56.
114. Soliman S.M.A., Colombeau L., Nouvel C., Babin J., Six J.L. Amphiphilic photosensitive dextran-g-poly (o-nitrobenzyl acrylate) glycopolymers. *Carbohyd. Polym.* 2016; 136:598–608.

115. Torrieri G., Fontana F., Figueiredo P., Liu Z., Ferreira M.P., Talman V., et al. Dual-peptide functionalized acetalated dextran-based nanoparticles for sequential targeting of macrophages during myocardial infarction. *Nanoscale* 2020; 12:2350–2358.
116. Sakaguchi M., Makino M., Ohura T., Yamamoto K., Enomoto Y., Takase H. Surface modification of Fe_3O_4 nanoparticles with dextran via a coupling reaction between naked Fe_3O_4 mechano-cation and naked dextran mechano-anion: A new mechanism of covalent bond formation. *Adv. Powder Technol.* 2019; 30:795–806.
117. Unterweger H., Dezsi L., Matuszak J., Janko C., Poettler M., Jordan, et al. Dextran-coated superparamagnetic iron oxide nanoparticles for magnetic resonance imaging: Evaluation of size-dependent imaging properties, storage stability and safety. *Int. J. Nanomed.* 2018; 13:1899–1915.
118. Wang Z., Shen Y., Shi Q.H., Sun Y. Insights into the molecular structure of immobilized protein A ligands on dextran-coated nanoparticles: Comprehensive spectroscopic investigation. *Biochem. Eng. J.* 2019; 146:20–30.
119. Hu Q., Lu Y., Luo Y. Recent advances in dextran-based drug delivery systems: From fabrication strategies to applications. *Carbohydr. Polym.* 2021; 264:117999.
120. Alibolandi M., Alabdollah F., Sadeghi F., Mohammadi M., Abnous K., Ramezani M., et al. Dextran-b-poly (lactide-co-glycolide) polymersome for oral delivery of insulin: In vitro and in vivo evaluation. *J. Control. Release* 2016; 227:58–70.
121. Jamwal S., Ram B., Ranote S., Dharela R., Chauhan G.S. New glucose oxidase-immobilized stimuli-responsive dextran nanoparticles for insulin delivery. *Int. J. Biol. Macromol.* 2019; 123:968–978.
122. Zion T.C., Henry H.T., Jackie Y.Y. Glucose-sensitive nanoparticles for controlled insulin delivery. 2003. http://hdl.handle.net/1721.1/3783.
123. Chalasani K.B., Russell-Jones G.J., Yandrapu S.K., Diwan P.V., Jain S.K. A novel vitamin B12-nanosphere conjugate carrier system for peroral delivery of insulin. *J. Control. Release* 2007; 117:421–429.
124. Reis C.P., Veiga F.J., Ribeiro A.J., Neufeld R.J., Damge C. Nanoparticulate biopolymers deliver insulin orally eliciting pharmacological response. *J. Pharm. Sci.* 2008; 97:5290–5305.
125. Souto E.B., Müller R.H. Lipid nanoparticles (SLN and NLC) for drug delivery. In: *Nanoparticles for Pharmaceutical Applications.* Stevenson Ranch, CA: American Scientific Publishers. 2007; 103–122.
126. Muller R.H., Runge S., Ravelli V. Oral bioavailability of cyclosporine: Solid lipid nanoparticles (SLN) versus drug nanocrystals. *Int. J. Pharm.* 2006; 317:82–89.
127. Olbrich C., Muller R.H. Enzymatic degradation of SLN-effect of surfactant and surfactant mixtures. *Int. J. Pharm.* 1999; 180:31–39.
128. Lukowski G., Kasbohm J., Pflegel P. Crystallographic investigation of cetylpalmitate solid lipid nanoparticles. *Int. J. Pharm.* 2000; 196:201–205.
129. Sarmento B., Ribeiro A., Veiga F., Ferreira D., Neufeld R. Oral bioavailability of insulin contained in polysaccharide nanoparticles. *Biomacromolecules* 2007; 8:3054–3060.
130. Zhang N., Ping Q., Huang G., Xu W., Cheng Y., Han X. Lectin-modified solid lipid nanoparticles as carriers for oral administration of insulin. *Int. J. Pharm.* 2006; 327:153–159.
131. Zhang Z., Lv H., Zhou J. Novel solid lipid nanoparticles as carriers for oral administration of insulin. *Pharmazie* 2009; 64:574–578.
132. Yang R., Gao R., Li F., He H., Tang X. The influence of lipid characteristics on the formation, in vitro release, and in vivo absorption of protein-loaded SLN prepared by the double emulsion process. *Drug Dev. Ind. Pharm.* 2011; 37:139–148.

133. Woodward S.C., Herrmann J.B., Cameron J.L., Brandes G., Pulaski E.J., Leonard F. Histotoxicity of cyanoacrylate tissue adhesive in the rat. *Ann. Surg.* 1965; 162:113–122.
134. Lenaerts V., Couvreur P., Christiaens-Leyh D., Joiris E., Roland M., Rollman B., et al. Degradation of poly (isobutyl cyanoacrylate) nanoparticles. *Biomater.* 1984; 5:65–68.
135. Alonso M.J., Couvreur P. Historical view of the design and development of nanocarriers overcoming biological bar- riers. In: Alonso MJ, Csaba NS, editors. *Nanostructured Bio-materials for Overcoming Barriers.* Dorchester (UK): RSC Publishing 2012; 3–36.
136. Vauthier C. A journey through the emergence of nanomedicines with poly(alkylcyanoacrylate) based nanoparticles. *J. Drug Target.* 2019; 27:1–24.
137. Damage C., Michel C., Aprahamian M., Couvreur P. New approach for oral administration of insulin with polyalkylcyanoacrylatenanocapsules as drug carrier *Diabetes*, 1988; 37(2):246–25.
138. Kafka A.P., Kleffmann T., Rades T., McDowell A. Characterization of peptide polymer interactions in poly(alkylcyanoacrylate) nanoparticles: A mass spectrometric approach. *Curr. Drug Deliv.* 2010; 7:208–215.
139. Graf A., Rades T., Hook S.M. Oral insulin delivery using nanoparticles based on microemulsions with different structure-types: Optimisation and in vivo evaluation. *Eur. J. Pharm. Sci.* 2009; 37:53–61.
140. Aboubakar M., Puisieux F., Couvreur P., Deyme M., Vauthier C. Study of the mechanism of insulin encapsulation in poly(isobutylcyanoacrylate) nanocapsules obtained by interfacial polymerization. *J. Biomed. Mater. Res.* 1999; 47(4):568–576.
141. Behan N., O'Sullivan C., Birkinshaw C. Synthesis and In-vitro drug release of insulin-loaded poly(n-butyl cyanoacrylate) nanoparticles. *Macromol. Biosci.* 2002; 2(7):336–340.
142. Cheng H., Zhang X., Qin L., Huo Y., Cui Z., Liu C., et al. Design of self-polymerized insulin loaded poly(n-butylcyanoacrylate) nanoparticles for tunable oral delivery. *J. Control. Release* 2020; 10(321):641–653.

11 Magnetic Digital Microfluidics

Promising Technology for Point of Care Diagnostics: Recent Developments

Nishant Nair, Vishakha Dave, Megha Pandya, Snehal Jani, Sushma Dave, and Medha Pandya

11.1 INTRODUCTION

Microfluidic systems based on droplets have been used to control discrete fluid volumes with immiscible phases. A paradigm change in mixing, sorting, encapsulating, sensing, and developing high-throughput devices for biomedical applications has been brought about by the microscale production of fluid droplets [1]. A subclass of microfluidic devices called droplet-based microfluidics or digital microfluidics use active or passive ways to produce droplets in their devices [2]. The active method for producing droplets uses an outside force, such as an electric field, to produce droplets [3]. Droplet microfluidics has created numerous opportunities in the fields of cell biology, molecular detection, drug administration, and microparticle production [4]. Many biological and chemical applications use passive and active microfluidic chips to support fluid mixing, particle manipulation, and signal detection. The applications of passive microfluidic devices are somewhat constrained and geometry-dependent. Sensors or detectors that convert chemical, biological, and physical changes into electrical or optical signals are referred to as active microfluidic devices [2,5,6]. Additionally, they are very adaptable microfluidic tools for disease diagnostics and organ modeling as well as transduction devices for the detection of biological and chemical changes in biomedical applications [7,8]. A variety of methods, including molding, etching, three-dimensional printing, and nanofabrication, are used to create microfluidic devices. Their wide range of applications include cancer disease modeling; diagnosis and treatment of neurological, cardiovascular, hepatic, and pulmonary disorders; and the identification of diagnostic biomarkers and organ-on-chip techniques [9]. Point of care testing is possible with biosensor applications using assays based on enzymes, nanozymes, antibodies, or nucleic acids (DNA or RNA) [10].

DOI: 10.1201/9781003316435-11

The field's predicted advancement includes the refinement of methods for creating microfluidic devices from biocompatible materials. These advancements will broaden the scope of biomedicine, lower diagnostic expenses, and reduce the time of microfluidics technology diagnosis. Microfluidics devices have emerged as promising tools for the diagnosis and treatment of infectious diseases [11]. These devices utilize microscale channels and chambers to manipulate small volumes of fluids, allowing for precise control of biochemical reactions and analysis of biological samples [12]. In recent years, there has been a growing interest in the development of microfluidics devices for infectious disease detection and management, driven by the need for rapid, sensitive, and cost-effective diagnostic tools in resource-limited settings. Several microfluidic-based platforms have been developed for the detection of infectious diseases, including viral, bacterial, and parasitic infections. These devices employ various techniques, such as nucleic acid amplification, immunoassays, and cell-based assays, to detect specific pathogens or antibodies in patient samples. Microfluidic devices have also been used for drug screening and personalized medicine, enabling the rapid screening of potential drug candidates and the optimization of therapeutic regimens. The potential of microfluidics devices for infectious disease management has been demonstrated in several studies, including the detection of HIV, malaria, and tuberculosis [11]. These devices offer several advantages over traditional diagnostic methods, including faster turnaround time, reduced sample volume and cost, and higher sensitivity and specificity. It is now possible to downsize traditional biochemical laboratory protocols into a microchannel networking system thanks to recent developments in the design and development of microfluidics (MFs) devices [5]. This system has shown to be an effective and affordable instrument. Biomedical microdevices comprise integrated structures made up of several tiny integrated devices, such as micro- and nanosized ones, where a variety of operations, such as particle manipulation and sensing, are carried out on the platform. Although various microfluidic devices can carry out similar functions in biomedical applications, passive systems are more frequently used to manipulate particles and mix liquids, whereas active systems are more frequently used to trap particles and perform sensing [13–15].

11.2 MAGNETIC DIGITAL MICROFLUIDICS

11.2.1 An Overview

Digital microfluidics, similar to continuous-flow droplet microfluidics, lays the foundation for droplet-based microfluidics. Continuous-flow droplet microfluidics deals with very small droplets, usually of pico- to nanoliter volume that are generated continuously in a closed microfluidic network. Manipulation of such droplets happens inside closed microchannels using controlled syringe pumps. As they are continuously generated in large quantities, individual manipulation of these droplets is not possible [2,16–18]. The main advantage of continuous-flow, droplet-based microfluidics is the high-throughput parallel reactions such as digital polymerase chain reaction (PCR) and sequencing library preparation. Contrary to this, digital microfluidics deals with droplets of similar volume, but discrete in nature [4,6,14]. The droplets are manipulated on a plain substrate with partial or no confinement. These discrete droplets on an open-surface platform are usually individually controlled and act as virtual reaction chambers. The major advantage of this approach is in applications related to point of care diagnostics that require complex sample preparation [19–26] or in on-demand synthesis of hazardous materials [13,26,27].

Depending on the actuation mechanism, digital microfluidics can be divided into three major parts: (i) electrowetting on dielectric (EWOD) [4,14,28–30], (ii) magnetic [22,31–34], and (iii) surface acoustic waves (SAW) and other types [18,21,35,36]. Other methods include manipulation using light, sound waves, temperature, and mechanical stress, but these methods are currently at an early stage and less practical. Currently, EWOD is the most popular actuation concept, followed by magnetic and SAW. For the manipulation of droplets, EWOD is very useful and provides very precise and automated control over the droplet. The convenience in splitting and dispensing the droplets is the highlight of this method. With time, many relevant difficulties have been overcome due to the latest developments in EWOD. This technique can now be applied to intricate bioassays and more complex platforms. A lot of literature is currently available explaining various aspects of EWOD-based digital microfluidics in detail [4,14,29,30]. Compared to this method, magnetic actuation can be a better alternative if we consider the difficulties and technical expertise required to set up a strong electric field. Magnetic actuation, although less popular, is a promising candidate owing to its easier and cost-effective ways to produce external magnetic fields. There are several ways in which magnetism and magnetic particles may be used for manipulation of droplets on an open substrates, which we will discuss from here. Magnetic digital microfluidics usually requires controlling magnetic particles in the droplet and permanent magnets or electromagnets to manipulate the droplets. The actuated magnetic particles drag the droplet along with them. As the magnetic particles are included inside the droplet, they can also provide a functional solid substrate for molecule adsorption as an extra advantage. This adds another dimension to the magnetic digital microfluidics and increases its advantages for the required applications. Recently, silica-functionalized magnetic particles were used to bind DNA molecules for solid-phase DNA extraction as well as control droplet motion which clearly demonstrated the dual use of these magnetic particles in this case [20,22,32,37]. Instead of using magnetic particles, if the substrate itself is magnetic, then adjusting the shape of the substrate by adding small defects using permanent magnets can allow us to add mobility to a stationary nonmagnetic droplet. Other than magnetic particles or magnetic substrate, magnetic fluids may also be used for this purpose. Magnetic fluids or ferrofluids contain superparamagnetic nanoparticles coated with a suitable surfactant, which renders the fluid responsive to external magnetic stimuli. Using this, nonmagnetic immiscible droplets can be controlled as well as layers of such ferrofluids on the open substrate can alter the surface energy interaction of the droplet with the substrate. Detailed description of these methods and recent reports of them are provided in the following subsections.

11.2.2 Magnetic Nanoparticles

Magnetic nanoparticles are superior in terms of their physical properties, such as their mechanical strength, chemical activity, and resistance to corrosion. The ferrite particles are typically soft and exhibit superparamagnetism in their natural state. As the particle size decreases, they display distinct changes in their magnetic behavior. The grain size of magnetic particles shifts from multi-domain to single domain as this causes a change in the coercivity of the particles. In regions with a single domain, it will reach a critical grain size value at which point the required coercive field will become zero. It is at this point that the particles begin to behave in a superparamagnetic manner. Figure 11.1 shows a list of some of the many useful qualities that magnetic nanoparticles (MNPs) possess [38,39].

With the assistance of an externally applied magnetic field, magnetic particles can be moved to a new location or kept in one spot for an extended period of time. Their movement can be controlled from a distance. When the field is removed, the magnetism leaves the object. The temperature of the particles can be altered by applying an alternating magnetic field with the appropriate frequency. Due to the fact that the single-domain particles behave like very small magnets, a magnetic field of a moderate strength is required.

An emerging application of magnetic digital microfluidics is the manipulation of particles and droplets by using magnetic fluid that contains magnetic nanoparticles on a scale of less than 10 nm. It is possible to use it for a variety of biomedical applications *in vivo* and *in vitro* due to its unique chemical and physical properties, such as hyperthermia, drug release, tissue engineering, biomagnetic

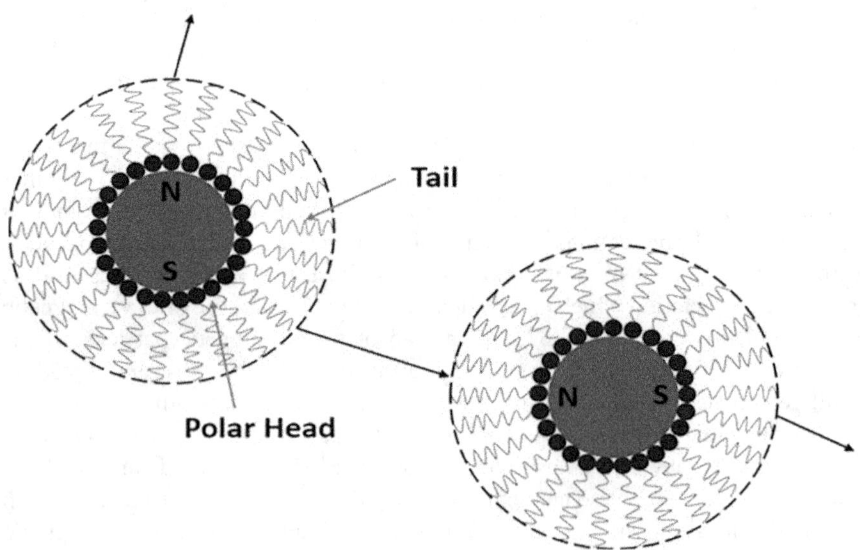

FIGURE 11.1 A schematic illustration of coated, tiny magnetic particles in magnetic nanofluids.

separation of biomolecules, and magnetic resonance imaging (MRI) as contrast agents. The following are some of the qualities of MNPs that make them a potentially useful tool in the field of biomedical applications. Magnetic nanoparticles are smaller in size compared to a cell, a gene, or a protein. They are able to be coated with biomolecules such as protein, silane, and starch. Because of this, it is easier to interact with a biological entity or bind it to something. Hence, it is possible to tag or label a biomolecule of interest. It has a relatively low toxic potential.

Magnetic nanofluids, or ferrofluids, are typically stable suspensions of single-domain magnetic nanoparticles. It is made up of a ferro- or ferrimagnetic material, primarily iron oxide. Magnetic nanoparticles are frequently coated with polymers, surfactants, or charged compounds to stabilize them by steric and/or electrostatic repulsion in order to create a stable colloidal suspension. They remain liquid in the presence of a magnetic field and exhibit a variety of physical phenomena such as Rosensweig instability, phase transitions, nonmagnetic material levitation, magneto-viscous effects, and magneto-optical effects. Chemical co-precipitation and size reduction are two common methods for preparing magnetic fluids [40].

The magnetic fluid contains a number of different forces, including the van der Waals force, the dipole–dipole force, and the gravitational force. These forces cause the particles in a carrier liquid to clump together and eventually settle at the bottom of the container. The criteria is to maintain particle size in the range of 8–10 nm in order to achieve the stability of particles against magnetic field gradients, gravitational forces, and dipole–dipole interactions. It is dependent on the amount of thermal contribution as well as the equilibrium between attractive and repulsive forces. Coating particles with polar group adsorption (Figure 11.1) or by adsorbing the opposite charges on the surface can create steric repulsive and electrostatic repulsive forces. Both of these methods can be used to coat particles (Figure 11.2).

The properties of magnetic nanoparticles, liquid carriers, and stabilizers can all be altered. Magnetic fluids are commonly used in technological and material

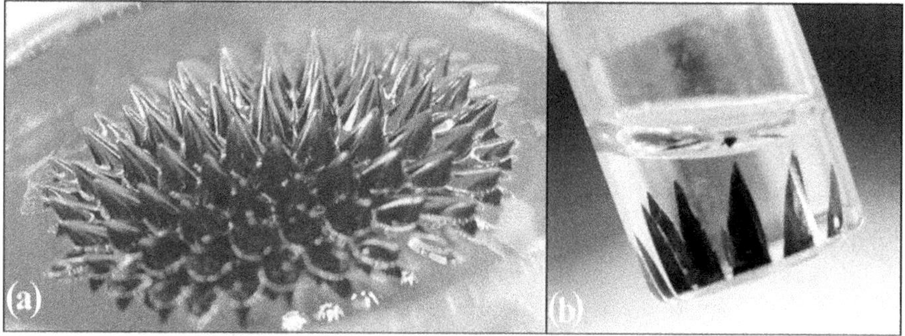

FIGURE 11.2 (a) The typical spike pattern/interfacial instability produced in a kerosene-based magnetic fluid under the influence of a magnetic fluid perpendicular to the fluid–air interface. (b) The same magnetic fluid immersed in an immiscible fluid.

science applications, such as material separation, magnetic domain detection, pressure-tight rotary-shaft sealing, and damping and cooling agents for loudspeakers [41,42].

11.2.3 Magnetic Fluid in Digital Microfluidics: Enabling Precise Droplet Manipulation

Magnetic fluid, also known as ferrofluid, is a liquid that contains very small, magnetic particles suspended within it. When a magnetic field is applied to the fluid, the particles align with the field, creating a fluid that can be manipulated using magnetic forces. This makes magnetic fluid an important component in magnetic digital microfluidics, a technology that uses magnetic fields to manipulate droplets of liquid on a chip or surface. One of the key advantages of using magnetic fluid in magnetic digital microfluidics is its ability to precisely control the movement and positioning of droplets. By applying different magnetic fields, droplets can be moved, split, merged, and even sorted based on the magnetic properties of the particles within them. This level of precision is important for applications such as lab-on-a-chip devices for biological and chemical analyses, where accurate manipulation of small volumes of liquid is necessary.

Another advantage of magnetic fluid is that it can be used in a wide range of applications. For example, magnetic digital microfluidics can be used in drug discovery to screen large numbers of compounds quickly and efficiently. It can also be used in cell sorting, where magnetic particles are used to label and sort cells based on their surface markers. Additionally, magnetic digital microfluidics can be used in DNA analysis, where droplets can be used to amplify and detect specific sequences of DNA. Magnetic fluid is also relatively easy to work with compared to other microfluidic techniques. It does not require any external energy source to manipulate droplets, as the magnetic fields can be generated using simple, low-cost magnets. Additionally, magnetic fluid can be used with a wide range of liquids, including water, organic solvents, and even blood. In summary, magnetic fluid is an important component in magnetic digital microfluidics because it allows for precise manipulation of droplets using magnetic fields. This precision and control is important for a wide range of applications, including drug discovery, cell sorting, and DNA analysis, and it is relatively easy to work with compared to other microfluidic techniques.

11.2.4 Magnetic Particle–Based Manipulation

Some of the ways in magnetic digital microfluidics using which particles and droplets can be manipulated are discussed here. In the most common method for magnetic manipulation, magnetic particles are added to the droplet to serve as the actuator. A permanent magnet or an electromagnetic setup is used to apply an external magnetic field from below the substrate which is hydrophobic. By moving the permanent magnet or by applying spatio-temporal variation in the magnetic field of the electromagnet, the droplet can be manipulated on the substrate.

These magnetic particles can be ferromagnetic, paramagnetic, or superparamagnetic in nature. Depending on the type of magnetic particle, the number density of particles in the droplets as well as the strength of the external magnetic field can be selected. It is to be noted that the substrates used in such cases are carefully rendered hydrophobic by applying a layer of low-surface-energy materials. This reduces the wetting of droplets, resulting in low friction and better mobility.

Using magnetic particle–laden droplets, many groups have shown their use as virtual reaction chambers for complex bioanalytical assays on magnetic digital microfluidic platforms. Pipper et al demonstrated the detection of highly pathogenic avian influenza virus H5N1 in a throat swab sample by using magnetic forces to manipulate a free droplet containing superparamagnetic particles [20]. Sequentially, the viral RNA was isolated, purified, preconcentrated by 50,000%, and subjected to ultrafast real-time RT-PCR. Their bioassay is 440% faster and 2,000%–5,000% cheaper compared to commercially available tests. Similarly, magnetic digital microfluidics is also suitable for assays that require washing such as ELISA. Shikida et al. and a few other groups presented particle-based ELISA on a magnetic digital microfluidic platform [43–47]. Magnetic particles were first functionalized with antibodies to capture the target molecules and then used for ELISA. By moving the droplet, extracting the magnetic particles, and merging the particles with another droplet, target recognition and particle washing could be realized.

To increase the throughput, parallel manipulation of multiple droplets using an array of magnetics was demonstrated in several studies. Ohashi et al. used a linear array of magnets to cycle droplets between three temperature zones for parallel PCR [47]. Okochi and Shi both used magnetic particles for parallel RNA extraction from multiple samples in a droplet array [48,49]. Park et al. used a magnetic droplet array to demonstrate particle-based ELISA in parallel [43]. In most cases, the permanent magnet was located below the open substrate, but Tsuchiya et al. performed droplet manipulation in an open channel using a permanent magnet placed in a second channel near the droplet channel in the same plane [48].

Other than using permanent magnets, arrays of electromagnets containing microcoils can also be used for droplet manipulation. In such a case, a droplet containing magnetic particles is placed on a substrate below which microcoils are placed. These microcoils function as electromagnets with controllable strength and direction, creating a small magnetic field gradient to displace the magnetic particles and along with it the droplet (Figure 11.3). Many previous studies have shown microcoil-enabled magnetic droplet manipulation and systematically investigated the underlying principles [50–53]. Optimization of microcoil patterns was done to facilitate efficient 2D droplet operation [50,53]. Lehmann et al. demonstrated DNA purification by a similar procedure [34] to those of Pipper et al. and Chiou et al., who demonstrated both DNA purification and PCR-based detection [31,34,37].

If hydrophobic or amphiphilic micro-/nanoparticles are used to encapsulate a water droplet, then it is called a liquid marble which also shows good promise for magnetic digital microfluidics [1,54–56]. In this case, a liquid droplet rolls across

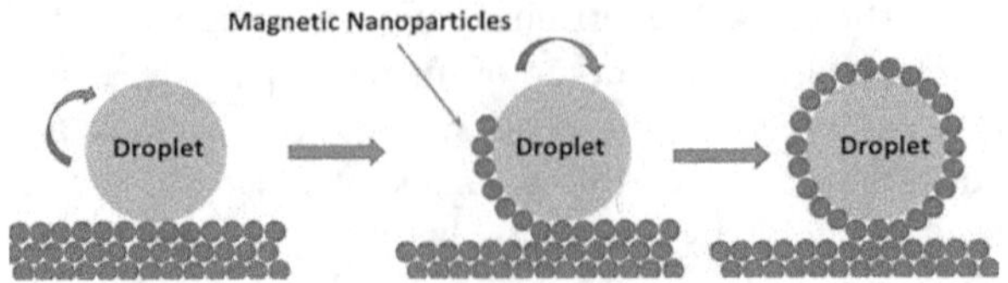

FIGURE 11.3 A liquid droplet rolls across the particles, which adhere to the droplet surface, creating a soft sphere at the liquid–vapor interface.

the particles, which adhere to the droplet surface, creating a soft sphere at the liquid–vapor interface as shown in the schematic representation in Figure 11.3. Using magnetic micro-/nanoparticles here makes the manipulation of liquid marbles easy via magnetic fields. The underlying physics of liquid marble formation and motion is studied in great detail recently [57]. But as the particles remain at the droplet interface, these magnetic particles cannot serve as a sloid-phase substrate for binding of molecules but can only serve as droplet actuator which significantly reduces their applicability in magnetic digital microfluidics.

11.2.5 Magnetically Controlled Flexible Substrate for Droplet Manipulation

Usually, droplet manipulation in magnetic digital microfluidics happens on a rigid substrate. The substrate does not play any role other than providing a low-energy surface for support. Recently, a novel technique was proposed to manipulate droplets on a flexible substrate. The flexible substrate can be easily deformed and creates a dent on the surface. The droplets simply roll toward the dent where the potential energy is minimum as shown in Figure 11.4. Hence, the movement of the droplet can be effectively controlled by deforming and shifting the location of the dent on the flexible substrate. Magnetic force is one of the most effective methods for deforming a flexible substrate. The flexible substrate is impregnated with magnetic materials, and bringing a magnet close to the surface attracts a part of the substrate toward it, creating a dent. Seo et al. mixed magnetic particles with polydimethylsiloxane (PDMS) [58]. After preparing the flexible substrate, magnetic materials were included in it, demonstrating droplet transport and merging on the proposed platform. Biswas et al. explained a different method for deforming a flexible substrate using magnetic force [59] by embedding individual steel balls into PDMS.

When a permanent magnet was brought closer to the steel ball below the surface, the substrate deformed and formed a dent for droplet control. They demonstrated transport and merging of droplet by sequentially attracting and releasing the steel balls at different nodes.

If a flexible substrate is coated with magnetic nanostructures, magnetic field can be used to control its morphology. It is known that altering the morphology of a surface and thereby its roughness can increase the apparent contact

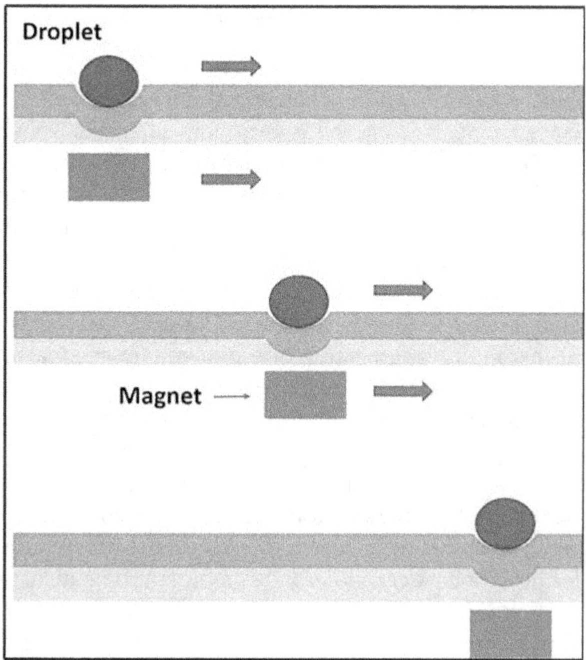

FIGURE 11.4 Principle of droplet actuation using a magnetically deformable substrate.

angle [60]. Carefully tailoring nanostructures on the surface can help control the surface roughness. If the micro-/nanostructures are made of flexible and magnetic materials, magnetic force can be used to tune the surface roughness. Zhou et al. deposited magnetic nanoparticles on a track-etched polycarbonate membrane that served as a sacrificial supporting material [61]. This sacrificial material was removed by plasma etching, and the deposition formed rough nanostructures on the surface. The droplet deposited on the surface stayed in the Cassie–Baxter state with a large contact angle, but when an external magnetic field was applied, the magnetic nanostructures collapsed, reducing the surface roughness and hence the apparent contact angle. Wang et al. also fabricated a magnetically tunable rough surface [62]. Nanometer-sized hair-like structures were grown on an array of micro-sized walls made of elastomers impregnated with magnetic particles. When a permanent magnet was placed beside the substrate, the micrometer-sized walls tilted toward the direction of the magnet. Initially, the droplet deposited on this substrate stayed on top of these microwalls in the Cassie–Baxter state. When the magnet pulled the wall, the droplet traveled toward the direction of pulling. Although manipulating droplets on a magnetically deformable substrate is very useful in magnetic digital microfluidics, the involvement of costly and complicated methods in fabricating such magnetically controllable flexible substrates remains an issue which as of now is not disadvantageous for sample-to-answer analysis for point of care diagnostics in low-resource environments.

11.2.6 Ferrofluid-Based Magnetic Droplet Manipulation

Ferrofluid is a colloidal suspension containing magnetic nanoparticles coated with a surfactant and dispersed in a suitable carrier liquid [40]. The synthesis of magnetic nanoparticles is done by a very convenient and popular chemical route called the chemical co-precipitation technique [40]. The size of the magnetic particles synthesized by this method is in the nanometer range, and they are superparamagnetic in nature. The carrier liquid can either be aqueous or oil-based, depending on the application [63]. Similar to magnetic particle–based manipulation, ferrofluid-based magnetic droplet manipulation involves the use of these surfactant-coated magnetic particle containing fluids. The advantage in this case is that there is no aggregation of the magnetic nanoparticles under the influence of magnetic field. Due to the stable dispersion of magnetic nanoparticles in the liquid, ferrofluids have been used to induce wetting and fluid deformation [15,50,63,64]. Mixing ferrofluid with an aqueous solution disturbs the stability of this colloidal suspension. Therefore, the unique chemical composition of ferrofluids is incompatible with the environment of an aqueous buffer in many bioanalytical assays. The ferrofluid is generally only used as the actuator to move the droplet cargo for liquid-phase reactions and does not participate in the solid-phase biochemical reactions [5].

If the ferrofluid is immiscible in the droplet phase, it can conveniently work as an actuator. This will be similar to the case of magnetic particle–based manipulation but in a more stable form. Figure 11.5 shows a schematic representation of the use of ferrofluid for droplet deformation, transportation, merging, mixing, and particle extraction. The disadvantage in this case is the inability to use ferrofluid for surface functionalization as the nanoparticles are coated with surfactant. Instead of using ferrofluids inside the droplet for controlling them, droplets can be placed on a pool or layer of ferrofluid prepared on a solid substrate. Nair et al. used an active surface, which is a carefully prepared layer of kerosene-based ferrofluid on a plane glass substrate via spin coating [3,65]. When a water droplet is placed on such a layer, due to the effect of surface tension, a complete encapsulation of the water droplet is done by the ferrofluid layer (Figure 11.6). This encapsulation of the water droplet happens because of a positive spreading coefficient, which is governed by the surface tension of water and ferrofluid. Upon placing a permanent magnet below and also from beside the substrate, the ferrofluid layer

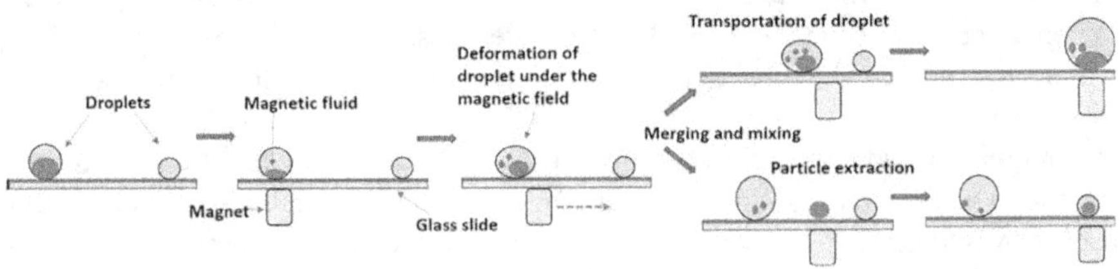

FIGURE 11.5 Schematic representation of a droplet actuated by ferrofluid and permanent magnet.

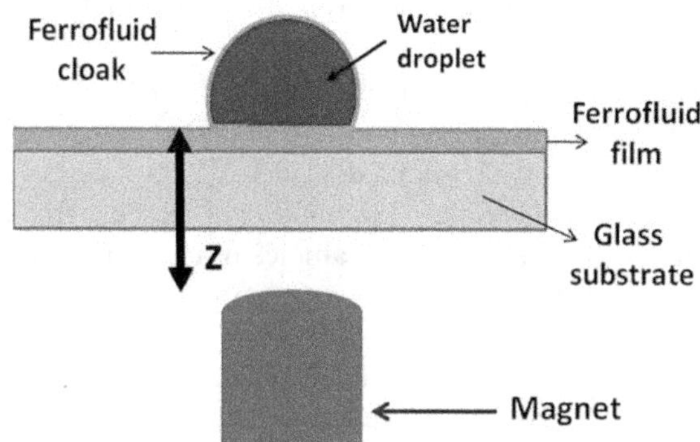

FIGURE 11.6 Active surface made of kerosene-based ferrofluid used to manipulate water droplet using permanent magnet.

easily transports the droplet in the desired direction. Bringing the magnet from the top of the droplet created deformities in the shape of the drop.

11.3 APPLICATIONS IN POINT OF CARE DIAGNOSTICS

Magnetic digital microfluidics is a fast-expanding discipline that combines microfluidics with magnetics principles to generate a potent diagnostic tool. These devices use magnetic particle manipulation in a fluidic environment to perform diagnostic procedures such as nucleic acid detection, protein identification, and cell analysis. Because of its compact size, mobility, and low cost, the technology is particularly well suited for point of care applications [66].

Essential components of a magnetic digital microfluidic device are a microfluidic chip and a magnetic field generator. A set of channels and chambers on the microfluidic chip are utilized to regulate the flow and movement of magnetic particles. The channels and chambers are often constructed of glass, silicon, or polymers and are created using processes like photolithography, soft lithography, or laser ablation. To manipulate the magnetic particles within the chip, a magnetic field generator, which might be a pair of magnets or an electromagnetic coil, is utilized.

Magnetic particles, commonly referred to as magnetic beads, are an important component in magnetic digital microfluidics. These particles are generally made up of a magnetic core (iron oxide) and a surface coating (polymeric or biological substance). The surface coating is intended to attach to a specific target molecule or cell, such as a cancer cell's genetic mutation or a viral particle [9]. Different kinds of magnetic particles can be utilized for various diagnostic procedures, allowing for the identification of many targets at the same time.

The capacity to do multiplexed assays, in which numerous diagnostic tests may be performed on a single sample, is one of the primary benefits of magnetic digital microfluidics. This is accomplished by the use of various magnetic particles, each of which is carefully engineered to attach to a certain target molecule or cell. The magnetic field generator is used to modify the magnetic particles within the microfluidic chip, allowing for the selective separation and detection of various particle kinds.

One of the key advantages of magnetic beads–based microfluidics devices is their ability to perform multiple operations, such as separation, concentration, and purification, in a single, integrated device. This can save time and reduce the amount of sample required compared to traditional methods that require multiple steps and separate instruments. Some examples of magnetic beads–based microfluidics devices include the following:

- Magnetic bead–based DNA and RNA purification systems.
- Magnetic bead–based cell separation systems.
- Magnetic bead–based protein purification systems.
- Magnetic bead–based immunoassays.
- Magnetic bead–based sample preparation systems for mass spectrometry.

Magnetic beads, for example, can be coated with specialized probes that bind to a target DNA or RNA sequence in the case of nucleic acid detection. After being introduced to a sample containing the target nucleic acid, the magnetic beads are captured in the magnetic digital microfluidic chip. The collected beads are subsequently identified using fluorescence, chemiluminescence, or colorimetry methods. Shao et al. showed the application of magnetic digital microfluidics to detect Epstein-Barr virus in clinical samples, with a detection limit of 10 viral copies per response [67]. Magnetic beads can be coated with particular antibodies that bind to a target protein in the case of protein detection. The magnetic beads are then introduced to a target protein-containing sample and captured in the magnetic digital microfluidic chip. The collected beads are subsequently identified using fluorescence, chemiluminescence, or colorimetry methods. Chen et al. used magnetic digital microfluidics to detect prostate-specific antigen (PSA) in blood samples, with a sensitivity and specificity of 96.8% and 94.1%, respectively [68–72]. Magnetic beads can be coated with particular antibodies that bind to cell surface indicators in the case of cell analysis. The magnetic beads are then mixed with a sample containing target cells.

In summary, magnetic microfluidic devices are an effective tool for studying infectious illnesses because they produce extremely sensitive and precise findings with low sample volume and reagent use. They are commonly employed for cell and pathogen isolation and purification, as well as the detection and quantification of infectious agents. While the technology has limits, future magnetic microfluidic devices are projected to play an increasingly essential role in the detection, treatment, and prevention of infectious illnesses.

REFERENCES

1. Zhao Y, Xu Z, Niu H, Wang X, Lin T. Magnetic liquid marbles: Toward "Lab in a Droplet." *Adv Funct Mater.* 2015 Jan;25(3):437–44.
2. Teh SY, Lin R, Hung LH, Lee AP. Droplet microfluidics. *Lab Chip.* 2008;8(2):198.

3. Nair N, Dave V, Jani S. Active manipulation of droplets on glass substrate using ferrofluid. *Mater Today Proc.* 2020;29:258–66.
4. Fair RB. Digital microfluidics: is a true lab-on-a-chip possible? *Microfluid Nanofluidics.* 2007 Jun 8;3(3):245–81.
5. Hang Koh W, Seng Lok K, Nguyen NT. A digital micro magnetofluidic platform for lab-on-a-chip applications. *J Fluids Eng.* 2013 Feb 1;135(2):021302.
6. Jebrail MJ, Bartsch MS, Patel KD. Digital microfluidics: A versatile tool for applications in chemistry, biology and medicine. *Lab Chip.* 2012;12(14):2452.
7. Shen HH, Fan SK, Kim CJ, Yao DJ. EWOD microfluidic systems for biomedical applications. *Microfluid Nanofluidics.* 2014 May 30;16(5):965–87.
8. Angelakeris M. Magnetic nanoparticles: A multifunctional vehicle in modern theranostics applications. doi: 10.1016/j.bbagen.2017.02.022.
9. Nayak S, Blumenfeld NR, Laksanasopin T, Sia SK. Point-of-care diagnostics: Recent developments in a connected age. *Anal Chem.* 2017 Jan 3;89(1):102–23.
10. Shah S, Maharshi A, Pandya M, Dhanalakshmi M, Das K. Nucleic acid based biosensor as a cutting edge tool for point of care diagnosis. In: *Biosensors for Emerging and Re-Emerging Infectious Diseases.* Elsevier; 2022. p. 265–301. doi: 10.1016/B978-0-323-88464-8.00014-2.
11. Chin CD, Laksanasopin T, Cheung YK, Steinmiller D, Linder V, Parsa H, et al. Microfluidics-based diagnostics of infectious diseases in the developing world. *Nat Med.* 2011 Aug 31;17(8):1015–9.
12. Chen F, Hu Q, Li H, Xie Y, Xiu L, Zhang Y, et al. Multiplex detection of infectious diseases on microfluidic platforms. *Biosensors (Basel).* 2023 Mar 21;13(3):410.
13. Keng PY, Chen S, Ding H, Sadeghi S, Shah GJ, Dooraghi A, et al. Micro-chemical synthesis of molecular probes on an electronic microfluidic device. *Proc Natl Acad Sci.* 2012 Jan 17;109(3):690–5.
14. Choi K, Ng AHC, Fobel R, Wheeler AR. Digital microfluidics. *Annu Rev Anal Chem.* 2012 Jul 19;5(1):413–40.
15. Nguyen NT, Wu Z. Micromixers-a review. *J Micromech Microeng.* 2005 Feb 1;15(2):R1–16.
16. Guo MT, Rotem A, Heyman JA, Weitz DA. Droplet microfluidics for high-throughput biological assays. *Lab Chip.* 2012;12(12):2146.
17. Joensson HN, Andersson Svahn H. Droplet microfluidics-a tool for single-cell analysis. *Angew Chem Int Ed.* 2012 Dec 3;51(49):12176–92.
18. Wang Z, Zhe J. Recent advances in particle and droplet manipulation for lab-on-a-chip devices based on surface acoustic waves. *Lab Chip.* 2011;11(7):1280.
19. Choi K, Ng AHC, Fobel R, Chang-Yen DA, Yarnell LE, Pearson EL, et al. Automated digital microfluidic platform for magnetic-particle-based immunoassays with optimization by design of experiments. *Anal Chem.* 2013 Oct 15;85(20):9638–46.
20. Pipper J, Inoue M, Ng LFP, Neuzil P, Zhang Y, Novak L. Catching bird flu in a droplet. *Nat Med.* 2007 Oct 23;13(10):1259–63.
21. Guttenberg Z, Müller H, Habermüller H, Geisbauer A, Pipper J, Felbel J, et al. Planar chip device for PCR and hybridization with surface acoustic wave pump. *Lab Chip.* 2005;5(3):308–17.
22. Zhang Y, Wang TH. Full-range magnetic manipulation of droplets via surface energy traps enables complex bioassays. *Adv Mater.* 2013 Jun 4;25(21):2903–8.
23. Huang CY, Shih PH, Tsai PY, Lee IC, Hsu HY, Huang HY, et al. AMPFLUID: Aggregation magnified post-assay fluorescence for ultrasensitive immunodetection on digital microfluidics. *Proc IEEE.* 2015 Feb;103(2):225–35.
24. Ng AHC, Chamberlain MD, Situ H, Lee V, Wheeler AR. Digital microfluidic immunocytochemistry in single cells. *Nat Commun.* 2015 Jun 24;6(1):7513.

25. Royal MW, Jokerst NM, Fair RB. Integrated sample preparation and sensing: Polymer microresonator sensors embedded in digital electrowetting microfluidic systems. *IEEE Photonics J.* 2012 Dec;4(6):2126–35.
26. Fiel SA, Yang H, Schaffer P, Weng S, Inkster JAH, Wong MCK, et al. Magnetic droplet microfluidics as a platform for the concentration of [18 F]Fluoride and radiosynthesis of Sulfonyl [^{18}F] Fluoride. *ACS Appl Mater Interfaces.* 2015 Jun 17;7(23):12923–9.
27. Javed MR, Chen S, Lei J, Collins J, Sergeev M, Kim HK, et al. High yield and high specific activity synthesis of [^{18}F] fallypride in a batch microfluidic reactor for micro-PET imaging. *Chem Commun.* 2014;50(10):1192–4.
28. Nelson WC, Kim CJ. Droplet actuation by electrowetting-on-dielectric (EWOD): A review. *J Adhes Sci Technol.* 2012 Sep 1;26(12–17):1747–71.
29. Cho SK, Moon H, Kim C-J. Creating, transporting, cutting, and merging liquid droplets by electrowetting-based actuation for digital microfluidic circuits. *J Microelectromech Syst.* 2003 Feb;12(1):70–80.
30. Miller EM, Wheeler AR. A digital microfluidic approach to homogeneous enzyme assays. *Anal Chem.* 2008 Mar 1;80(5):1614–9.
31. Chiou CH, Jin Shin D, Zhang Y, Wang TH. Topography-assisted electromagnetic platform for blood-to-PCR in a droplet. *Biosens Bioelectron.* 2013 Dec;50:91–9.
32. Zhang Y, Park S, Liu K, Tsuan J, Yang S, Wang TH. A surface topography assisted droplet manipulation platform for biomarker detection and pathogen identification. *Lab Chip.* 2011;11(3):398–406.
33. Shin DJ, Wang TH. Magnetic droplet manipulation platforms for nucleic acid detection at the point of care. *Ann Biomed Eng.* 2014 Nov 10;42(11):2289–302.
34. Lehmann U, Hadjidj S, Parashar VK, Vandevyver C, Rida A, Gijs MAM. Two-dimensional magnetic manipulation of microdroplets on a chip as a platform for bioanalytical applications. *Sens Actuators B Chem.* 2006 Oct;117(2):457–63.
35. Ding X, Li P, Lin SCS, Stratton ZS, Nama N, Guo F, et al. Surface acoustic wave microfluidics. *Lab Chip.* 2013;13(18):3626.
36. Yeo LY, Friend JR. Surface acoustic wave microfluidics. *Annu Rev Fluid Mech.* 2014 Jan 3;46(1):379–406.
37. Pipper J, Zhang Y, Neuzil P, Hsieh TM. Clockwork PCR including sample preparation. *Angew Chem Int Ed.* 2008 May 13;47(21):3900–4.
38. Mehta R. Impact of magnetic nanomaterials on biotechnology and biomedicine. *Modern Appl Bioequivalence Bioavailability.* 2017 Sep 22;2(2):555581.
39. Mehta RV. Synthesis of magnetic nanoparticles and their dispersions with special reference to applications in biomedicine and biotechnology. *Mater Sci Eng C.* 2017 Oct;79:901–16.
40. Rosensweig RE. *Ferrohydrodynamic.* Cambridge: Cambridge University Press; 1985.
41. Mehta RV, and Upadhyay RV. Science and technology of ferrofluids. *Curr Sci.* 1999;76(3):305.
42. Raj K, Moskowitz B, Casciari R. Advances in ferrofluid technology. *J Magn Magn Mater.* 1995 Aug;149(1–2):174–80.
43. Park MC, Kim M, Lim GT, Kang SM, An SSA, Kim TS, et al. Droplet-based magnetic bead immunoassay using microchannel-connected multiwell plates (μCHAMPs) for the detection of amyloid beta oligomers. *Lab Chip.* 2016;16(12):2245–53.
44. Kim JA, Kim M, Kang SM, Lim KT, Kim TS, Kang JY. Magnetic bead droplet immunoassay of oligomer amyloid β for the diagnosis of Alzheimer's disease using micro-pillars to enhance the stability of the oil-water interface. *Biosens Bioelectron.* 2015 May;67:724–32.

45. Shikida M, Takayanagi K, Honda H, Ito H, Sato K. Development of an enzymatic reaction device using magnetic bead-cluster handling. *J Micromech Microeng.* 2006 Sep 1;16(9):1875–83.
46. Shikida M, Takayanagi K, Inouchi K, Honda H, Sato K. Using wettability and interfacial tension to handle droplets of magnetic beads in a micro-chemical-analysis system. *Sens Actuators B Chem.* 2006 Jan;113(1):563–9.
47. Ohashi T, Kuyama H, Hanafusa N, Togawa Y. A simple device using magnetic transportation for droplet-based PCR. *Biomed Microdevices.* 2007 Aug 23;9(5):695–702.
48. Tsuchiya H, Okochi M, Nagao N, Shikida M, Honda H. On-chip polymerase chain reaction microdevice employing a magnetic droplet-manipulation system. *Sens Actuators B Chem.* 2008 Mar;130(2):583–8.
49. Shi X, Chen CH, Gao W, Chao S, Meldrum DR. Parallel RNA extraction using magnetic beads and a droplet array. *Lab Chip.* 2015;15(4):1059–65.
50. Beyzavi A, Nguyen NT. Modeling and optimization of planar microcoils. *J Micromech Microeng.* 2008 Sep 1;18(9):095018.
51. Nguyen NT, Ng KM, Huang X. Manipulation of ferrofluid droplets using planar coils. *Appl Phys Lett.* 2006 Jul 31;89(5):052509.
52. Rida A, Fernandez V, Gijs MAM. Long-range transport of magnetic microbeads using simple planar coils placed in a uniform magnetostatic field. *Appl Phys Lett.* 2003 Sep 22;83(12):2396–8.
53. Beyzavi A, Nguyen NT. One-dimensional actuation of a ferrofluid droplet by planar microcoils. *J Phys D Appl Phys.* 2009 Jan 7;42(1):015004.
54. Aussillous P, Quéré D. Liquid marbles. *Nature.* 2001 Jun;411(6840):924–7.
55. McHale G, Newton MI. Liquid marbles: Principles and applications. *Soft Matter.* 2011;7(12):5473.
56. Zhao Y, Xu Z, Parhizkar M, Fang J, Wang X, Lin T. Magnetic liquid marbles, their manipulation and application in optical probing. *Microfluid Nanofluidics.* 2012 Oct 10;13(4):555–64.
57. Ooi CH, Nguyen NT. Manipulation of liquid marbles. *Microfluid Nanofluidics.* 2015 Sep 23;19(3):483–95.
58. Seo KS, Wi R, Im SG, Kim DH. A superhydrophobic magnetic elastomer actuator for droplet motion control. *Polym Adv Technol.* 2013 Dec;24(12):1075–80.
59. Biswas S, Pomeau Y, Chaudhury MK. New drop fluidics enabled by magnetic-field-mediated elastocapillary transduction. *Langmuir.* 2016 Jul 12;32(27):6860–70.
60. Wenzel RN. Surface roughness and contact angle. *J Phys Colloid Chem.* 1949 Sep 1;53(9):1466–7.
61. Zhou Q, Ristenpart WD, Stroeve P. Magnetically induced decrease in droplet contact angle on nanostructured surfaces. *Langmuir.* 2011 Oct 4;27(19):11747–51.
62. Wang L, Zhang M, Shi W, Hou Y, Liu C, Feng S, et al. Dynamic magnetic responsive wall array with droplet shedding-off properties. *Sci Rep.* 2015 Jun 10;5(1):11209.
63. Zhang Y, Nguyen NT. Magnetic digital microfluidics - a review. *Lab Chip.* 2017;17(6):994–1008.
64. Manukyan S, Schneider M. Experimental investigation of wetting with magnetic fluids. *Langmuir.* 2016 May 24;32(20):5135–40.
65. Nair N, Jani S. Magnetically controlled contact angle of ferrofluid encapsulated water droplet. *J Nanofluids.* 2018 Feb 1;7(1):26–9.
66. Sharma S, Bhatia V. Magnetic nanoparticles in microfluidics-based diagnostics: An appraisal. *Nanomedicine.* 2021 Jun;16(15):1329–42.

67. Shi X, Shao C, Luo C, Chu Y, Wang J, Meng Q, et al. Microfluidics-based enrichment and whole-genome amplification enable strain-level resolution for airway metagenomics. *mSystems.* 2019 Aug 27;4(4):e00198.
68. Chen H, Chen C, Bai S, Gao Y, Metcalfe G, Cheng W, et al. Multiplexed detection of cancer biomarkers using a microfluidic platform integrating single bead trapping and acoustic mixing techniques. *Nanoscale.* 2018;10(43):20196–206.
69. Churi HS, Dave S. Strategic synthesis of diagnostic novel materials against infectious diseases. In *Point-of-Care Biosensors for Infectious Diseases.* 2023 (pp. 209–33). Wiley-VCH GmbH.
70. Santhamoorthy M, Thirupathi K, Krishnan S, Guganathan L, Dave S, Phan TTV and Kim SC. Preparation of Magnetic Iron Oxide Incorporated Mesoporous Silica Hybrid Composites for pH and Temperature-Sensitive Drug Delivery. *Magnetochemistry* 2023;9(3):81.
71. Dave S, Dave S, Mathur A, Das J. Biological synthesis of magnetic nanoparticles. In *Nanobiotechnology* (pp. 225–234). Elsevier, 2021.
72. Dave S, Das Jayshankar. *Advanced Nanomaterials for Point of Care Diagnosis and Therapy.* Elsevier, 2022. https://doi.org/10.1016/C2020-0-02584-3.

12 Wearable Sensors and Their Advancement Using Nanotechnology

Barkha Tiwari and Sushma Dave

12.1 INTRODUCTION

An emerging trend in the human health management is the recent rapid advancements in the wearable and flexible functional devices, which have promoted monitoring human activities and improved traditional medical diagnosis with combined features like wearability, remote operation, comfortability, timely feedback, etc. Wearable devices for monitoring human activities could be utilized for the continuous, non-invasive, comfortable health assessment and vital real-time diagnosis to maintain their health regime. Measurement of various health-related signs such as muscle movement, body motion, heart rate, pulse rate, respiratory rate, skin and breath moisture, body temperature, electrophysiological signals (e.g., electrocardiogram (ECG), electromyogram (EMG), electroencephalogram (EEG) and electroglottogram (EGG)), and biochemical constituents (such as electrolytes) places huge demands on the development of conformal and flexible sensing devices [1,2]. Consequently, different kinds of wearable and flexible sensing devices are produced, such as strain/pressure sensors, humidity/temperature sensors, electrochemical sensors and integrated sensing platforms for the detection of health status [3–7]. Besides, electronic power devices have been integrated to wearable sensing devices as power sources through stretchable and flexible conductive wires as interconnection components. To be fixed on a human body or integrated with goods like textiles, the devices should be wearable, so their components should be highly flexible, i.e., stretchable, lightweight, human friendly and mechanically robust [8]. To develop such devices with stretchable and flexible properties, two important strategies have to be kept in mind, i.e., deformable structures and flexible materials [9–15]. Various materials incur this flexible property such as metal nanomaterials, advanced carbon materials and conductive polymers. Hence, these materials are used in the manufacturing of wearable electronic devices [16,17].

The advanced carbon materials when introduced in this chapter have been referred to carbon materials consisting of the crystal-like honeycomb structure that are formed using sp^2-bonded carbon atoms, like graphene, graphene oxide (GO), carbon nanotubes (CNTs), reduced graphene oxide (rGO) and other

DOI: 10.1201/9781003316435-12

materials of carbon such as carbon black, graphite and bio-derived natural carbon. When comparison is made among these materials, advanced carbon possesses some unique properties like good electrical conductivity, high thermal and chemical stability, low toxicity and ease of use, endowing them a great potential for the applications in flexible/wearable electronics [18,19]. Table 12.1 shows comparison of the basic properties in the metal materials and advanced materials. On the basis of the unique features of such materials, advanced carbon materials have been used widely as functional materials in stretchable and flexible biochemical and physical sensors and energy electronics for producing various smart flexible/wearable devices. In this chapter, we will focus on the progress in the controlled design preparation of various carbon materials with desired structures for various applications in high-performing, stretchable and flexible devices for the production of smart wearable gadgets. The macroscopic forms of carbon materials like fiber, film and foam are explained in this chapter for the applications of flexible and wearable devices.

The fabrication, design, function of design mechanism and its performance for various kinds of carbon-based materials that are stretchable/flexible were discussed in detail in this chapter, including temperature sensors, pressure/strain sensors, electrochemical sensors, humidity sensors and power devices. The applications that monitor human activities, health-related biomarkers, electrophysiological signals and other health-related signs are described in this chapter. Furthermore, integration of several sensors with energy storage and conversion devices through stretchable or flexible wires in multifunctional smart systems of wearable devices is also described. Finally, the challenges that exist and future perspectives in the field of carbon materials in the applications of wearable flexible healthcare systems have been discussed in this chapter [20]. Compared to the recent research done in this field that incorporated the fabrication of advanced carbon materials having varied morphologies to the development of physiological

TABLE 12.1
Comparison of Basic Properties of Advanced Carbon Materials and Metal Materials

	Electrical Conductivity	Chemical/ Thermal Stability	Chemical Modification	Metallic or Semiconductive	Morphology Variety	Lightweight
Advanced carbon materials	$0.17^{-2} \times 10^7$ S/m (CNTs) ~10^8 S/m (graphene)	Superior	Yes	Metallic, semi-metallic, semiconductive	Rich	Good
Metal materials	6.3×10^7 S/m (Ag bulk) 5.96×10^7 S/m (Cu bulk)	Inferior	No	Metallic	Poor	Poor

sensors, this chapter aims to fully review this new field for making an understanding of the design and unique features of carbon materials in the applications of flexible smart systems, including stretchable sensors like biochemical sensors and physiological sensors, flexible electrodes and power devices that are integrated as multifunctional wearable electronics.

The wearable devices have been expected to play an important role in monitoring human health in the field of medicine as they can continuously and even closely monitor an individuals' physical health status by identifying their activities. Their stretchability, high flexibility and conformability made these devices an ideal platform for designing future advanced healthcare devices. The emerging trends in materials science and nanotechnology have led to the development of smart wearable flexible devices in the field of medicine as shown in Figure 12.1. On this account, we would focus only on the new trends in the application of wearable devices for both chemical and physical sensing in this chapter.

In the following sections, we will mention the innovation of materials, fabrication of wearable device, design and integration of sensing systems to non-invasive devices for their flexible and wearable properties. Finally, the challenges and different opportunities in creating flexible devices that can be mounted on the skin for personalized health monitoring are also discussed in this chapter.

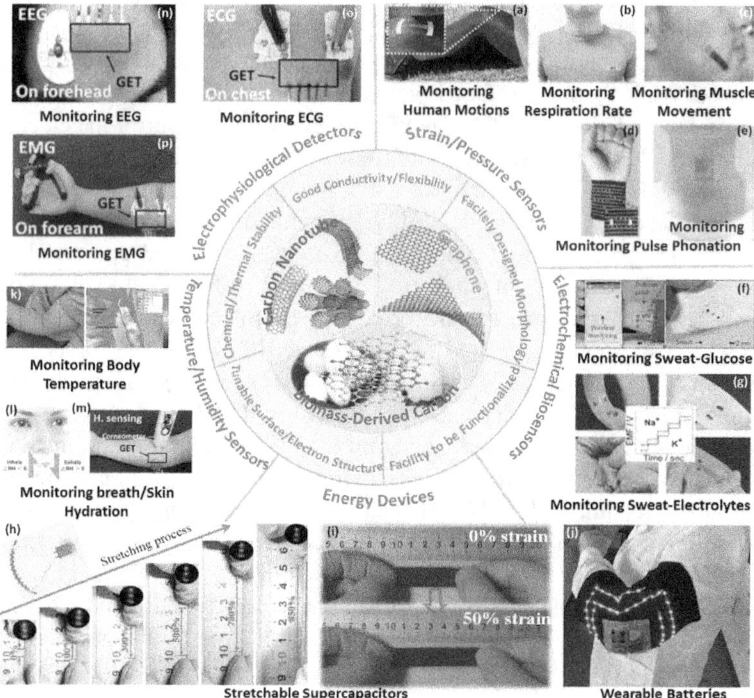

FIGURE 12.1 Materials and its applications in flexible and wearable devices for physical and chemical sensing.

12.2 MATERIALS AND DEVICE FABRICATION

As illustrated in Figure 12.1, main components in the typical configuration of a wearable device are the active layer, the interface layer between the components, and the substrate. The substrate for developing a device is usually a base, the active layer involves certain materials to add different functionalities, and the interface layer is important to some extent for keeping active layer or inside the base substrate. The layers of these devices must be well designed for the set target. The main layer, that is, active layer, is composed of electrical components or materials on its surface to add functionalities that are necessary for constructing the electronic devices on the wearable flexible substrate [21]. One of the widely explored flexible device materials are organic materials. In contrast to organic materials, inorganic materials have good physiochemical properties, high hole/electron mobility, mechanical strength, and chemical durability, so these can even be used as an active layer material to construct wearable flexible devices through physical lithography techniques. For example, graphene [23] and carbon nanotubes (CNTs) [22] are used as materials for active layer in the transistors and sensors, and semiconducting nanowires show very high performance as field-effect transistors on wearable substrates [24–26]. The composite materials like Ag nanoparticle and carbon nanotubes can be used in active conductive layer on wearable and flexible substrates [27]. To form an effective interface layer, the active layer between the substrate is very important, especially for operation of field-effect transistors. In the case of metal oxide semiconductor and single-walled carbon nanotube (SWCNT), the interface is very important to achieve gate controllability [28]. Thin layer of single SWCNT network is required to control the electrostatic operation of field-effect transistor, and these are gained only when SWCNTs and the substrate interlink in an attractive condition on the interface layer [29].

Because of their excellent flexibility, stretchability and conductivity, liquid metals are designed to initiate uniform coating on soft and curved electronic device surfaces because of their exceptional flexibility, stretchability, and conductivity. [30]. Gallium metal alloys and Galinstan (Ga/In/Sn) are among the most widely applicable liquid metals in electrodes and sensors as electrical components. These are ideal materials in structuring a wearable and flexible electronic skin device. Under extreme stretching, bending and twisting, other than contacts based on polymers and solid metals, the liquid metal interconnections can act as a "self-healing" wire to maintain good performance in electrical devices due to its fluidity [31–34]. As the process of preparing the components for the active layers is a prerequisite for the process of putting an active layer onto the substrate's surface. As defined in literature, physical transfer and the solution processes have been analyzed in this chapter. Nanowires directly get contacted to the substrate and then transferred in an aligned manner in the physical transfer method. For example, germanium nanowires are grown vertically onto the flat donor substrates that can be transferred through the mechanical shearing on to acceptor or germanium nanowires substrate that have been grown on a roller that can be transferred on to the substrate using a mechanical roller [35].

Such nanowire arrangements can be patterned using the photolithography technique and lift-off processes. Nanowire arrays showed high optoelectronic performance as a flexible polyimide substrate [36]. By means of van der Waals' and electrostatic interaction forces, the nanowires could be transferred on to the substrate surface which is flexible and stretchable. Uniform nanowires form an active layer that can serve as a high-mobility transistor to design and develop electronic skin devices.

To construct the active layers for a wearable device, solution transfer processes have been used widely because of its low temperature and greater suitability in the mass-production printing technology [37–39]. To form a printing ink, nanomaterials are mixed with organic materials to target the surface. SWCNT solutions were synthesized as the inks for printing applications. It is unavoidable to take into consideration that SWCNTs were rolled with surfactants to forbid aggregation in the printing ink solution. The design of the interaction between the substrate and the surfactant is critical to effectively form an active layer. To assemble field-effect transistor grade SWCNT networks, the percolation limit between the electrodes in less than the areal density of the randomly deposited SWCNTs [40]. Because of the bundled SWCNTs which shows a metallic behavior, the SWCNTs must be a single-layer thin carbon sheet. Otherwise, it is difficult to modulate the carriers to operate field-effect transistors. One of the effective deposition techniques was developed via cholate surfactants, like sodium cholate, to prepare SWCNT inks in combination with a designed substrate that was modified using amine-terminated interlayers, like poly-l-lysine (PLL) and 3-aminopropyl trimethoxy silane (APTES). For the design of sodium cholate surfactant and the interlayer of aminate which facilitates the assembly of SWCNTachieving around 90% effective coverage. However, alkyl chain-based surfactants can also scatter SWCNTs in an ink produced on a PLL-modified surface with poor assembly. As a result, the combined effect of the sodium cholate surfactant and the amine-terminated interlayer route is one of the effective ways to assemble SWCNTs quickly [41–43].

SWCNT network on polyethylene terephthalate (PET) is demonstrated as a substrate in this chapter at a scale of 1 m in length.

12.3 CARBON MATERIALS FOR WEARABLE STRAIN/PRESSURE SENSORS

Wearable electromechanical sensors, like strain and pressure sensors, that could be used to measure the pressure change and deformations by detecting pressure-incorporated electrical signals have attracted lot of attention due to their potential usage in monitoring human body movements such as joint motions and physiological signals like pulse, muscle and breathe rate [44–46]. The working mechanism of wearable pressure/strain sensors could be divided into four important types: capacitance-type, triboelectric-type, resistance-type and piezoelectric-type sensors. When we compare the sensors based on the above mechanism system, resistance-type sensors have double benefits of simple systems for reading out signals and simplicity in device fabrication, and meanwhile capacitance-type sensors have superior merits like linear and fast response that makes them attract a lot of research interest. The transduction mechanism along with development of wearable triboelectric-type pressure/strain and piezoelectric-type sensors has been researched and designed by some scientists [47,48]. Here, we will only summarize the advances in the usage of carbon-based materials that are flexible and wearable with resistance- or capacitance-type pressure/strain sensors.

Flexible, wearable, resistance-type pressure/strain sensors are mainly composed of certain electrically conductive elements for sensing that are coupled with elastic polymers and some other wearable stretchable substrates like fibers, yarns and textiles. Strain and pressure changes would incorporate the fluctuations of contact resistance between the conductive elements that could be detected by measuring systems of electrical devices, and similarly the detection of pressure and strain stimuli could be easily realized. Wearable capacitance-type pressure/strain sensors exhibit two flexible conductive layers that are well separated by an elastomer dielectric layer. The capacitance denoted in this case by C is related to area of the two conductive layers, thickness of the elastomer dielectric and the relative permittivity. When stimuli of pressure/strain are applied to the sensors, S or d changes, so the capacitance value also changes, thus enabling the detection of pressure/strain. The overall performance of wearable strain sensors is usually calculated via few important parameters, including sensitivity that is also known as gauge factor (GF), response time, sensing range and long-term stability. The GF is defined as the data obtained from the plots of relative capacitance/resistance change with respect to applied mechanical stimuli. The higher the GF, the higher the sensitivity. Wearable and conductive materials are desired in both capacitance-type and resistance-type pressure/strain sensors. Different types of nanomaterials such as metal nanowires/nanoparticles [49–53], graphene [54–60], carbon materials, graphite [61–67], natural biomaterial–derived carbon materials [74–76], carbon black [68,69] and their composites [70,71] have been applied to the sensing components for producing flexible resistance-type pressure/strain sensors due to their outstanding electrical and mechanical conductive properties. Metal nanoparticles/nanowires, graphene and carbon nanotubes have been excessively used and explored as the conductive layers for wearable capacitance-type sensors. Besides, elastomers that have low modulus, like polydimethylsiloxane PDMS and Ecoflex, and they have been designed as elastomeric dielectric materials. Compared to other metal nanomaterials [72–74], carbon materials have superior qualities like good flexibility, high stability, excellent electrical conductivity, and ability to have various morphologies, which benefit their applications in wearable pressure/strain sensors.

In the following, flexible pressure and strain sensors based on carbon materials like CNTs [77–79], graphite and graphene [80–83] as in the various macroscopic forms have been discussed. The details of important features of wearable capacitance-type and resistance-type pressure/strain sensors based on various active materials are presented in Tables 12.2 and 12.3. Carbon nanotubes have the

TABLE 12.2
Summary of Important Features of Wearable Capacitance-Type and Resistance-Type Strain Sensors

Active Materials	Working Mechanism	Strain Range	Sensitivity (GF)	Response Time (ms)	Ref.
Silver NWs	Resistance type	<70%	2–14	tunable H200	[45]
Platinum NPs	Resistance type	<2%	16 at 2% strain	—	[52]
Aligned SWCNT films	Resistance type	<280%	0.82 strain of 0%–40%, 60%–200%	14	[54]
Thickness-gradient CNT film	Resistance type	<150%	161 within 2% strain, 9.8, 0.58 within strain of 2%–15%, 5%–150%	—	[57]
Dry-spun CNT fiber	Resistance type	<960%	0.54 within 400% strain, 64 within strain of 400%–960%	10	[58]
Graphene mesh	Resistance type	<8%	500 within 2% strain, 10,000 at 8%	—	[56]
CNT-PDMS composite	Resistance type	<120%	27.8, 1084, 9617 within strain of 0%–40%, 40%–90%, 90%–120%	58	[88]
CNTs/PDMS/CNTs	Capacitance type	<300%	1.01	100	[80]
SWCNTs/silicone/SWCNTs	Capacitance type	<100%	0.99	—	[73]
Silver NWs/PDMS/Silver NWs	Capacitance type	<30%	–2	—	[77]
Silver NWs/PDMS/Silver NWs	Capacitance type	<50%	0.7	40	[78]
Crumpled/wrinkled graphene film	Resistance type	<70%	0.76, 1.67, 2.55 at 10%, 40%, 70% strain	—	[89]
Fish-scale linker rGO layer	Resistance type	<80%	16.2	—	[86]
rGO-based fiber	Resistance type	0.2%–100%	10, 3.7 within 1%,	< 100	[62]
Active Materials	**Working Mechanism**	**Strain Range**	**Sensitivity (GF)**	**Response Time (ms)**	**Ref.**
Carbonized silk fabric	Resistance type	<500%	9.6 within 250% strain, 37.5 within strain of 250%–500%	<70	[14]
Carbon black-PDMS composite	Resistance type	<80%	5.5, 1.8 within strain of 0%–10%, 10%–80%	—	[74]
3D graphene foam/CNT composite	Resistance type	<85%	2, 20.5 at 5%, 85% strain	30	[63]
Pencil-drawn graphite	Resistance type	–0.62% to 0.62%	150.5, 60.5, 53.6 within strain –0.62% to 0.32%	110	[66]

TABLE 12.3
Summary of Some Important Features of Wearable Capacitance-Type and Resistance-Type Pressure Sensors

Active Materials	Working Mechanism	Pressure Range	Sensitivity (GF)	Response Time (ms)	Ref.
Silver NWs	Resistance type	13 Pa–50 kPa	1.14 kPa	17	[50]
Au-coated PDMS micropillar/polyaniline	Resistance type	15 Pa–3.5 kPa	2 kPa^{-1} below 0.22 kPa	50	[52]
SWCNT film/micropatterned PDMS	Resistance type	0.6 Pa–1.2 kPa	1.8 kPa^{-1} below 0.3 kPa	<10	[54]
CNT-PDMS composite with microdome arrays	Resistance type	0.2 Pa–59 kPa	15.1 kPa^{-1} below 0.5 kPa	40	[57]
Hierarchically structured graphene	Resistance type	1 Pa–12 kPa	8.5 kPa^{-1}	40	[58]
Fingerprint-like 3D graphene film	Resistance type	0.2 Pa–75 kPa	110 kPa^{-1} below 200 Pa	30	[56]
CNT-graphene composite film	Resistance-type	0.6 Pa–6 kPa	19.8 kPa^{-1} below 0.3 kPa	16.7	[59]
rGO-coated polyureathane (PU) foam	Resistance type	<10 kPa	0.26 kPa^{-1} below 2 kPa	—	[65]
CNT-coated textile/Ni-coated textile	Resistance type	6 Pa–20 kPa	14.4 kPa^{-1} below 3.5 kPa	24	[62]
3D carbonized cotton sponge	Resistance type	<700 kPa	Ma. 6.04 kPa^{-1}	—	[86]
Carbonized silk nanofiber membrane	Resistance type	0.8 Pa–5 kPa	34.47 kPa^{-1} at 0.8–400 Pa	16.7	[63]
Silver NP-SBS composite/PDMS	Capacitance type	<20 kPa	0.21 kPa^{-1} below 2 kPa, 0.064 kPa^{-1} above 2 kPa	40	[66]
Silver NWs/PDMS	Capacitance type	<1.4 MPa	1.62 MPa^{-1} below 0.5 MPa, 0.57 MPa^{-1} above 0.5 MPa	40	[74]
CNT-Ecoflex composite film/microporous Ecoflex	Capacitance type	0.1 Pa–130 kPa	0.601 $kMPa^{-1}$ below 5 kPa, 0.077 kPa^{-1} at 30–130 kPa	—	[94]
CNT fiber/Ecoflex	Capacitance type	0.38 Pa–25 kPa	0.034–0.05 kPa^{-1} below 0.1 kPa	63	[77]

most promising properties as materials for highly wearable strain sensors due to their excellent electrical conductivity, outstanding flexibility and extremely large aspect ratio. CNTs (carbon nanotubes) having various formats like aligned CNT arrays, CNT films and CNT fibers are produced through wet or dry approaches. For example, a highly wearable [84] and stretchable strain sensor on the basis of thin film of aligned SWCNTs has been obtained directly due to its vertically aligned SWCNT array [85]. When tensile strain is applied, interstices and islets would grow throughout the SWCNT film along with the islets bridged via interconnection of SWCNT bundles. The stable and unique island-gap morphology provides the strain sensor a tolerable strain of nearly 280%, fast response and good durability, but low relative sensitivity (GF of 0.06 within strain of 60%–200% and 0.82 within strain of 0%–40%). Moreover, carbon nanotube fibers that could be directly dry spun from the super-aligned CNT arrays [86] are used for fabrication of strain sensors. By attaching a carbon nanotube fiber on a prestressed elastic substrate (Ecoflex), a CNT-based flexible or wearable strain sensor with high sensitivity, fast response, ultrahigh stretchability (bearable strain of H900%) and high durability can be produced. Such types of devices have relatively low reproduction quality and high cost. In future, when we will realize large-scale designing of carbon nanotubes along with controlled structures for developing new device fabrication with low cost, these strategies may promote the overall performance and practical applications of CNT-based strain sensors. Graphene, which contains exemplary flexibility with very good electrical conductivity, is one of the important materials for production of wearable strain sensors. There are two categories of graphene materials that have been endowed for wearable strain sensors: graphene grown by chemical vapor deposition (CVD) [87] and graphene grown from exfoliated graphite [88]. For pure graphene that is grown using CVD, the tolerable strain due to the corresponding strain sensors are usually smaller than the value of 1% [89] that limits its usage in wearable devices. In order to foster a wearable stretchability, graphene designed in different structures like graphene ripples, graphene films [91], crumpled/wrinkled graphene meshes [90] and 3D graphene interconnected foams has been synthesized. As compared to graphene grown using CVD method, the graphene exfoliated from pristine graphite has merits of mass production at low cost with benefiting practical applications. Including graphene materials that are derived from GO solutions could be produced in various formats like ribbons, fibers, sponges and films. When easily combined with some other materials, it can have various applications. The designed fabrication methods for forming various GO and rGO formats have been referred as an important part mentioned in this chapter. For example, a high performance with good efficiency of strain sensor with a fish-scale-like rGO film due to the sensing layer could be fabricated by adhering an rGO film onto a wearable-type substrate. The fish-scale type of microstructure provides the strain sensor added merits including a broad sensing range of 82% strain, excellent cycling stability and high sensitivity with a GF of 1.62.

From the above, wearable sensors like strain sensors based on carbon nanotubes and graphene normally show wide sensing range with low sensitivity or small sensing range with high sensitivity. Combining the 2D graphene with 1D nanomaterials that are conductive in nature like carbon nanotubes and Ag nanowires is an effective approach to improve the overall performance of strain sensors on the basis of mono nanocarbon materials. All the carbon interconnected network has been synthesized using techniques that consist of a 3D graphene–like network in foam form with carbon nanotubes grown on the graphene skeleton which could be utilized as wearable strain sensors. The cooperation of 1D carbon nanotubes in addition to the 3D graphene foam provide the strain sensors of 3D graphene foam/CNTs with huge sensing range near to 85% strain and endows high sensitivity than the pure 3DGF. Apart from carbon nanotubes and graphene, other types of carbon materials like carbon black, graphite and natural biomaterial–derived carbon with relatively low cost are also applied as a wearable strain sensor. For example, the carbon form graphite could be easily deposited on wearable flexible substrates via drawing by using a pencil that could further be applied for fabricating of flexible strain sensors. On the basis of the reversible disconnection in the graphite flakes of the paper, such graphite-based strain sensor can be used to detect bending-induced compressive/tensile strain with a very high sensitivity (GF of 150.5, 60.6 and 536.6 in the strain range from –0.62% to +0.32%, –0.22% to 0.22% and 0.32%, respectively). Besides, carbon black and graphite powder could even be combined with polymers to make conductive inks which could be used to fabricate wearable strain sensors via printing technique [92]. In order to create patterned graphite thin films for wearable, stretchable strain sensors, glue, like graphite, is made of methylcellulose and graphite that were printed on a wearable, flexible paper.

Neatly designed or patterned large-scale graphite films with different sizes and shapes (morphologies) could be facilely procured via printing. Due to the micro/nano-cracked contact reversible effect, strain sensors show fast response and high sensitivity to compression and tension deformations. Various naturally occurring biomaterials like silk, corncobs [93], cotton and mushrooms [94] could also be used as carbon materials. Naturally occurring bio-derived carbon materials have certain merits such as renewable resource, low-cost production, large-scale capability with human benignity and environmentally friendliness. But certain demerits and limitations are also there in using biomaterials to synthesize carbon materials like low carbon yield and the relatively low quality, which usually result in low electrical conductivity and mechanical property [96]. However, the versatile structures of hierarchical morphologies of natural biomaterials provide plenty of room for synthesizing materials like carbon with desired microstructures, thus allowing the naturally derived biomaterial carbon to emerge as active sensing components for strain sensors. The hierarchical structures, i.e., yearns, which are actually composed of twisted or paralleled microfibers of the fabrics like knitted fabrics and woven fabrics, play a pivotal role in achieving very high performance of strain sensors. The sensing performance of such wearable strain sensors could be tuned by selecting various woven structures that are desired for practical usage. For example, the wearable flexible strain sensors derived from plain weave silk fabric have shown high sensitivity and ultra-stretchability with tolerable strain

>500% and a GF of 9.6 within 250% strain [95]. On the contrary, wearable strain sensors having carbonized silk georgette, both warp yarns and weft are collected of highly twisted fibers and act as an active material consisting ultralow detection limit 0.01% strain and superior sensitivity but with smaller range of sensing GF of 29.7 within 40% strain. Apart from the fabric derived from hierarchically structured carbon, flexible and transparent nanostructured carbon derived from electrospun membranes of silk nanofibers [98] has also been researched for flexible and wearable strain sensors with extremely high sensitivity and transparency [97]. The previous work or research already shows the immense potential of bio-derived natural materials like carbon for high performance of strain sensors. However, still several other possibilities of natural biomaterial–derived carbon that has unique microstructures shows potential but have not been yet researched for wearable flexible strain sensors. Capacitance-type strain sensors designed using carbon materials have also been synthesized. Typically, resistance-type, carbon-based strain sensors have hysteresis and irreversibility under fast and linear response, in contrast to capacitance-type strain sensors which have superior fast and linear response. Wearable stretchable electrodes of the capacitance-type strain sensors show great promise due to the extremely high length to diameter ratio, mechanical robustness, and interlinking between macro-assemblies of carbon nanotubes and carbon nanotubes, such as CNT films and networks.

A pioneer work utilizing carbon materials that are stretchable/wearable/flexible conductive electrodes reported that networks of SWCNTs were sprayed on PDMS substrates to design a capacitive strain sensor in the form of skin-like structures with a tolerable range of strain up to 50% and a GF value of 0.969. Compared to the carbon nanotube films that were fabricated using spraying and then filtration techniques, CNT films obtained from the floating catalyst CVD show more interlinking and curvilinear attributes. This makes CNT films suitable for producing stretchable and transparent devices. By joining carbon nanotubes films with silicone elastomers, superstretchable, transparent, capacitance-type strain sensors were fabricated, which detect maximum strain up to 300% and reveal a linear response in all the whole range of sensing with a GF of nearly 1.0. Graphene and some other types of carbon materials have been rarely studied for usage in wearable and flexible capacitance-type strain sensors because of the lack of intrinsic stretchability.

12.4 WEARABLE ELECTRONIC DEVICES

The tremendous growth in the flexible sensor devices have seen hindrance due to the lack of anatomically compliant power sources [99,100]. Innovative efforts have been done in the past years that have led to the demonstration of implantable BFCs (BIO FUEL CELLS) in different organisms [101]. But the difficulties faced by implantable BFCs would lead to recent explorations of non-invasive flexible BFCs that gather energy from biofuels [100]. The old platform merging an enzymatic BFCs with flexible technologies is a very attractive method for harvesting energy via human perspiration. Based on a bioanode along with cathode that is printed on a temporary tattoo for the first epidermal BFC used in extracting bioenergy from sweat lactate during exercising pattern [102]. Such devices mostly relied on the oxidation process of the lactate biofuel, mediated by tetrathiafulvalene (TTF) and catalyzed by lactate oxidase (LOx). The electron shuffling between the electrode and LOx was enhanced using an electron-acceptor and electron-donor TTF/CNT interface. Non-penetrating operation that is demonstrated by attaching the BFC tattoo on human subjects in the process of exercise enables power densities nearly 70 $\mu W/cm^2$. Such concept was analyzed further on substrates of textiles, and this could lead to a light emitting diode using an integrated DC/DC converter [103].

Several mechanical stresses are experienced by epidermal BFCs during its practical applications which lead to the deteriorated performance as the conductive support is cracked that anchors the enzyme. To address such challenges, researchers have designed screen-printable flexible inks that involve mechanical and electrochemical properties of carbon nanotubes along with the flexible properties of a binder, i.e., polyurethane, with a free-standing design of serpentine. Now interfacing these stress-enduring inks with the serpentine configuration thus offers an additional degree of flexibility, which represents the first platform for the flexible/stretchable enzymatic BFCs. Now enhancing the overall power density is attained by wearable BFCs thus require optimization of the quantity of incorporated enzyme, conductive components and mediator [104]. To boost the loading levels of these components, compressed bioanode pellets have been developed. Since such approaches might compromise with the mechanical properties, efforts need to be made to create flexible island-bridge microstructures combined with the high enzyme loading of pellet islands along with the stretchable serpentine bridge interconnects [105]. Such unique kind of architectures thus result in a soft device known as bioelectronic skin for getting relatively very high energy due to the human perspiration, thus leading to a power density of 1.2 mW. Such skin-worn flexible BFCs thus give an outcome power of ~1 mW during the fitness routine/exercise which is sufficient to power an electronic device. Including all this, we describe that the first and foremost example of very high flexible textile-based BFCs could be applied as self-powered sensors, thus extracting electrical signal/power from sweat lactose and glucose [106]. Scavenged bioenergy prepared using the wearer's sweat itself could be utilized directly to determine the metabolic levels, thus minimizing the demand for external energy sources.

Unlike precedented BFCs that are based on oxygen reduction cathodes which may fall into an anaerobic condition, the textile BFC was dependent on an Ag_2O/Ag cathode. Such type of electrode "cathode" is independent of the oxygen reduction, thus allowing generation of power under the fluctuation of oxygen-rich concentrations. Alternatively, for the operation under severe oxygen-deficit conditions, we can possibly use oxygen-rich cathode [107]. A minimally spread, microneedle-based BFC was analyzed via integration of enzyme carbon pastes inside a hollow microneedle. This type of system shows glucose level–dependent outputs of power toward utility in self-powered uniform glucose observation without limitation of battery life. Due to its high selectivity against interferences of electroactive, carbon paste offers favorable storage life and stability as the enzymes confined in a hydrophobic matrices of carbon paste minimize overall protein mobility [108]. Such a small quantity invasive system thus needs critical assessment for biocompatibility. Redox mediators are dependent on many BFCs that shuttle electrons between electrode and the enzyme-active site. The usage of mediators gives rise to several concerns for production of flexible electronic devices, including instability and no safety due to leaching and toxicity. An alternative environmentally friendly approach is based on the usage of edible electrode components with inclusion of plant and mushroom extracts as biocatalyst BFC system [109].

The system relies on oxygen and ethanol-oxidation reduction biocatalytic systems coupled with natural mediators. This system has the potential to be further applicable as a self-powered flexible ethanol biosensing in particular for applications with biocompatibility.

REFERENCES

1. Choi S., Lee H., Ghaffari R., Hyeon T., Kim D. H. Recent advances in flexible and stretchable bio-electronic devices integrated with nanomaterials. *Adv. Mater.* 2016; 28:4203. Available from: https://onlinelibrary.wiley.com/doi/10.1002/adma.201504150. doi: 10.1002/adma.201504150.
2. Khan Y., Ostfeld A. E., Lochner C. M., Pierre A., Arias A. C. Monitoring of vital signs with flexible and wearable medical devices. *Adv. Mater.* 2016; 28:4373. Available from: https://onlinelibrary.wiley.com/doi/10.1002/adma.201504366. doi: 10.1002/adma.201504366.
3. Zang Y., Zhang F., Di C., Zhu D. Advances of flexible pressure sensors toward artificial intelligence and health care applications. *Mater. Hariz* 2015; 2:140. Available from: https://pubs.rsc.org/en/content/articlelanding/2015/mh/c4mh00147h. doi: 10.1039/C4MH00147H.
4. Kim S. Y., Park S., Park H. W., Park D. H., Jeong Y., Kim D. H. Highly sensitive and multimodal all-carbon skin sensors capable of simultaneously detecting tactile and biological stimuli. *Adv. Mater.* 2015; 27:4178. Available from: https://onlinelibrary.wiley.com/doi/10.1002/adma.201501408. doi: 10.1002/adma.201501408.
5. Han S., Kim M. K., Wang B., Wie D. S., Wang S., Lee C. H. Mechanically reinforced skin-electronics with networked nanocomposite elastomer. *Adv. Mater.* 2016; 28:10257. Available from: https://onlinelibrary.wiley.com/doi/10.1002/adma.201603878. doi: 10.1002/adma.201603878.
6. Hong S. Y., Lee Y. H., Park H., Jin S. W., Jeong Y. R., Yun J., You I., Zi G., Ha J. S. Stretchable active-matrix temperature sensor array of polyaniline nanofibers for electronic skin. *Adv. Mater.* 2016; 28:930. Available from: https://onlinelibrary.wiley.com/doi/10.1002/adma.201504659. doi: 10.1002/adma.201504659.
7. Windmiller J. R., Wang J. Wearable electrochemical sensors and biosensors: A review. *Electroanalysis.* 2013; 25:29. Available from: https://analyticalsciencejournals.onlinelibrary.wiley.com/doi/10.1002/elan.201200349. doi: 10.1002/elan.201200349.
8. Kim D.-H., Rogers J. A. Stretchable electronics: materials strategies and devices. *Adv. Mater.* 2008; 20:4887. Available from: https://onlinelibrary.wiley.com/doi/abs/10.1002/adma.200801788. doi: 10.1002/adma.200801788.

9. Chortos A., Koleilat G. I., Pfattner R., Kong D., Lin P., Nur R., Lei T., Wang H., Liu N., Lai Y. C. Mechanically durable and highly stretchable transistors employing carbon nanotube semiconductor and electrodes. *Adv. Mater.* 2016; 28:4441. Available from: https://onlinelibrary.wiley.com/doi/10.1002/adma.201501828. doi: 10.1002/adma.201501828.
10. Chortos A., Zhu C., Oh J. Y., Yan X., Pochorovski I., To J. W.-F., Liu N., Kraft U., Murmann B., Bao Z. Stretchable self-healing polymeric dielectrics cross-linked through metal-ligand coordination. *ACS Nano* 2017; 11:7925. Available from: https://pubs.acs.org/doi/10.1021/jacs.6b02428. doi: 10.1021/jacs.6b02428.
11. Liu N., Chortos A., Lei T., Jin L., Kim T. R., Bae W.-G., Zhu C., Wang S., Pfattner R., Chen X. Ultra-transparent and stretchable graphene electrodes. *Chem. Sci. Adv.* 2017; 3:1700159. Available from: https://www.science.org/doi/10.1126/sciadv.1700159. doi:10.1126/sciadv.1700159.
12. Wang Y., Zhu C., Pfattner R., Yan H., Jin L., Chen S., Molina-Lopez F., Lissel F., Liu J., Rabiah N. I. A highly stretchable, transparent and conductive polymer. *Sci. Adv.* 2017; 3:1602076. Available from: https://www.science.org/doi/10.1126/sciadv.1602076. doi: 10.1126/sciadv.1602076.
13. Xu J., Wang S., Wang G.-J. N., Zhu C., Luo S., Jin L., Gu X., Chen S., Feig V. R., To J. W. Design of intrinsically stretchable and highly conductive polymers for fully stretchable electrochromic devices. *Science* 2017; 355:59. Available from: https://www.nature.com/articles/s41598-020-73259-x. doi: 10.1038/s41598-020-73259-x.
14. Wang C., Zhang M., Xia K., Gong X., Wang H., Yin Z., Guan B., Zhang Y. Flexible and highly sensitive pressure sensors based on bionic hierarchical structures. *ACS Appl. Mater. Interfaces* 2017; 9:1333. Available from: https://onlinelibrary.wiley.com/doi/abs/10.1002/adfm.201606066. doi: 10.1002/adfm.201606066.
15. Zhang M., Wang C., Liang X., Yin Z., Xia K., Wang H., Jian M., Zhang Y. Advanced carbon for flexible and wearable electronics. *Adv. Electron Mater.* 2017;3:201700193. Available from: https://onlinelibrary.wiley.com/doi/abs/10.1002/adma.201801072. doi: 10.1002/adma.201801072.
16. Gong S., Cheng W. One-dimensional nanomaterials for soft electronics. *Adv. Electron. Mater.* 3:1600314. Available from: https://onlinelibrary.wiley.com/doi/10.1002/aelm.201600314. doi: 10.1002/aelm.201600314.
17. Yao S., Swetha P., Zhu Y. (2018) Nanomaterial-enabled wearable sensors for healthcare. *Adv. Healthcare Mater.* 2017; 7:1700889. Available from: https://onlinelibrary.wiley.com/doi/10.1002/adhm.201700889. doi: 10.1002/adhm.201700889.
18. Chen K., Gao W., Emamineiad S., Kiriya D., Ota H., Nyein H. Y. Y., Takei K., Jayey A. Fully integrated wearable sensor arrays for multiplexed in situ perspiration analysis. *Adv. Mater.* 2016; 28:4397. Available from: https://www.nature.com/articles/nature16521. doi: 10.1038/nature16521.
19. Jang H., Park Y. J., Chen X., Das T., Kim M. S., Ahn J. H. Graphene based flexible and stretchable electronics. *Adv. Mater.* 2016; 28:4184. Available from: https://onlinelibrary.wiley.com/doi/10.1002/adma.201504245. doi: 10.1002/adma.201504245.
20. Jian M., Wang C., Wang Q., Wang H., Xia K., Yin Z., Zhang M., Liang X., Zhang Y. Extremely black vertically aligned carbon nanotube arrays for solar steam generation. *Sci. China Mater.* 2017; 60:1026. Available from: https://pubs.acs.org/doi/10.1021/acsami.7b08619. doi: 10.1021/acsami.7b08619.
21. Takahashi T., Takei K., Adabi E., Fan Z., Nikneiad A. M., Jayey A. Parallel array InAs nanowire transistor for mechanically bendable, ultrahigh frequency electronics. *ACS Nano.* 2010; 4:5855. Available from: https://pubs.acs.org/doi/10.1021/nn1018329. doi: 10.1021/nn1018329.

22. Fan Z., Ho J. C., Takahashi T., Yerushalmi R., Takei K., Ford A. C., Chueh Y. L., Jayey A. Toward the development of printable nanowire electronics and sensors. *Adv. Mater.* 2009; 21:3730. Available from: https://onlinelibrary.wiley.com/doi/10.1002/adma.200900860. doi: 10.1002/adma.200900860.
23. Nomura K., Ohta H., Takagi A., Kamiya T., Hirano M., Hosono H. Room temperature fabrication of transparent flexible thin film transistors using amorphous oxide semiconductors. *Nature.* 2004; 432:488. Available from: https://www.nature.com/articles/nature03090. doi: 10.1038/nature03090.
24. Takei K., Yu Z., Zheng M., Ota H., Takahashi T., Jayey A. Highly sensitive electronic whiskers based on patterned carbon nanotube and silver nanoparticle composite films. *Proc. Natl. Acad. Sci. USA.* 2014; 111:1703. Available from: https://www.pnas.org/doi/full/10.1073/pnas.1317920111. doi: 10.1073/pnas.1317920111.
25. Takahashi T., Takei K., Gillies A. G., Fearing R. S., Jayey A. Carbon nanotube active-matrix backplanes for conformal electronics and sensors. *Nano Lett.* 2011; 11:5408. Available from: https://pubs.acs.org/doi/10.1021/nl203117h. doi: 10.1021/nl203117h.
26. Sangwan V. K., Oritz R. P., Alabison J. M. P., Emery J. D., Bedzyk M. J., Lauhon L. J., Marks T. J., Hersam M. C. Fundamental performance limits of carbon nanotube thin-film transistors achieved using hybrid molecular dielectrics. *ACS Nano.* 2012; 6:7480. Available from: https://pubs.acs.org/doi/10.1021/nn302768h. doi: 10.1021/nn302768h.
27. Kiriya D., Chen K., Ota H., Lin Y. J., Zhao P. D., Yu Z. B., Ha T. J., Jayey A. A design of surfactant substrate interaction for roll-to-roll assembly of carbon nanotubes for thin-film transistors. *J. Am. Chem. Soc.* 2014; 136:11188. Available from: https://pubs.acs.org/doi/10.1021/ja506315j. doi: 10.1021/ja506315j.
28. Daeneke T., Khoshmanesh K., Mahmood N., de Castro I. A., Esrafilzadeh D., Barrow S. J., Dickey M. D., Kalantar Zadeh K. Liquid metals: fundamental and applications in chemistry. *Chem. Soc. Rev.* 2018; 47:4073. Available from: https://pubs.rsc.org/en/content/articlelanding/2018/CS/C7CS00043J. doi: 10.1039/C7CS00043J.
29. Ota H., Chen K., Lin Y., Kiriya D., Shiraki H., Yu Z., Ha T. J., Jayey A. Highly deformable liquid state heterojunction sensors. *Nat. Commun.* 2014; 5:5032. Available from: https://www.nature.com/articles/ncomms6032. doi: 10.1038/ncomms6032.
30. Gao Y., Ota H., Schaler E. W., Chen K., Zhao A., Gao W., Fahad H. M., Leng Y., Zheng A., Xiong F., Zhang C., Tai L. C., Zhao P., Fearing R. S., Jayey A. Wearable microfluidic diaphragm pressure sensor for health and tactile touch monitoring. *Adv. Mater.* 2017; 29:1701985. Available from: https://onlinelibrary.wiley.com/doi/10.1002/adma.201701985. doi: 10.1002/adma.201701985.
31. Ota H., Emaminejad S., Gao Y., Zhao A., Wu E., Challa S., Chen K., Fahad H. M., Jha A. K., Kiriya D., Gao W., Shiraki H., Morioka K., Ferguson A. R., Healy K. E., Davis R. W., Jayey A. Application of 3 D printing for smart objects with embedded electronic sensors and systems. *Adv. Mater. Technol.* 2016; 1:1600013. Available from: https://onlinelibrary.wiley.com/doi/abs/10.1002/admt.201600013. doi: 10.1002/admt.201600013.
32. Ota H., Chao M., Gao Y., Wu E., Tai L. C., Chen K., Matsuoka Y., Iwai K., Fahad H. M., Gao W., Nyein H. Y. Y., Lin L., Jayey A. 3D printed "earable" smart devices for real-time detection of core body temperature. *ACS Sens.* 2017; 2:990. Available from: https://pubs.acs.org/doi/10.1021/acssensors.7b00247. doi: 10.1021/acssensors.7b00247.

33. Park Y. L., Chen B. R., Wood R. J. Design and fabrication of soft artificial skin using embedded microchannels and liquid conductors. *IEEE Sens. J.* 2012; 12:2711. Available from: https://ieeexplore.ieee.org/document/6203551. doi: 10.1109/JSEN.2012.2200790.
34. Yerushalmi R., Jacobson Z. A., Ho J. C., Fan Z., Jayey A. Large scale, highly ordered assembly of nanowire parallel arrays by differential roll printing. *Appl. Phys. Lett.* 2007; 91:203104. Available from: https://pubs.aip.org/aip/apl/article/91/20/203104/325171/Large-scale-highly-ordered-assembly-of-nanowire. doi: 10.1063/1.2813618.
35. Fan Z., Ho J. C., Jacobson Z. A., Razayi H., Jayey A. Large scale, heterogeneous integration of nanowire arrays for iamge sensor circuitry. *Proc. Natl. Acad. Sci. USA*. 2008; 105:11066. Available from: https://www.pnas.org/doi/full/10.1073/pnas.0801994105. doi: 10.1073/pnas.0801994105.
36. Arias A. C., Mackenzie J. D., McCulloch I., Riynay J., Sallen A. Materials and applications for large area electronics: Solution-based approaches. *Chem. Rev.* 2010; 110:3. Available from: https://pubs.acs.org/doi/10.1021/cr900150b. doi: 10.1021/cr900150b.
37. Fujisaki Y., Koga H., Nakajima Y., Nakata M., Tsuji H., Yamamoto T., Kurita T., Nogi M., Shimidzu N. Transparent nanopaper based flexible organic thin-film transistor array. *Adv. Funct. Mater.* 2014; 24:1657. Available from: https://onlinelibrary.wiley.com/doi/abs/10.1002/adfm.201303024. doi: 10.1002/adfm.201303024.
38. Yeom C., Chen K., Kiriya D., Yu Z., Cho G., Jayey A. Large-area compliant tactile sensors using printed carbon nanotube active-matrix backplanes. *Adv. Mater.* 2015; 27:1561. Available from: https://onlinelibrary.wiley.com/doi/10.1002/adma.201404850. doi: 10.1002/adma.201404850.
39. Sangwan V., Behman A., Ballarotto V., Fuhrer M., Ural A., Williams E. Optimizing transistor performance of percolating carbon nanotube networks. *Appl. Phys. Lett.* 2010; 97:043111. Available from: https://pubs.aip.org/aip/apl/article/97/4/043111/986861/Optimizing-transistor-performance-of-percolating. doi: 10.1063/1.3469930.
40. Takei K., Takahashi T., Ho J. C., Ko H., Gillies A. G., Leu P. W., Fearing R. S., Jayey A. Nanowire active-matrix circuitry for low voltage macroscale artificial skin. *Nat. Mater.* 2010; 9:821. Available from: https://www.nature.com/articles/nmat2835. doi: 10.1038/nmat2835.
41. Wang C., Hwang D., Yu Z., Takei K., Park J., Chen T., Ma B., Jayey A. User interactive electronic skin for instantaneous pressure visualization. *Nat. Mater.* 2013; 12:899. Available from: https://www.nature.com/articles/nmat3711. doi: 10.1038/nmat3711.
42. Harada S., Honda W., Arie T., Akita S., Takei K. Fully printed, highly sensitive multifunctional artificial electronic whisker arrays integrated with strain and temperature sensors. *ACS Nano* 2014; 8:3921. Available from: https://pubs.acs.org/doi/10.1021/nn500845a. doi: 10.1021/nn500845a.
43. Yamamoto Y., Harada S., Yamamoto D., Honda W., Arie T., Akita S., Takei K. Printed multifunctional flexible device with an integrated motion sensor for health care monitoring. *Sci. Adv.* 2016; 2:1601473. Available from: https://www.science.org/doi/10.1126/sciadv.1601473. doi: 10.1126/sciadv.1601473.
44. Yang T., Xie D., Li Z., Zhu H. Recent advances in wearable tactile sensors: Materials, sensing mechanisms and device performance. *Mater. Sci. Eng.* 2017; 115:1. Available from: https://www.sciencedirect.com/science/article/abs/pii/S0927796X16301231. doi: 10.1016/j.mser.2017.02.001.

45. Amjadi M., Kyung K. U., Park I., Sitti M. Stretchable, skin-mountable and wearable strain sensors and their potential applications: A review. *Adv. Funct. Mater.* 2016; 26:1678. Available from: https://onlinelibrary.wiley.com/doi/abs/10.1002/adfm.201504755. doi: 10.1002/adfm.201504755.
46. Liu M., Pu X., Jiang C., Liu T., Huang X., Chen L., Du C., Sun J., Hu W., Wang Z. L. Large-area all textile pressure sensors for monitoring human motion and physiological signals. *Adv. Mater.* 2017; 29:1703700. Available from: https://onlinelibrary.wiley.com/doi/10.1002/adma.201703700. doi: 10.1002/adma.201703700.
47. Wang X., Dong L., Zhang H., Yu R., Pan C., Wang Z. L. Photocatalytic organic pollutants degradation in metal-organic frameworks. *Adv. Sci.* 2015; 2:1500169. Available from: https://pubs.rsc.org/en/content/articlelanding/2014/ee/c4ee01299b. doi: 10.1039/C4EE01299B.
48. Tran Quang T., Lee N. E. Flexible and stretchable physical sensor integrated platforms for wearable human- activity monitoring and personal healthcare. *Adv. Mater.* 2016; 28:4338. Available from: https://onlinelibrary.wiley.com/doi/10.1002/adma.201504244. doi: 10.1002/adma.201504244.
49. Pang C., Lee G. Y., Kim T., Kim S. M., Kim H. N., Ahn S. H., Suh K. Y. A flexible and highly sensitive strain-gauge sensor using reversible interlocking of nanofibers. *Nat. Mater.* 2012; 11:795. Available from: https://www.nature.com/articles/nmat3380. doi: 10.1038/nmat3380.
50. Amjadi M., Pichtipajongkit A., Lee S., Ryu S., Park I. Highly stretchable and sensitive strain sensor based on silver nanowire-elastomer nanocomposite. *ACS Nano* 2014; 8:5154. Available from: https://pubs.acs.org/doi/10.1021/nn501204t. doi: 10.1021/nn501204t.
51. Gong S., Schwalb W., Wang Y., Chen Y., Tang Y., Si J., Shirinzadeh B., Cheng W. A wearable and highly sensitive pressure sensor with ultrathin gold nanowires. *Nat. Commun.* 2014; 5:3132. Available from: https://www.nature.com/articles/ncomms4132. doi: 10.1038/ncomms4132.
52. Park B., Kim J., Kang D., Jeong C., Kim K. S., Kim J. U., Yoo P. J., Kim T. I. Dramatically enhanced mechanosenstivity and signal-to-noise ratio of nanoscale crack-based sensors: Effect of crack depth. *Adv. Mater.* 2016; 28:8130. Available from: https://onlinelibrary.wiley.com/doi/10.1002/adma.201602425. doi: 10.1002/adma.201602425.
53. Su M., Li F., Chen S., Huang Z., Qin M., Li W., Zhang X., Song Y. Nanoparticle based curve arrays for multirecognition flexible electronics. *Adv. Mater.* 2016; 28:1369. Available from: https://onlinelibrary.wiley.com/doi/10.1002/adma.201504759. doi: 10.1002/adma.201504759.
54. Yamada T., Hayamizu Y., Yamamoto Y., Yomogida Y., Izadi Najafabadi A., Futaba D. N., Hata K. A stretchable carbon nanotube strain sensor for human motion detection. *Nat. Nanotechnol.* 2011; 6:296. Available from: https://www.nature.com/articles/nnano.2011.36/. doi: 10.1038/nnano.2011.36.
55. Steven E., Saleh W. R., Lebedev V., Acquah S. F., Laukhin V., Alamo R. G., Brooks J. S. Carbon nanotubes on a spider silk scaffold. *Nat. Commun.* 2013; 4:2435. Available from: https://www.mendeley.com/catalogue/2feb6595-a231-3a2d-b8b7-ec1f144a7077/. doi: 10.1038/ncomms3435.
56. Park J., Lee Y., Hong J., Lee Y., Ha M., Jung Y., Lim H., Kim S. Y., Ko H. Tactile-direction-sensitive and stretchable skins based on human-skin-inspired interlocked microstructures. *ACS Nano* 2014; 8:12020. Available from: https://pubs.acs.org/doi/10.1021/nn505953t. doi: 10.1021/nn505953t.

57. Liu Z., Qi D., Guo P., Liu Y., Zhu B., Yang H., Liu Y., Li B., Zhang C., Yu J. Thickness gradient films for high gauge factor stretchable strain sensors. *Adv. Mater.* 2015; 27:6230. Available from: https://onlinelibrary.wiley.com/doi/10.1002/adma.201503288. doi: 10.1002/adma.201503288.
58. Ryu S., Lee P., Chou J. B., Xu R., Zhao R., Hart A. J., Kim S. G. Extremely elastic wearable carbon nanotube fiber strain sensor for monitoring of human motion. *ACS Nano* 2015; 9:5929. Available from: https://pubs.acs.org/doi/10.1021/acsnano.5b00599. doi: 10.1021/acsnano.5b00599.
59. Wang Y., Yang R., Shi Z., Zhang L., Shi D., Wang E., Zhang G. Super elastic graphene ripples for flexible strain sensors. *ACS Nano* 2011; 5:3645. Available from: https://pubs.acs.org/doi/10.1021/nn103523t. doi: 10.1021/nn103523t.
60. Boland C. S., Khan U., Backes C., O'Neil A., McCauley J., Duane S., Shanker R., Liu Y., Jurewicz I., Dalton A. B. Sensitive, high-strain, high-rate bodily motion sensors based on graphene-rubber composites. *ACS Nano* 2014; 8:8819. Available from: https://pubs.acs.org/doi/10.1021/nn503454h. doi: 10.1021/nn503454h.
61. Yan C., Wang J., Kang W., Cui M., Wang X., Foo C. Y., Chee K. J., Lee P. S. Highly stretchable piezoresistive graphene nanocellulose nanopaper for strain sensors. *Adv. Mater.* 2014; 26:2022. Available from: https://onlinelibrary.wiley.com/doi/10.1002/adma.201304742. doi: 10.1002/adma.201304742.
62. Cheng Y., Wang R., Sun J., Gao L. A stretchable and highly sensitive graphene-based fibre for sensing tensile strain, bending, and torsion. *Adv. Mater.* 2015; 27:7365. Available from: https://pubmed.ncbi.nlm.nih.gov/26479040/. doi: 10.1002/adma.201503558.
63. Liu Q., Zhang M., Huang L., Li Y., Chen J., Li C., Shi G. High quality graphene ribbons prepared from graphene oxide hydrogels and their applications for strain sensors. *ACS Nano* 2015; 9:12320. Available from: https://pubmed.ncbi.nlm.nih.gov/26481766/. doi: 10.1021/acsnano.5b05609.
64. Qin Y., Peng Q., Ding Y., Lin Z., Wang C., Li Y., Xu F., Li J., Yuan Y., He X. Lightweight mechanically flexible and thermally superinsulating rGO/polyimide nanocomposite foam with an anisotropic microstructure. *ACS Nano* 2015; 9:8933. Available from: https://pubs.rsc.org/en/content/articlehtml/2019/na/c9na00444k. doi: 10.1039/C9NA00444K.
65. Yang T., Wang W., Zhang H., Li X., Shi J., He Y., Zheng Q. S., Li Z., Zhu H. Tactile sensing system based on arrays of graphene woven microfabrics: electromechanical behaviour and electronic skin application. *ACS Nano* 2015; 9:10867. Available from: https://pubs.acs.org/doi/10.1021/acsnano.5b03851. doi: 10.1021/acsnano.5b03851.
66. Liao X., Liao Q., Yan X., Liang Q., Si H., Li M., Wu H., Cao S., Zhang Y. Flexible and highly sensitive strain sensors fabricated by pencil drawn for wearable monitor. *Adv. Funct. Mater.* 2015; 25:2395. Available from: https://onlinelibrary.wiley.com/doi/abs/10.1002/adfm.201500094. doi: 10.1002/adfm.201500094.
67. Amjadi M., Turan M., Clementson C. P., Sitti M. Parallel microcracks-based ultrasensitive and highly stretchable strain sensors. *ACS Appl. Mater. Interfaces* 2016; 8:5618. Available from: https://pubmed.ncbi.nlm.nih.gov/26842553/. doi: 10.1021/acsami.5b12588.
68. Kanaparthi S., Badhulika S. Solvent-free fabrication of a biodegradable all-carbon paper-based field effect transistor for human motion detection through strain sensing. *Green Chem.* 2016; 18:3640. Available from: https://pubs.rsc.org/en/content/articlelanding/2016/gc/c6gc00368k. doi: 10.1039/C6GC00368K.
69. Liao X., Zhang Z., Liao Q., Liang Q., Qu Y., Xu M., Li M., Zhang G., Zhang Y. Flexible and printable paper-based strain sensors for wearable and large-area green electronics. *Nanoscale* 2016; 8:13025. Available from: https://pubs.rsc.org/en/content/articlelanding/2016/nr/c6nr02172g. doi: 10.1039/C6NR02172G.

70. Toan D., Hoang-Phuong P., Qamar A., Nam-Trung N., Dzung Viet D. Flexible and multifunctional electronics fabricated by a solvent-free and user-friendly method. *RSC Adv.* 2016; 6:77267. Available from: https://pubs.rsc.org/en/content/articlelanding/2016/ra/c6ra14646e/unauth#. doi: 10.1039/C6RA14646E.
71. Zhang M., Wang C., Wang Q., Jian M., Zhang Y. Quantitative evaluation of pseudo strain signals caused by yarn structural deformation. *ACS Appl. Mater. Interfaces* 2016; 8:20894. Available from: https://link.springer.com/article/10.1007/s42765-021-00101-y. doi: 10.1007/s42765-021-00101-y.
72. Toan D., Hoang Phuong P., Tuan Khoa N., Qamar A., Woodfield P., Zhu Y., Nam Trung N., Dzung Viet D Environment-friendly carbon nanotube based flexible electronics for non-invasive and wearable healthcare. *Appl. Phys.* 2017; 50:215401. Available from: https://pubs.rsc.org/en/content/articlelanding/2016/tc/c6tc02708c#!. doi: 10.1039/C6TC02708C.
73. Cohen D. J., Mitra D., Peterson K., Maharbiz M. M. A highly elastic, capacitive strain gauge based on percolating nanotube networks. *Nano Lett.* 2012; 12:1821. Available from: https://pubs.acs.org/doi/10.1021/nl204052z. doi: 10.1021/nl204052z.
74. Kong J. H., Jang N. S., Kim S. H., Kim J. M. Simple and rapid micropatterning of conductive carbon composites and its applications to elastic strain sensors. *Carbon* 2014; 77:199. Available from: https://www.sciencedirect.com/science/article/abs/pii/S000862231400462X. doi: 10.1016/j.carbon.2014.05.022.
75. Jeon J. Y., Ha T. J. Waterproof electronic-bandage with tunable sensitivity for wearable strain sensors. *ACS Appl. Mater. Interfaces* 2016; 8:2866. Available from: https://pubs.acs.org/doi/10.1021/acsami.5b12201. doi: 10.1021/acsami.5b12201.
76. Shi J., Li X., Cheng H., Liu Z., Zhao L., Yang T., Dai Z., Cheng Z., Shi E., Yang L. Strain sensing: Graphene reinforced carbon nanotube networks for wearable strain sensors. *Adv. Funct. Mater.* 2016; 26:2038. Available from: https://onlinelibrary.wiley.com/doi/10.1002/adfm.201670078. doi: 10.1002/adfm.201670078.
77. Yao S., Zhu Y. Wearable multifunctional sensors using printed stretchable conductors made of silver nanowires. *Nanoscale* 2014; 6:2345. Available from: https://pubs.rsc.org/en/content/articlelanding/2014/nr/c3nr05496a. doi: 10.1039/C3NR05496A.
78. Kim S. R., Kim J. H., Park J. W. Wearable and transparent capacitive strain sensor with highly sensitivity based on patterned Ag nanowire networks. *ACS Appl. Mater. Interfaces* 2017; 9:26407. Available from: https://pubs.acs.org/doi/10.1021/acsami.7b06474. doi: 10.1021/acsami.7b06474.
79. Lee J., Kwon H., Seo J., Shin S., Koo J. H., Pang C., Son S., Kim J. H., Jang Y. H., Kim D. E., Lee T Conductive fibre based ultrasensitive textile pressure sensor for wearable electronics. *Adv. Mater.* 2015; 27:2433. Available from: https://onlinelibrary.wiley.com/doi/10.1002/adma.201500009. doi: 10.1002/adma.201500009.
80. Lipomi D. J., Vosgueritchian M., Tee B. C. K., Hellstrom S. L., Lee J. A., Fox C. H., Bao Z. Skin-like pressure and strain sensors based on transparent elastic films of carbon nanotubes. *Nat. Nanotechnol.* 2011; 6:788. Available from: https://www.nature.com/articles/nnano.2011.184. doi: 10.1038/nnano.2011.184.
81. Cai L., Song L., Luan P., Zhang Q., Zhang N., Gao Q., Zhao D., Zhang X., Tu M., Yang F., Zhou W., Fan Q., Luo J., Zhou W., Ajayan P. M., Xie S. Super-stretchable, transparent carbon nanotube-based capacitive strain sensors for human motion detection. *Sci. Rep.* 2013; 3:3402. Available from: https://www.nature.com/articles/srep03048. doi: 10.1038/srep03048.
82. Wang X., Li T., Adam J., Yang J. Transparent, stretchable, carbon-nanotube-inlaid conductors enabled by standard replication technology for capacitive pressure, strain and touch sensors. *J. Mater. Chem.* 2013; 1:3580. Available from: https://pubs.rsc.org/en/content/articlelanding/2013/ta/c3ta00079f. doi: 10.1039/C3TA00079F.

83. Park S., Kim H., Vosgueritchian M., Cheon S., Kim H., Koo J. H., Kim T. R., Lee S., Schwartz G., Chang H., Bao Z. Stretchable energy-harvesting tactile electronic skin capable of differentiating multiple mechanical stimuli modes. *Adv. Mater.* 2014; 26:7324. Available from: https://onlinelibrary.wiley.com/doi/10.1002/adma.201402574. doi: 10.1002/adma.201402574.
84. Kwon D., Lee T. I., Shim J., Ryu S., Kim M. S., Kim S., Kim T. S., Park I. Highly sensitive, flexible, wearable pressure sensor based on a giant piezocapacitive effect of three-dimensional microporous elastomeric dielectric layer. *ACS Appl. Mater. Interfaces* 2016; 8:16922. Available from: https://pubmed.ncbi.nlm.nih.gov/27286001/. doi: 10.1021/acsami.6b04225.
85. Filippidou M. K., Tegou E., Tsouti V., Chatzandroulis S. A flexible strain sensor made of graphene nanoplatelets/polydimethylsiloxane nanocomposite. *Microelectron. Eng.* 2015; 142:7. Available from: https://www.sciencedirect.com/science/article/abs/pii/S0167931715300149. doi: 10.1016/j.mee.2015.06.007.
86. Kang M., Kim J., Jang B., Chae Y., Kim J. H., Ahn J. H. Graphene based three-dimensional capacitive touch sensor for wearable electronics. *ACS Nano* 2017; 11:7950. Available from: https://pubmed.ncbi.nlm.nih.gov/28727414/. doi: 10.1021/acsnano.7b02474.
87. Zhu S. E., Ghatkesar K. M., Zhang C., Janssen G. Graphene based piezoresistive pressure sensor. *Appl. Phys. Lett.* 2013; 102:161904. Available from: https://www.semanticscholar.org/paper/Graphene-based-piezoresistive-pressure-sensor-Zhu-Ghatkesar/0a2ecd35e249a2599b77b62357ef5691e9a8e7ce. doi: 10.1063/1.4802799.
88. Wang Y., Wang L., Yang T., Li X., Zang X., Zhu M., Wang K., Wu D., Zhu H. Wearable and highly sensitive graphene strain sensors for human motion monitoring. *Adv. Funct. Mater.* 2014; 24:4666. Available from: https://onlinelibrary.wiley.com/doi/abs/10.1002/adfm.201400379. doi: 10.1002/adfm.201400379.
89. Yang T., Jiang X., Zhong Y., Zhao X., Lin S., Li J., Li X., Xu J., Li Z., Zhu H. A wearable and highly sensitive graphene strain for precise home-based pulse wave monitoring. *ACS Sens.* 2017; 2:967. Available from: https://onlinelibrary.wiley.com/doi/abs/10.1002/adfm.201400379.
90. Han J., Lee J. Y., Lee J., Yeo S. Highly stretchable and reliable, transparent and conductive entangled graphene mesh networks. *Adv. Mater.* 2018; 30:1704626. Available from: https://onlinelibrary.wiley.com/doi/10.1002/adma.201704626. doi: 10.1002/adma.201704626.
91. Lu N., Lu C., Yang S., Rogers J. Highly sensitive skin-mountable strain gauges based entirely on elastomers. *Adv. Funct. Mater.* 2012; 22:4044. Available from: https://onlinelibrary.wiley.com/doi/10.1002/adfm.201200498. doi: 10.1002/adfm.201200498.
92. Karnan M., Subramani K., Srividhya P. K., Sathish M. Electrochemical studies on corncob derived activated porous carbon for supercapacitors application in aqueous and non-aqueous electrolytes. *Electrachim. Acta* 2017; 228:586. Available from: https://www.sciencedirect.com/science/article/abs/pii/S0013468617300956. doi: 10.1016/j.electacta.2017.01.095.
93. Xu N., Hu X., Xu W., Li X., Zhou L., Zhu S., Zhu J. Mushrooms as efficient solar steam-generation devices. *Adv. Mater.* 2017; 29:1606762. Available from: https://onlinelibrary.wiley.com/doi/abs/10.1002/adma.201606762. doi: 10.1002/adma.201606762.
94. Wang C., Xia K., Jian M., Wang H., Zhang M., Zhang Y. Carbonized silk georgette as an ultrasensitive wearable strain sensor for full range human activity monitoring. *J. Mater. Chem. C* 2017; 5:7604. Available from: https://pubmed.ncbi.nlm.nih.gov/27168096/. doi: 10.1002/adma.201601572.

95. Zhang M., Wang C., Wang H., Jian M., Hao X., Zhang Y. Carbonized cotton fabric for high-performance wearable strain sensors. *Adv. Funct. Mater.* 2017; 27:1604795. Available from: https://link.springer.com/article/10.1007/s10570-019-02432-x. doi: 10.1007/s10570-019-02432-x.
96. Wang C., Xia K., Zhang M., Jian M., Zhang Y. An all silk-derived dual mode e-skin for simultaneous temperature-pressure detection. *ACS Appl. Mater. Interfaces* 2017; 9:39484. Available from: https://pubmed.ncbi.nlm.nih.gov/29065259/. doi: 10.1021/acsami.7b13356.
97. Wang C., Wu S., Jian M., Xie J., Xu L., Yang X., Zheng Q., Zhang Y. Silk nanofibers as highly efficient and light weight air filter. *Nano Res.* 2016; 9:2590. Available from: https://link.springer.com/article/10.1007/s12274-016-1145-3. doi: 10.1007/s12274-016-1145-3.
98. Park J., Lee Y., Hong J., Ha M., Jung Y. D., Lim H., Kim S. Y., Ko H. Giant tunnelling piezoresistance of composite elastomers with interlocked microdome arrays for ultrasensitive and multimodal electronic skins. *ACS Nano* 2014; 8:4689. Available from: https://pubmed.ncbi.nlm.nih.gov/24592988/. doi: 10.1021/nn500441k.
99. Stoppa M., Chiolerio A. Wearable electronics and smart textiles: A critical review. *Sensors* 2014; 14:11957. Available from: https://www.mdpi.com/1424-8220/14/7/11957. doi: 10.3390/s140711957.
100. Bandodkar A. J., Wang J. Wearable biofuel cells: A review. *Electroanalysis* 2016; 28:1188. Available from: https://analyticalsciencejournals.onlinelibrary.wiley.com/doi/abs/10.1002/elan.201600019. doi: 10.1002/elan.201600019.
101. Katz E., MacVittie K. Implanted biofuel cells operating in vivo-methods, applications and perspectives-feature article. *Energy Environ. Sci.* 2013; 6:2791. Available from: https://pubs.rsc.org/en/content/articlelanding/2013/ee/c3ee42126k#!. doi: 10.1039/C3EE42126K.
102. Dave S, Das Jayshankar. *Advanced Nanomaterials for Point of Care Diagnosis and Therapy.* Elsevier, 2022. https://doi.org/10.1016/C2020-0-02584-3.
103. Berchmans S., Bandodkar A. J., Jia W., Ramrez J., Meng Y. S., Wang J. An epidermal alkaline rechargeable Ag-Zn printable tattoo battery for wearable electronics. *J. Mater. Chem. A* 2014; 2:15788. Available from: https://pubs.rsc.org/en/content/articlelanding/2014/ta/c4ta03256j. doi: 10.1039/C4TA03256J.
104. Zebda A., Gondran C., Cinquin P., Cosnier S. Glucose biofuel cell construction based on enzyme, graphite particle and redox mediator compression. *Sens. Actuators B* 2012; 173:760. Available from: https://www.sciencedirect.com/science/article/abs/pii/S0925400512007824. doi: 10.1016/j.snb.2012.07.089.
105. Bandodkar A. J., You J. M., Kim N. H., Gu Y., Kumar R., Mohan A. M. V., Kurniawan J., Imani S., Nakagawa T., Parish B., Parthasarathy M., Mercier P. P., Xu S., Wang J. Soft, stretchable, high power density electronic skin-based biofuel cells for scavenging energy from human sweat. *Energy Environ. Sci.* 2017; 10:1581. Available from: https://pubs.rsc.org/en/content/articlelanding/2017/ee/c7ee00865a. doi: 10.1039/C7EE00865A.
106. Ieerapan I., Sepionatto J. R., Pavinatto A., You J. M., Wang J. Stretchable biofuel cells as wearable textile-based self-powered sensors. *J. Mater. Chem. A* 2016; 4:18342. Available from: https://pubs.rsc.org/en/content/articlelanding/2016/ta/c6ta08358g. doi: 10.1039/C6TA08358G.
107. Santhamoorthy M, Thirupathi K, Krishnan S, Guganathan L, Dave S, Phan TTV and Kim SC. Preparation of Magnetic Iron Oxide Incorporated Mesoporous Silica Hybrid Composites for pH and Temperature-Sensitive Drug Delivery. *Magnetochemistry* 2023; 9(3):81.

108. Dave S, Dave S, Mathur A, Das J. Biological synthesis of magnetic nanoparticles. In *Nanobiotechnology* (pp. 225–234). Elsevier, 2021.
109. Wang J., Liu J., Cepra G. Thermal stabilization of enzymes immobilized within carbon paste electrodes. *Anal. Chem.* 1997; 69:3124. Available from: https://pubmed.ncbi.nlm.nih.gov/21639334/. doi: 10.1021/ac9702305.

Index

www.ingramcontent.com/pod-product-compliance
Lightning Source LLC
LaVergne TN
LVHW020659110826
845149LV00012B/2056

* 9 7 8 1 0 3 2 3 2 7 2 9 7 *